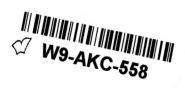
W9-AKC-558

Sexually Transmitted Diseases
SOURCEBOOK

SEVENTH EDITION

Health Reference Series

Sexually Transmitted Diseases

SOURCEBOOK

SEVENTH EDITION

Basic Consumer Health Information about Sexual Health and the Screening, Diagnosis, Treatment, and Prevention of Common Sexually Transmitted Diseases (STDs), Including Chancroid, Chlamydia, Gonorrhea, Herpes, Hepatitis, Human Immunodeficiency Virus/ Acquired Immunodeficiency Syndrome (HIV/AIDS), Human Papillomavirus (HPV), Syphilis, and Trichomoniasis

Along with Facts about Risk Factors and Complications, Trends and Disparities in Infection Rates, Tips for Discussing Sexually Transmitted Diseases with Sexual Partners, a Glossary of Related Terms, and Resources for Additional Help and Information

OMNIGRAPHICS

615 Griswold, Ste. 520, Detroit, MI 48226

Bibliographic Note
Because this page cannot legibly accommodate all the copyright notices, the Bibliographic Note portion of the Preface constitutes an extension of the copyright notice.

* * *

OMNIGRAPHICS
Angela L. Williams, *Managing Editor*
* * *

Library of Congress Cataloging-in-Publication Data
Names: Omnigraphics, Inc., issuing body.

Title: Sexually transmitted diseases sourcebook: basic consumer health information about sexual health and the screening, diagnosis, treatment, and prevention of common sexually transmitted diseases (STDs), including chancroid, chlamydia, gonorrhea, herpes, hepatitis, human immunodeficiency virus/acquired immunodeficiency syndrome (HIV/AIDS), human papillomavirus (HPV), syphilis, and trichomoniasis; along with facts about risk factors and complications, trends and disparities in infection rates, tips for discussing stds with sexual partners, a glossary of related terms, and resources for additional help and information.

Description: Seventh edition. | Detroit, MI: Omnigraphics, [2019] | Series: Health reference series | Includes index.

Identifiers: LCCN 2018061734 (print) | LCCN 2019000435 (ebook) | ISBN 9780780816923 (ebook) | ISBN 9780780816916 (hard cover: alk. paper)

Subjects: LCSH: Sexually transmitted diseases--Popular works.

Classification: LCC RC200.2 (ebook) | LCC RC200.2.S387 2019 (print) | DDC 616.95/1--dc23

LC record available at https://lccn.loc.gov/2018061734

Table of Contents

Part II: Types of Sexually Transmitted Diseases

vii

Part III: Complications That May Accompany Sexually Transmitted Disease Infection

ix

Part IV: Sexually Transmitted Diseases Testing and Treatment Concerns

Part V: Sexually Transmitted Diseases Risks and Prevention

Part VI: Living with Sexually Transmitted Diseases

Part VII: Additional Help and Information

Preface

About This Book

Every year, more than 20 million people in the United States are diagnosed with sexually transmitted diseases (STDs), and the Centers for Disease Control and Prevention (CDC) reports that diagnosing, treating, and preventing these potentially life-threatening STDs is one of the greatest public-health challenges today. For some STDs, such as the easily treatable chlamydia, the rates of reported cases are on the rise, especially among adolescent girls and young women. The diagnosis rates of other STDs, such as human immunodeficiency virus (HIV), have decreased in recent years due to increased education and prevention efforts. Regardless of prevalence or severity, all STDs have significant health consequences if they are not diagnosed and treated.

Sexually Transmitted Diseases Sourcebook, Seventh Edition offers basic information about sexual health and the screening, diagnosis, treatment, and prevention of common sexually transmitted diseases, including chancroid, chlamydia, gonorrhea, herpes, hepatitis, HIV, acquired immunodeficiency syndrome (AIDS), human papillomavirus (HPV), syphilis, and trichomoniasis. It discusses trends in STD rates, developments in STD vaccine research, tips on talking to doctors and sexual partners, a glossary of related terms, and resources for additional help and information.

How to Use This Book

This book is divided into parts and chapters. Parts focus on broad areas of interest. Chapters are devoted to single topics within a part.

Part I: Introduction to Sexually Transmitted Diseases identifies the parts of the male and female reproductive system and discusses trends in STD rates in the United States and worldwide. It also examines the impact of these diseases on women, men, children and teens, and older adults. The part concludes with statistical information on minorities disproportionately affected by STDs and recent STD research findings.

Part II: Types of Sexually Transmitted Diseases identifies the symptoms, diagnoses, and treatments of common types of STDs, including chancroid, chlamydia, donovanosis, gonorrhea, herpes, hepatitis, HPV, lymphogranuloma venereum, syphilis, and trichomoniasis. The part also includes information on how HIV causes AIDS and the disease's transmission, testing, and treatment, as well as strategies for living with HIV and paying for medical care.

Part III: Complications That May Accompany Sexually Transmitted Disease Infection provides information about infections and syndromes that may develop after sexual contact, such as bacterial vaginosis, cytomegalovirus, yeast infection, intestinal parasites, molluscum contagiosum, sexually transmitted gastrointestinal syndromes, pubic lice, and scabies. The part also provides information about conditions related to STDs that can cause long-term health complications for men and women, including cervicitis, epididymitis, infertility and pregnancy complications, pelvic inflammatory disease, and vaginitis.

Part IV: Sexually Transmitted Diseases Testing and Treatment Concerns offers information about how medical professionals test patients for STDs and addresses common issues associated with STD testing, such as maintaining confidentiality and discussing STDs with healthcare providers. Information about unproven STD treatment products is also included.

Part V: Sexually Transmitted Diseases Risks and Prevention discusses sexual behaviors that increase the likelihood of STD transmission, such as choosing high-risk partners and using illegal substances. The part also offers tips on talking to sexual partners and adolescents about STDs and addresses the effectiveness of sexual and abstinence education as forms of STD prevention. The part concludes with information about preventing STDs by using safer sex and barrier methods such as condoms, by using medication after a known exposure to STDs, by preventing the transmission of these diseases from a pregnant woman to her child, and by using STD vaccines and microbicides.

Part VI: Living with Sexually Transmitted Diseases discusses about how to have a conversation about HIV status, social stigma associated with HIV, and ways to overcome it. It also deals with STD medication and vaccines, and offers insights on how STD patients can cope physically and mentally.

Part VII: Additional Help and Information provides a glossary of important terms related to sexually transmitted diseases and a directory of organizations that offer information to people with STDs or their sexual partners.

Bibliographic Note

This volume contains documents and excerpts from publications issued by the following U.S. government agencies: Centers for Disease Control and Prevention (CDC); *Eunice Kennedy Shriver* National Institute of Child Health and Human Development (NICHD); Genetic and Rare Diseases Information Center (GARD); National Cancer Institute (NCI); National Institute of Allergy and Infectious Diseases (NIAID); National Institute of Neurological Disorders and Stroke (NINDS); National Institute on Deafness and Other Communication Disorders (NIDCD); National Institutes of Health (NIH); *NIH News in Health*; Office of Disease Prevention and Health Promotion (ODPHP); Office of the Surgeon General (OSG); Office on Women's Health (OWH); U.S. Department of Health and Human Services (HHS); and U.S. Food and Drug Administration (FDA).

It may also contain original material produced by Omnigraphics and reviewed by medical consultants.

About the Health Reference Series

The *Health Reference Series* is designed to provide basic medical information for patients, families, caregivers, and the general public. Each volume takes a particular topic and provides comprehensive coverage. This is especially important for people who may be dealing with a newly diagnosed disease or a chronic disorder in themselves or in a family member. People looking for preventive guidance, information about disease warning signs, medical statistics, and risk factors for health problems will also find answers to their questions in the *Health*

Reference Series. The *Series*, however, is not intended to serve as a tool for diagnosing illness, in prescribing treatments, or as a substitute for the physician/patient relationship. All people concerned about medical symptoms or the possibility of disease are encouraged to seek professional care from an appropriate healthcare provider.

A Note about Spelling and Style

Health Reference Series editors use *Stedman's Medical Dictionary* as an authority for questions related to the spelling of medical terms and the *Chicago Manual of Style* for questions related to grammatical structures, punctuation, and other editorial concerns. Consistent adherence is not always possible, however, because the individual volumes within the *Series* include many documents from a wide variety of different producers, and the editor's primary goal is to present material from each source as accurately as is possible. This sometimes means that information in different chapters or sections may follow other guidelines and alternate spelling authorities. For example, occasionally a copyright holder may require that eponymous terms be shown in possessive forms (Crohn's disease vs. Crohn disease) or that British spelling norms be retained (leukaemia vs. leukemia).

Medical Review

Omnigraphics contracts with a team of qualified, senior medical professionals who serve as medical consultants for the *Health Reference Series*. As necessary, medical consultants review reprinted and originally written material for currency and accuracy. Citations including the phrase "Reviewed (month, year)" indicate material reviewed by this team. Medical consultation services are provided to the *Health Reference Series* editors by:

Dr. Vijayalakshmi, MBBS, DGO, MD
Dr. Senthil Selvan, MBBS, DCH, MD
Dr. K. Sivanandham, MBBS, DCH, MS (Research), PhD

Our Advisory Board

We would like to thank the following board members for providing initial guidance on the development of this series:

- Dr. Lynda Baker, Associate Professor of Library and Information Science, Wayne State University, Detroit, MI

- Nancy Bulgarelli, William Beaumont Hospital Library, Royal Oak, MI

- Karen Imarisio, Bloomfield Township Public Library, Bloomfield Township, MI

- Karen Morgan, Mardigian Library, University of Michigan-Dearborn, Dearborn, MI

- Rosemary Orlando, St. Clair Shores Public Library, St. Clair Shores, MI

Health Reference Series *Update Policy*

The inaugural book in the *Health Reference Series* was the first edition of *Cancer Sourcebook* published in 1989. Since then, the *Series* has been enthusiastically received by librarians and in the medical community. In order to maintain the standard of providing high-quality health information for the layperson the editorial staff at Omnigraphics felt it was necessary to implement a policy of updating volumes when warranted.

Medical researchers have been making tremendous strides, and it is the purpose of the *Health Reference Series* to stay current with the most recent advances. Each decision to update a volume is made on an individual basis. Some of the considerations include how much new information is available and the feedback we receive from people who use the books. If there is a topic you would like to see added to the update list, or an area of medical concern you feel has not been adequately addressed, please write to:

Managing Editor
Health Reference Series
Omnigraphics
615 Griswold, Ste. 520
Detroit, MI 48226

Part One

Introduction to Sexually Transmitted Diseases

Chapter 1

Overview of Sexual Health and the Reproductive System

Chapter Contents

3

Section 1.1

Overview and Impact

This section includes text excerpted from "Reproductive and Sexual Health," Office of Disease Prevention and Health Promotion (ODPHP), U.S. Department of Health and Human Services (HHS), February 11, 2019.

An estimated 19 million new cases of sexually transmitted diseases (STDs) are diagnosed each year in the United States—almost half of them among young people ages 15 to 24. An estimated 1.1 million Americans are living with the human immunodeficiency virus (HIV), and 1 out of 5 people with HIV do not know they have it. Untreated STDs can lead to serious long-term health consequences, especially for adolescent girls and young women, including reproductive-health problems and infertility, fetal and perinatal-health problems, cancer, and further sexual transmission of HIV.

For many, reproductive and sexual-health services are the entry point into the medical care system. These services improve health and reduce costs by not only covering pregnancy prevention, HIV and STD testing and treatment, and prenatal care, but also by screening for intimate partner violence (IPV) and reproductive cancers, providing substance-abuse treatment referrals, and counseling on nutrition and physical activity. Each year, publicly funded family-planning services help prevent 1.94 million unintended pregnancies, including 400,000 teen pregnancies. For every $1 spent on these services, nearly $4 in Medicaid expenditures for pregnancy-related care is saved.

Improving reproductive and sexual health is crucial to eliminating health disparities, reducing rates of infectious diseases and infertility, and increasing educational attainment, career opportunities, and financial stability.

Health Impact of Reproductive and Sexual Health

Reproductive and sexual health is a key component to the overall health and quality of life (QOL) for both men and women. Reproductive and sexual-health services can:

- **Prevent unintended pregnancies.** Nearly half of all pregnancies are unintended. Risks associated with unintended pregnancy include low birth weight, postpartum depression, delays in receiving prenatal care, and family stress.

- **Prevent adolescent pregnancies.** More than 400,000 teen girls ages 15 to 19 give birth each year in the United States.

- **Detect health conditions early.** Prenatal care can detect gestational diabetes or preeclampsia before it causes problems, and taking prenatal vitamins can prevent birth defects of the brain and spinal cord.

- **Increase the detection and treatment of STDs.** Untreated STDs can lead to serious long-term health consequences, especially for adolescent girls and young women.

- **Decrease rates of infertility.** The Centers for Disease Control and Prevention (CDC) estimates that undiagnosed and untreated STDs cause at least 24,000 women in the United States each year to become infertile.

- **Slow the transmission of HIV through testing and treatment.** People living with HIV who receive antiretroviral therapy are 92 percent less likely to transmit HIV to others.

Section 1.2

Life Stages and Determinants

This section includes text excerpted from "Reproductive and Sexual Health," Office of Disease Prevention and Health Promotion (ODPHP), U.S. Department of Health and Human Services (HHS), February 11, 2019.

The major function of the reproductive system is to ensure the survival of the species. An individual may live a long, healthy, and happy life without producing offspring, but if the species is to continue, at least some individuals must produce offspring. Within the context of producing offspring, the reproductive system has four functions:

- To produce egg and sperm cells
- To transport and sustain these cells
- To nurture the developing offspring
- To produce hormones

These functions are divided between the primary and secondary, or accessory, reproductive organs.

- Primary reproductive organs, or gonads—consist of the ovaries and testes that are responsible for producing egg and sperm cells with gametes and hormones. These hormones function in the maturation of the reproductive system, the development of sexual characteristics, and the regulation of the normal physiology of the reproductive system.

- All other organs, ducts, and glands in the reproductive system are considered secondary, or accessory, reproductive organs. These structures transport and sustain the gametes and nurture the developing offspring.

Reproductive and Sexual Health across the Life Stages

Reproductive and sexual health is an important part of an individual's overall health, particularly during childbearing years.

Infants

Babies of mothers who do not get prenatal care are three times more likely to have a low birth weight and five times more likely to die than those born to mothers who do get prenatal care.

Adolescents

Sexually transmitted diseases (STDs) are a risk to adolescents' health and fertility. Nearly half of new STD infections are among young people age 15 to 24.

Adolescents who become pregnant are much less likely to complete their education. About 50 percent of teen mothers get a high-school diploma by age 22, compared with 90 percent of teen girls who do not give birth. Only 50 percent of teen fathers who have children before age 18 finish high school or get their general education development (GED) by age 22.

Older Adults

People age 50 and over account for decreasing numbers of new human immunodeficiency virus (HIV) diagnoses, and older adults may not consider themselves to be at risk of HIV infection. However, many older adults are sexually active, including those living with HIV, and may have the same HIV risk factors as younger people. Consider the following:

- People age 50 and over accounted for 17 percent of the new HIV diagnoses in 2015 in the United States.

- 45 percent of Americans living with diagnosed HIV are over age 50.

- Older women may be especially at risk for HIV infection due to age-related thinning and dryness of vaginal tissue.

- Some older adults, compared with those who are younger, may be less knowledgeable about HIV, and therefore, less likely to protect themselves. Many do not perceive of themselves as at risk for HIV, do not use condoms, and are less likely than young people to get tested for HIV or to discuss sexual habits or drug use with their doctor.

- Older people in the United States are more likely than younger people to have late-stage HIV infection at the time of diagnosis.

Determinants of Reproductive and Sexual Health

Reproductive and sexual health, particularly the spread of sexually transmitted diseases (STDs) including HIV and the prevalence of unintended pregnancy, are determined in part by social, economic, and behavioral factors. Stigma is still a major barrier to people accessing reproductive and sexual-health services. For example, the continued stigma around HIV and its association with men who have sex with men can prevent people from getting tested and knowing their serostatus.

Many other factors affect an individual's reproductive and sexual health decision-making, including access to medical care, social norms, educational attainment, age, income, geographic location, insurance status, sexual orientation, and dependency on alcohol or other drugs. Addressing these determinants is key to reducing health disparities and improving the health of all Americans.

Section 1.3

Facts on Reproductive and Sexual Health

This section includes text excerpted from "Reproductive and Sexual Health," Office of Disease Prevention and Health Promotion (ODPHP), U.S. Department of Health and Human Services (HHS), February 11, 2019.

Where We've Been and Where We're Going

Between 2006 to 2010 and 2011 to 2015, there was no statistically significant change in the percentage of sexually active females aged 15 to 44 years who received reproductive-health services in the past 12 months (78.6% in 2006 to 2010 and 77.8% in 2011 to 2015). From 2011 to 2015, several groups of women had the highest rate of receipt of reproductive-health services in their specific demographic categories, including nonHispanic Black females, those aged 18 to 24 years, those with family incomes 500 percent or more of the poverty threshold, those aged 20 to 44 years with a bachelor's degree, and those with private health insurance.

From 2010 to 2015, the estimated number of persons aged 13 years and over living with diagnosed or undiagnosed human immunodeficiency virus (HIV) increased approximately 11.6 percent, from 1,006,300 to 1,122,900. During the same period, the proportion of people living with HIV who were aware of their HIV infection increased by 2.9 percent, from 83.1 percent to 85.5 percent. In 2015, several population groups in specific demographic categories had the highest rate of awareness of their HIV infection, including women, the white population, older adults, and female injection-drug users.

Sexually Active Females Who Received Reproductive-Health Services (FP-7.1)

*   Healthy People 2020 objective FP-7.1 tracks the proportion of sexually active females aged 15 to 44 years who received reproductive-health services in the past 12 months.

*   HP2020 baseline: 78.6 percent of sexually active females aged 15 to 44 years received reproductive-health services in the past 12 months in 2006 to 2010.

*   HP2020 target: 86.5 percent, a 10 percent improvement over the baseline.

- Among racial/ethnic groups, sexually active nonHispanic Black women aged 15 to 44 years had the best (highest) rate of receipt of reproductive-health services in the past 12 months, 85.7 percent as reported in 2011 to 2015. Rates for women in other racial/ethnic groups were:

  - 76.2 percent among Hispanic or Latinx women; the best group rate was 12.5 percent higher

  - 77.2 percent among nonHispanic White women; the best group rate was 11.1 percent higher

- Females (sexually active) aged 18 to 24 years had the highest (best) level of receipt of reproductive-health services in the past 12 months among age groups, 84.9 percent as reported in 2011 to 2015. Rates for women in other age groups were:

  - 71.6 percent among females aged 15 to 17 years; the best group rate was 18.7 percent higher

  - 76.0 percent among females aged 25 to 44 years; the best group rate was 11.8 percent higher

- Females (sexually active) aged 15 to 44 years whose family income was at or above 500 percent of the poverty threshold had the highest (best) rate of receipt of reproductive-health services in the past 12 months, 82.5 percent as reported in 2011 to 2015. Rates for women in other income groups were:

  - 74.5 percent for those with incomes under the poverty threshold; the best group rate was 10.7 percent higher

  - 78.3 percent for those with incomes 100 to 199 percent of the poverty threshold; the best group rate was 5.2 percent higher

  - 76.5 percent for those with incomes 200 to 399 percent of the poverty threshold; the best group rate was 7.7 percent higher

  - 82.4 percent for those with incomes 400 to 499 percent of the poverty threshold; not significantly different than the best group rate

- Females (sexually active) aged 20 to 44 years with a 4-year college degree had the highest (best) rate of receipt of reproductive-health services in the past 12 months, 83.1 percent as reported in 2011 to 2015. Rates for women in other education groups were:

- 68.3 percent for those with less than a high-school education; the best group rate was 21.7 percent higher

- 68.9 percent for those with a high-school education or general educational development (GED); the best group rate was 20.6 percent higher

- 75.8 percent for those with some college education; the best group rate was 9.6 percent higher

- 79.5 percent for those with an associate's degree; not significantly different than the best group rate

- 79.9 percent for those with an advanced degree; not significantly different than the best group rate

Sexually Active Females Receiving Reproductive-Health Services by Educational Attainment, 2011 to 2015

In 2011–15, the proportion of sexually active females aged 20–44 years who received reproductive health services in the past 12 months generally **increased as education level increased.**

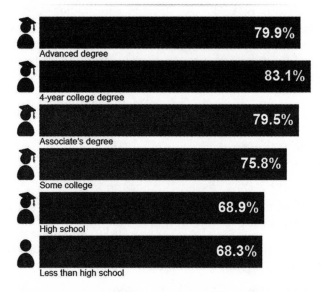

Figure 1.1. *Sexually Active Females Receiving Reproductive-Health Services by Educational Attainment, 2011 to 2015* (Source: National Survey of Family Growth (NSFG), Centers of Disease Control and Prevention/National Center for Health Statistics (CDC/NCHS).)

Females (sexually active) aged 15 to 44 years with private health insurance had the highest (best) rate of receipt of reproductive-health services in the past 12 months, 81.7 percent as reported in 2011 to 2015. Rates for women in other health insurance groups were:

• 60.9 percent for those with no health insurance; the best group rate was 34.0 percent higher

• 81.4 percent for those with public-health insurance; not significantly different than the best group rate

Awareness of Human Immunodeficiency Virus Infection Status (HIV-13)

• Healthy People 2020 objective HIV-13 tracks the proportion of persons aged 13 years and over living with HIV who are aware of their HIV infection.

   • HP2020 baseline: 83.1 percent of persons aged 13 years and over living with HIV were aware of their HIV infection in 2010.

   • HP2020 target: 90.0 percent, consistent with the National HIV/AIDS Strategy.

• Females aged 13 years and over had a higher rate of awareness of their HIV infection than males in 2015 (88.5% versus 84.6%).

• Among racial/ethnic groups, white persons aged 13 years and over with HIV had the highest (best) rate of awareness of HIV infection (88.1%) in 2015. This rate was 9.6 percent higher than the lowest rate, which was among Asian persons with HIV (80.4%). The rates for other race/ethnic groups were:

   • 81.3 percent among American Indian and Alaska Native persons; the best group rate was 8.4 percent higher

   • 82.2 among Native Hawaiian or Other Pacific Islander persons; the best group rate percent was 7.2 percent higher

   • 83.5 percent among Hispanic or Latinx persons; the best group rate was 5.5 percent higher

   • 84.9 percent among Black persons

   • 85.6 percent among persons of two or more races

11

- Persons aged 55 years and over with HIV had the highest (best) rate of HIV infection awareness (95.1%) in 2015. This rate was twice the lowest rate, which was among persons aged 13 to 24 years (48.6%). The rates for other age groups were:

  - 71.4 percent among persons aged 25 to 34 years; the best group rate was 33.2 percent higher

  - 85.2 percent among persons aged 35 to 44 years; the best group rate was 11.6 percent higher

  - 91.9 percent among persons aged 45 to 54 years

Section 1.4

Recommendations for Better Reproductive and Sexual Health

. This section includes text excerpted from "Reproductive and Sexual Health," Office of the Surgeon General (OSG), February 12, 2019.

Healthy reproductive and sexual practices can play a critical role in enabling people to remain healthy and actively contribute to their community. Planning and having a healthy pregnancy is vital to the health of women, infants, and families, and is especially important in preventing teen pregnancy and childbearing, which will help raise educational attainment, increase employment opportunities, and enhance financial stability. Access to quality health services and support for safe practices can improve physical and emotional well-being and reduce teen and unintended pregnancies, human immunodeficiency virus (HIV)/acquired immunodeficiency syndrome (AIDS), viral hepatitis, and other sexually transmitted infections (STIs).

Recommendations

- Increase use of preconception and prenatal care.

- Support reproductive and sexual-health services and support services for pregnant and parenting women.

- Provide effective sexual health education, especially for adolescents.

- Enhance early detection of HIV, viral hepatitis, and other STIs and improve linkage to care.

What Can State, Tribal, Local, and Territorial Governments Do?

- Increase access to comprehensive preconception and prenatal care, especially for low-income and at-risk women.

- Strengthen delivery of quality reproductive and sexual-health services (e.g., family planning, HIV/STI testing).

- Implement evidence-based practices to prevent teen pregnancy and HIV/STIs and ensure that resources are targeted to communities at highest risk.

- Use social marketing, support services, and policies to increase the number of people tested and linked to care for HIV, viral hepatitis, and other STIs.

What Can Businesses and Employers Do?

- Provide health coverage and employee assistance programs that include family planning and reproductive-health services.

- Provide time off for pregnant employees to access prenatal care.

- Implement and enforce policies that address sexual harassment.

What Can Healthcare Systems, Insurers, and Clinicians Do?

- Advise patients about factors that affect birth outcomes, such as alcohol, tobacco, and other drugs, poor nutrition, stress, lack of prenatal care, and chronic illness or other medical problems.

- Include sexual-health risk assessments as a part of routine care, help patients identify ways to reduce the risk for unintended pregnancy, HIV and other STIs, and provide recommended testing and treatment for HIV and other STIs to patients and their partners when appropriate.

- Provide vaccination for hepatitis B virus and human papillomavirus (HPV), as recommended by the Advisory Committee on Immunization Practices (ACIP).

- Offer counseling and services to patients regarding the range of contraceptive choices either onsite or through referral consistent with federal, state, and local regulations and laws.

- Implement policies and procedures to ensure culturally competent and confidential reproductive and sexual-health services.

What Can Early Learning Centers, Schools, Colleges, and Universities Do?

- Support medically accurate, developmentally appropriate, and evidence-based sexual health education.

- Support teen parenting programs and assist parents in completing high school, which can promote health for teen parents and children.

- Provide students with confidential, affordable reproductive and sexual-health information and services consistent with federal, state, and local regulations and laws.

- Implement mentoring or skills-based activities that promote healthy relationships and change social norms about teen dating violence.

What Can Community, Nonprofit, and Faith-Based Organizations Do?

- Support pregnant women obtaining prenatal care in the first trimester (e.g., transportation services, patient navigators).

- Educate communities, clinicians, pregnant women, and families on how to prevent infant mortality (e.g., nutrition, stress reduction, postpartum and newborn care).

- Promote and offer HIV and other STI testing and enhance linkages with reproductive and sexual-health services (e.g., counseling, contraception, HIV/STI testing and treatment).

- Provide information and educational tools to both men and women to promote respectful, nonviolent relationships.

- Promote teen-pregnancy prevention and positive youth development, support the development of strong communication skills among parents, and provide supervised after-school activities.

What Can Individuals and Families Do?

• Eat healthfully, take a daily supplement of folic acid, stay active, stop tobacco use and drinking alcohol, and see their doctor before and during pregnancy.

• Discuss their sexual-health history, get tested for HIV and other STIs, and discuss birth control options with potential partners.

• Notify their partner if they find out they have HIV or another STI.

• Discuss sexual-health concerns with their healthcare provider.

• Use recommended and effective prevention methods to prevent HIV and other STIs and reduce the risk for unintended pregnancy.

• Communicate with children regarding their knowledge, values, and attitudes related to sexual activity, sexuality, and healthy relationships.

• Make efforts to know where their children are and what they're doing and, make sure they are supervised by adults in the after-school hours.

Section 1.5

Female Reproductive System

This section contains text excerpted from the following sources: Text under the heading "Introduction to the Reproductive System" is excerpted from "Introduction to the Reproductive System," National Cancer Institute (NCI), January 29, 2019; Text under the heading "How the Female Reproductive System Works" is excerpted from "How the Female Reproductive System Works," girlshealth.gov, Office on Women's Health (OWH), April 15, 2014. Reviewed February 2019; Text under the heading "Female Sexual Response and Hormone Control" is excerpted from "Female Sexual Response and Hormone Control," Surveillance, Epidemiology and End Results Program (SEER), National Cancer Institute (NCI), September 7, 2016.

Introduction to the Reproductive System

The major function of the reproductive system is to ensure the survival of the species. An individual may live a long, healthy, and happy life without producing offspring, but if the species is to continue, at least some individuals must produce offspring. Within the context of producing offspring, the reproductive system has four functions:

- To produce egg and sperm cells

- To transport and sustain these cells

- To nurture the developing offspring

- To produce hormones

These functions are divided between the primary and secondary, or accessory, reproductive organs.

- **Primary reproductive organs, or gonads**—consist of the ovaries and testes that are responsible for producing egg and sperm cells with gametes and hormones. These hormones function in the maturation of the reproductive system, the development of sexual characteristics, and the regulation of the normal physiology of the reproductive system.

- **All other organs, ducts, and glands in the reproductive system** are considered secondary, or accessory, reproductive organs. These structures transport and sustain the gametes and nurture the developing offspring.

How the Female Reproductive System Works

The female reproductive system is all the parts of your body that help reproduce or have babies. Consider these two fabulous facts:

- A female body likely has hundreds and thousands of eggs that could grow into a baby, and they have them from the time they are born.

- Right inside each female is a perfect place for those eggs to meet with the sperm and grow into a whole human being!

What's inside the Female Reproductive System?

- **The ovaries**—two small organs. Before puberty, it's as if the ovaries are asleep. During puberty, they "wake up." The ovaries start making more estrogen and other hormones, which cause body changes. One important body change is that these hormones cause you to start getting your period, which is called "menstruating." Once a month, the ovaries release one egg (ovum). This is called "ovulation."

- **The fallopian tubes**—connect the ovaries to the uterus. The released egg moves along a fallopian tube.

- **The uterus**—or womb—is where a baby would grow. It takes several days for the egg to get to the uterus. As the egg travels, estrogen makes the lining of the uterus (called the "endometrium") thick with blood and fluid. This makes the uterus a good place for a baby to grow. One can become pregnant if a female has sex with a male without birth control and his sperm joins the egg (called "fertilization") on its way to the uterus. If the egg doesn't get fertilized, it will be shed along with the lining of the uterus during the next period (menses). But don't look for the egg—it's too small to see! The blood and fluid that leave the body during the period pass through the cervix and vagina.

- **The cervix**—a narrow entryway in between the vagina and uterus. The cervix is flexible so it can expand to let a baby pass through during childbirth.

- **The vagina**—a tube that can grow wider to deliver a baby that has finished growing inside the uterus.

- **The hymen**—covers the opening of the vagina. It is a thin piece of tissue that has one or more holes in it. Sometimes a hymen may be stretched or torn when a female uses a tampon or during a first sexual experience. If it does tear, it may bleed a little bit.

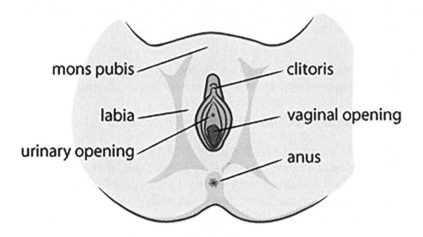

Figure 1.2. *External Reproductive System*

What's outside the Vagina?

The external reproductive system. The vulva covers the entrance to the vagina. The vulva has five parts:

- **Mons pubis:** The mons pubis is the mound of tissue and skin above the legs, in the middle. This area becomes covered with hair when a female goes through puberty.

- **Labia:** The labia are the two sets of skin folds (often called "lips") on either side of the opening of the vagina. The labia majora are the outer lips, and the labia minora are the inner lips. It is normal for the labia to look different from each other.

- **Clitoris:** The clitoris is a small, sensitive bump at the bottom of the mons pubis that is covered by the labia minora.

- **Urinary opening:** The urinary opening, below the clitoris, is where the urine (pee) leaves the body.

- **Vaginal opening:** The vaginal opening is the entry to the vagina and is found below the urinary opening.

Those are the basics of the female reproductive system.

Female Sexual Response and Hormone Control

The female sexual response includes arousal and orgasm. A woman may become pregnant without having an orgasm. Follicle-stimulating hormone (FSH), luteinizing hormone (LH), estrogen, and progesterone have major roles in regulating the functions of the female reproductive system.

At puberty, when the ovaries and uterus respond to certain stimuli, this causes the hypothalamus to secrete a gonadotropin-releasing hormone. This hormone enters the blood and goes to the anterior pituitary gland, where it stimulates the secretion of FSH and LH. These hormones, in turn, affect the ovaries and uterus and the monthly cycles begin. A woman's reproductive cycle lasts from menarche to menopause.

Menopause occurs when a woman's reproductive cycles stop. This period is marked by decreased levels of ovarian hormones and increased levels of pituitary FSH and LH. The changing hormone levels are responsible for the symptoms associated with menopause.

Section 1.6

Male Reproductive System

"The Male Reproductive System," © 2016 Omnigraphics.
Reviewed February 2019.

Like all living things, human beings reproduce. Reproduction is essential for the survival of a species. Most species have males and females for that purpose, with each sex having its own reproductive system.

What Are the Difference between the Male and Female Reproductive Systems?

There are many differences between male and female reproductive systems. Unlike the human female reproductive system, most of the parts of the male reproductive system are situated outside the body. Where the female reproductive system releases only one egg every month during the menstrual process, the male reproductive system can produce millions of sperm cells in a day. Each system also has a primary function which is unique to the reproduction process. The main function of the male reproductive system is to produce and deliver sperm as well as produce hormones such as testosterone, which is responsible for many of the important physical changes the male goes through during puberty. Testosterone is essential to the male reproductive system because it stimulates the ongoing production of sperm.

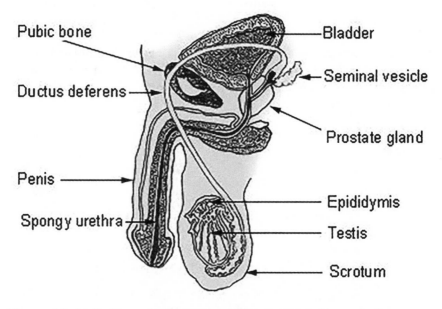

Figure 1.3. *Male Reproductive System* (Source: "Male Reproductive System," Centers for Disease and Control Prevention (CDC).)

Function of Male Reproductive System

- The external parts of the male reproductive system consist of the penis, scrotum, and testicles.

- The internal organs, or accessory glands, include the epididymis, vas deferens, seminal vesicles, urethra, prostate gland, bulbourethral glands, and the ejaculatory duct.

External Organs
Penis

The penis is the male organ used during intercourse. It consists of two main parts, the shaft, and the glans. The glans is a cone-shaped structure situated at the end of the penis and is covered by foreskin, which is a thin, loose layer of skin, which is sometimes removed by a medical procedure called circumcision. Circumcision is done for many reasons: for hygiene, social, religious, or cultural reasons. The tip of the penis contains the opening of the urethra, a tube that transports urine and semen. Inside, the penis consists of sponge-like tissues which absorb blood and makes the penis become erect for intercourse.

Scrotum

The scrotum is a bag-like structure that can be found behind the penis. It contains the testicles, which produce sperm, the male gamete, and sex hormones. The scrotum protects the testicles and adjusts the body temperature to ensure the survival of sperm. The scrotum contains special muscles in its wall which helps it to contract and relax according to the body temperature necessary for the proper functioning of the sperm.

Testicles

Also called "testes," the testicles are two oval organs inside the scrotum. Testicles produce hormones, including testosterone, and create sperm. The sperms are produced by seminiferous tubules inside the testes.

Accessory Glands
Urethra

The urethra is a long tube that carries urine from the urinary bladder. In boys, it also brings semen out of the body during ejaculation. During sexual intercourse, when the penis becomes erect, urine is blocked and only the semen is allowed to come out of the urethra.

Epididymis

One of the accessory organs of the male reproductive system, the epididymis is found inside the body. Before transporting the sperm to the vas deferens, the epididymis matures the sperm cells.

Vas Deferens

The vas deferens is a long muscular tube connecting the epididymis and the pelvic area. The vas deferens is the duct system that carries semen—the sperm-nourishing fluid—to the urethra.

Other accessory glands of the male reproductive system include the ejaculatory ducts, which empty semen into the urethra; the seminal vesicles responsible for producing the majority of the fluid found in semen; the prostate gland, which produces fluids that nourish and protect the sperm, and the bulbourethral or Cowper's glands which produce preejaculate to provide lubrication for semen to pass through the urethra.

What Does the Male Reproductive System Do?

All of the organs that make up the male reproductive system are designed to work in harmony to generate and release sperm into the female's vagina during sexual intercourse. Once released into the vagina, if a healthy sperm meets a mature egg conception can begin. In addition, the male reproductive system produces hormones that play a vital role in ensuring that a boy will develop into a sexually mature man who is capable of reproducing.

References

1. Dr. David T. Derrer, MD. "The Male Reproductive System," WebMD, February 27, 2014.

2. "Male Reproductive System," The Nemours Foundation/ KidsHealth, 2015.

3. "Male Reproductive System," PubMed Health Glossary, n.d.

4. "Bulbourethral Glands," Human Anatomy, 2012.

5. "The Male Reproductive System," The Cleveland Clinic Foundation, 2013.

Chapter 2

Understanding Sexually Transmitted Diseases

Chapter Contents

Section 2.1

What Is a Sexually Transmitted Disease?

This section includes text excerpted from documents published by two public domain sources. Text under the headings marked 1 are excerpted from "Sexually Transmitted Diseases (Stds)," *Eunice Kennedy Shriver* National Institute of Child Health and Human Development (NICHD), January 31, 2017; Text under the headings marked 2 are excerpted from "Sexually Transmitted Infections," Office on Women's Health (OWH), U.S. Department of Health and Human Services (HHS), January 31, 2019.

Sexually Transmitted Disease?[1]

Sexually transmitted diseases (STDs), also known as "sexually transmitted infections" (STIs), are typically caused by bacteria or viruses and are passed from person to person during sexual contact with the penis, vagina, anus, or mouth. The symptoms of STDs/STIs vary between individuals, depending on the cause, and many people may not experience symptoms at all.

Many STDs/STIs have significant health consequences. For instance, certain STIs can also increase the risk of getting and transmitting the human immunodeficiency virus (HIV)/acquired immune deficiency syndrome (AIDS) and alter the way the disease progresses. STIs can also cause long-term health problems, particularly in women and infants. Some of the health problems that arise from STIs include pelvic inflammatory disease (PID), infertility, tubal or ectopic pregnancy, cervical cancer, and perinatal or congenital infections in infants.

Who Gets Sexually Transmitted Diseases and Sexually Transmitted Infections[2]

Nearly 20 million people in the United States get an STI each year. These infections affect women and men of all backgrounds and economic levels. But half of all new infections are among young people 15 to 24 years old.

How Do You Get Sexually Transmitted Diseases or Sexually Transmitted Infections?[2]

STIs are spread in the following ways:

- Having unprotected (without a condom) vaginal, oral, or anal sex with someone who has an STI. It can be difficult to tell if someone has an STI. STIs can be spread even if there are no signs or symptoms.

- During genital touching. It is possible to get some STIs, such as syphilis and herpes, without having sex.

- Through sexual contact between women who have sex only with other women

- From a pregnant or breastfeeding woman to her baby

- Through men who only have sex with men

- Through unprotected heterosexual intercourse

What Causes Sexually Transmitted Diseases or Sexually Transmitted Infections[1]

There are three major causes of STDs/STIs:

- Bacteria, including chlamydia, gonorrhea, and syphilis

- Viruses, including HIV/AIDS, herpes simplex virus, human papillomavirus (HPV), hepatitis B virus, cytomegalovirus (CMV), and Zika

- Parasites, such as *Trichomonas vaginalis*, or insects such as crab lice or scabies mites

Any STI can be spread through sexual activity, including sexual intercourse, and some STIs spread through oral sex and other sexual activity. Ejaculation does not have to occur for an STI to pass from person to person.

In addition, sharing contaminated needles, such as those used to inject drugs, or using contaminated body piercing or tattooing equipment also can transmit some infections, such as HIV, hepatitis B, and hepatitis C. A few infections can be sexually transmitted and are also spread through nonsexual, close contact. Some of these infections, such as CMV, are not considered STIs even though they can be transmitted through sexual contact.

Regardless of how a person is exposed, once a person is infected by an STI, she or he can spread the infection to other people through oral, vaginal, or anal sex, even if no symptoms are apparent.

What Are the Symptoms of Sexually Transmitted Diseases or Sexually Transmitted Infections?[1]

People with STDs/STIs may feel ill and notice some of the following signs and symptoms:

- Unusual discharge from the penis or vagina
- Sores or warts on the genital area
- Painful or frequent urination
- Itching and redness in the genital area
- Blisters or sores in or around the mouth
- Abnormal vaginal odor
- Anal itching, soreness, or bleeding
- Abdominal pain
- Fever

In some cases, people with STIs have no symptoms. Over time, any symptoms that are present may improve on their own. It is also possible for a person to have an STI with no symptoms and then pass it on to others without knowing it.

If you are concerned that you or your sexual partner may have an STI, talk to your healthcare provider. Even if you do not have symptoms, it is possible you may have an STI that needs treatment to ensure your and your partners' sexual health.

Can Sexually Transmitted Diseases or Sexually Transmitted Infections Cause Health Problems?[2]

Yes. Each STI causes different health problems for both women and men. Certain types of untreated STIs can cause or lead to:

- Problems getting pregnant or permanent infertility
- Problems during pregnancy and health problems for the unborn baby
- Infection in other parts of the body
- Organ damage
- Certain types of cancer, such as cervical cancer

• Death

• Having certain types of STIs makes it easier for you to get HIV (another STI) if you come into contact with it.

How Do You Get Tested for Sexually Transmitted Diseases and Sexually Transmitted Infections?[2]

Ask your doctor or nurse about getting tested for STIs. Your doctor or nurse can tell you what test(s) you may need and how they are done. Testing for STIs is also called STI screening.

STI testing can include:

• **Pelvic and physical exam.** Your doctor looks for signs of infection, such as warts, rashes, or discharge.

• **Blood test.** A nurse will draw some blood to test for an STI.

• **Urine test.** You urinate (pee) into a cup. The urine is then tested for an STI.

• **Fluid or tissue sample.** Your doctor or nurse uses a cotton swab to take fluid or discharge from an infected place on your body. The fluid is looked at under a microscope or sent to a lab for testing.

How Are Sexually Transmitted Diseases and Sexually Transmitted Infections Treated?[2]

For some STIs, treatment may involve taking medicine by mouth or getting a shot. For other STIs that can't be cured, like herpes or HIV and AIDS, medicines can help reduce the symptoms.

Is There a Cure for Sexually Transmitted Diseases and Sexually Transmitted Infections?[1]

Viruses such as HIV, genital herpes, human papillomavirus, hepatitis, and cytomegalovirus cause STDs/STIs that cannot be cured. People with an STI caused by a virus will be infected for life and will always be at risk of infecting their sexual partners. However, treatments for these viruses can significantly reduce the risk of passing on the infection and can reduce or eliminate symptoms. STIs caused by bacteria, yeast, or parasites can be cured using appropriate medication.

disease, ectopic pregnancy (pregnancy outside of the uterus), infertility, and chronic pelvic pain.

- **Age disparities.** Young people ages 15 to 24 account for half of all new STDs, although they represent just 25 percent of the sexually experienced population. Adolescent females may have increased susceptibility to infection because of increased cervical ectopy.

- **Social, economic, and behavioral factors.** The spread of STDs is directly affected by social, economic, and behavioral factors. Such factors may cause serious obstacles to STD prevention due to their influence on social and sexual networks, access to and provision of care, willingness to seek care, and social norms regarding sex and sexuality. Among certain vulnerable populations, historical experience with segregation and discrimination exacerbates the influence of these factors. Social, economic, and behavioral factors that affect the spread of STDs include:

  - **Racial and ethnic disparities.** Certain racial and ethnic groups (mainly African American, Hispanic, and American Indian/Alaska Native populations) have high rates of STDs, compared with rates for Whites. Race and ethnicity in the United States are correlated with other determinants of health status, such as poverty, limited access to healthcare, fewer attempts to get medical treatment, and living in communities with high rates of STDs.

  - **Poverty and marginalization.** STDs disproportionately affect disadvantaged people and people in social networks where high-risk sexual behavior is common, and either access to care or health-seeking behavior is compromised.

  - **Access to healthcare.** Access to high-quality healthcare is essential for early detection, treatment, and behavior-change counseling for STDs. Groups with the highest rates of STDs are often the same groups for whom access to or use of health services is most limited.

  - **Substance abuse**. Many studies document the association of substance abuse with STDs. The introduction of new illicit substances into communities often can alter sexual behavior drastically in high-risk sexual networks, leading to the epidemic spread of STDs.

- **Sexuality and secrecy.** Perhaps the most important social factors contributing to the spread of STDs in the United States are the stigma associated with STDs and the general discomfort of discussing intimate aspects of life, especially those related to sex. These social factors separate the United States from industrialized countries with low rates of STDs.

- **Sexual networks.** Sexual networks refer to groups of people who can be considered "linked" by sequential or concurrent sexual partners. A person may have only one sex partner, but if that partner is a member of a risky sexual network, then the person is at higher risk for STDs than a similar individual from a lower-risk network.

Section 3.1

Trends in Sexually Transmitted Disease Infection in the United States

This section includes text excerpted from "Reported STDs in the United States, 2017—High Burden of STDs Threatens Millions of Americans," Centers for Disease Control and Prevention (CDC), September 26, 2018.

Sexually transmitted diseases (STDs) are a substantial health challenge facing the United States. Many cases of chlamydia, gonorrhea, and syphilis continue to go undiagnosed and unreported, and data on several additional STDs—such as human papillomavirus (HPV) and herpes simplex virus (HSV)—are not routinely reported to the Centers for Disease Control and Prevention (CDC). As a result, national surveillance data captures only a fraction of America's STD burden. However, the data presented in the 2017 STD Surveillance Report provides important insight into the scope, distribution, and trends in STD diagnoses in the country.

Table 3.1. Reported STDs in the United States, 2017

STDs	Cases Reported	Rate per 100,000 people
Chlamydia	1,708,569	529
Gonorrhea	555,608	172
Syphilis (primary and secondary)	30,644	10
Syphilis (congenital)	918	23
Total	2,295,739	

Sexually Transmitted Disease Prevention Challenges

Maintaining and strengthening core prevention infrastructure is essential to mounting an effective national response. Limited resources make it challenging to quickly identify and treat STDs. More than half of state and local STD program budgets have been cut, resulting in staff layoffs, reduced clinic hours, and increased patient co-pays that can limit access to essential diagnosis and treatment services. Antibiotics can cure chlamydia, gonorrhea, and syphilis. However, left untreated, they put men, women, and infants at risk for severe, lifelong health outcomes such as chronic pain, severe reproductive-health complications, and HIV. People who cannot get STD care remain vulnerable to short- and long-term health consequences and are more likely to transmit infections to others, further compounding America's STD burden.

Some Groups Are Uniquely Susceptible to the Health Consequences of STDs

Chlamydia Can Cause Lifelong Damage to Young Women

Chlamydia is the most commonly reported STD, with approximately 1.7 million cases reported in 2017. Young women (ages 15 to 24) account for nearly half (45%) of reported cases and face the most severe consequences of an undiagnosed infection. Untreated STDs, such as chlamydia and gonorrhea, put women at increased risk for pelvic inflammatory disease, which may result in chronic pelvic pain, infertility, and potentially life-threatening ectopic pregnancy. It is estimated that undiagnosed STDs cause infertility in more than 20,000 women each year.

Troubling Rise in Syphilis among Women and Newborns

While syphilis was nearly eliminated more than a decade ago, today it is on the rise. Diagnosis of primary and secondary syphilis, the most infectious stages of the disease, increased 76 percent from 2013 to 2017 (17,365 to 30,644). Increasing rates of syphilis among women have led to a sharp rise in congenital syphilis—which occurs when syphilis passes from mother to baby during pregnancy. More than 900 cases of congenital syphilis were reported in 2017, which resulted in a number of deaths and severe health complications among newborns. The disease is preventable through routine screening and timely treatment for syphilis among pregnant women.

STDs Accelerating among Men, Particularly Gay and Bisexual Men

- If not adequately treated, syphilis places a person at increased risk for HIV. The CDC estimates about half of MSM who have syphilis also have HIV.

35

- While gonorrhea increased among men and women in 2017, the steepest increases were seen among men (19%) from 170 cases per 100,000 men in 2016 to 203 cases per 100,000 in 2017. Research suggests that reported cases of gonorrhea have increased among MSM in recent years. The rise in gonorrhea nationally is particularly alarming in light of the growing threat of drug resistance to the last remaining recommended gonorrhea treatment. While medication for gonorrhea has been available for decades, the bacteria have grown resistant to nearly every drug ever used to treat it. In the United States as of now, only one recommended treatment option remains—a combination of the antibiotics azithromycin and ceftriaxone.

What Can Be Done?

Turning back the rise in STDs will require renewed commitment from all players:

- **The CDC** uses national-level information to detect and rapidly respond to evolving threats, trains frontline health workers, and provides STD-prevention resources to state and local health departments.

- **State and local health departments** should direct resources to STD investigation and clinical service infrastructure for rapid detection and treatment for people living in areas hardest hit by the STD epidemic.

- **Providers** should make STD screening and timely treatment a standard part of medical care, especially for pregnant women and MSM. They should also try to seamlessly integrate STD screening and treatment into prenatal care, as well as HIV prevention and care services to leverage pre-exposure prophylaxis (or PrEP) clinical guidelines.

- **Everyone** should talk openly about STDs, get tested regularly, and reduce risk by using condoms and dental dams or practicing mutual monogamy if sexually active.

Section 3.2

The Global Human Immunodeficiency Virus/Acquired Immunodeficiency Syndrome Epidemic

This section includes text excerpted from "Global HIV/AIDS Overview," HIV.gov, U.S. Department of Health and Human Services (HHS), November 20, 2018.

Human immunodeficiency virus (HIV), the virus that causes acquired immunodeficiency syndrome (AIDS), is one of the world's most serious public-health challenges, but there is a global commitment to stopping new HIV infections and ensuring that everyone living with HIV has access to HIV treatment.

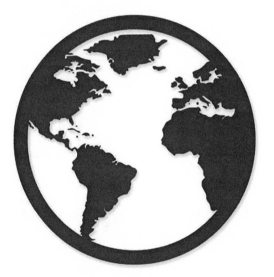

36.9 MILLION
people worldwide are currently living
with HIV/AIDS.

Figure 3.1. *Global HIV/AIDS*

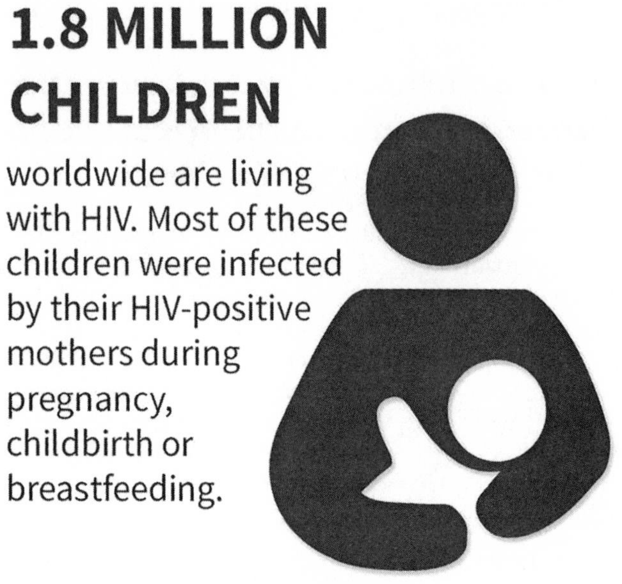

1.8 MILLION
CHILDREN

worldwide are living with HIV. Most of these children were infected by their HIV-positive mothers during pregnancy, childbirth or breastfeeding.

Figure 3.2. *Global HIV/AIDS in Children*

According to the Joint United Nations Programme on HIV and AIDS (UNAIDS):

- There are 36.9 million people worldwide who are currently living with HIV/AIDS and 2.1 million children worldwide are living with HIV.

- There were approximately 36.9 million people worldwide living with HIV/AIDS in 2017, of these, 1.8 million were children (<15 years old).

- An estimated 1.8 million individuals worldwide became newly infected with HIV in 2017, about 5,000 new infections per day. This includes 180,000 children (<15 years). Most of these children live in sub-Saharan Africa and were infected by their HIV-positive mothers during pregnancy, childbirth or breastfeeding.

- Approximately 75 percent of people living with HIV globally were aware of their HIV status in 2017. The remaining 25 percent (over 9 million people) still need access to HIV testing services. HIV testing is an essential gateway to HIV prevention, treatment, care, and support services.

- In 2017, 21.7 million people living with HIV (59%) were accessing antiretroviral therapy (ART) globally, an increase of 2.3 million since 2016 and up from 8 million in 2010.

- HIV treatment access is key to the global effort to end AIDS as a public-health threat. People living with HIV who are aware of their status, take ART daily as prescribed, and get and keep an undetectable viral load can live long, healthy lives. There is also a major prevention benefit. People living with HIV who adhere to HIV treatment and get and keep an undetectable viral load have effectively no risk of sexually transmitting HIV to their HIV-negative partners.

- AIDS-related deaths have been reduced by more than 51 percent since the peak in 2004. In 2017, 940 000 people died from AIDS-related illnesses worldwide, compared to 1.4 million in 2010 and 1.9 million in 2004.

- The vast majority of people living with HIV are in low- and middle-income countries.

- In 2017, there were 19.6 million people living with HIV (53%) in eastern and southern Africa, 6.1 million (16%) in western and central Africa, 5.2 million (14%) in Asia and the Pacific, and 2.2 million (6%) in Western and Central Europe and North America.

- Despite advances in our scientific understanding of HIV and its prevention and treatment, as well as years of significant effort by the global health community and leading government and civil society organizations, too many people living with HIV or at risk for HIV still do not have access to prevention, care, and treatment, and there is still no cure. However, effective treatment with antiretroviral drugs can control the virus so that people with HIV can enjoy healthy lives and reduce the risk of transmitting the virus to others.

- The HIV epidemic not only affects the health of individuals, it impacts households, communities, and the development and economic growth of nations. Many of the countries hardest hit by HIV also suffer from other infectious diseases, food insecurity, and other serious problems.

- Despite these challenges, there have been successes and promising signs. New global efforts have been mounted to address the epidemic, particularly in the last decade. The number of people newly infected with HIV has declined over the years. In addition, the number of people with HIV receiving treatment in resource-poor countries has dramatically increased in the past decade.

- Progress also has been made in preventing mother-to-child transmission of HIV and keeping mothers alive. In 2017, 80 percent (61 to >95%) of pregnant women living with HIV had access to antiretroviral medicines to prevent transmission of HIV to their babies, up from 47 percent in 2010.

- However, despite the availability of this widening array of effective HIV prevention tools and methods and a massive scale-up of HIV treatment in recent years, new infections among adults globally have not decreased sufficiently.

Section 3.3

U.S. Response to the Global Epidemic

This section includes text excerpted from "Global HIV/AIDS Overview," HIV.gov, U.S. Department of Health and Human Services (HHS), November 20, 2018.

What Is PEPFAR?

The U.S. President's Emergency Plan for AIDS Relief (PEPFAR) is the U.S. government's response to the global human immunodeficiency virus (HIV)/acquired immunodeficiency syndrome (AIDS) epidemic and represents the largest commitment by any nation to address a single disease in history. Through PEPFAR, the U.S. has supported a world safer and more secure from infectious-disease threats. It has demonstrably strengthened the global capacity to prevent, detect, and respond to new and existing risks, which ultimately enhances global health security and protects America's borders.

In addition, the National Institutes of Health (NIH) represents the largest public investment in HIV/AIDS research in the world. NIH is engaged in research around the globe to understand, diagnose, treat, and prevent HIV infection and its many associated conditions, and to find a cure.

U.S. Government Global HIV/AIDS Activities

A number of U.S. government agencies have come together in the common cause of turning the tide against the HIV/AIDS pandemic. They support a range of activities, from research to technical assistance and financial support to other nations, to combat the global HIV/AIDS pandemic. These global activities are coordinated with PEPFAR.

Department of State and Its Role

The U.S. Global AIDS Coordinator reports directly to the Secretary of State. At the direction of the Secretary, the U.S. Department of State's (DoS) support for the Office of the Global AIDS Coordinator (OGAC) includes:

- Providing human-resources services

- Tracking budgets within its accounting system

- Transferring funds to other implementing agencies

- Providing office space, communication, and information-technology services

Chiefs of mission provide essential leadership to interagency HIV/AIDS teams and, along with other U.S. officials, engage in policy discussions with host-country leaders to generate additional attention and resources for the pandemic and ensure strong partner coordination.

The U.S. Agency for International Development

The U.S. Agency for International Development (USAID) is an independent federal government agency that receives overall foreign policy guidance from the Secretary of State. USAID implemented its first HIV/AIDS programs in 1986 and currently supports the implementation of PEPFAR programs in nearly 100 countries, through direct in-country presence in 50 countries and through seven regional programs in the remaining countries. As a development agency, USAID has focused for many years on strengthening primary healthcare systems in order to prevent, and more recently to treat and care for, a number of communicable diseases, including HIV/AIDS.

U.S. Department of Defense

The U.S. Department of Defense (DoD) implements PEPFAR programs by supporting HIV/AIDS prevention, treatment, and care, strategic information, human-capacity development, and program and policy development in host militaries and civilian communities of 73 countries around the world. These activities are accomplished through direct military-to-military assistance, support to nongovernmental organizations and universities, and collaboration with other U.S. government agencies in the country. Members of the defense forces in 13 PEPFAR focus countries have been the recipients of DoD military-specific HIV/AIDS prevention programs designed to address their unique risk factors, in addition to treatment and care programs for their personnel.

U.S. Department of Commerce

The U.S. Department of Commerce (DoC) has provided and continues to provide in-kind support to PEPFAR, aimed at furthering private-sector engagement by fostering public–private partnerships. The U.S. Census Bureau, within the DoC, is also an important partner in PEPFAR. Activities include assisting with data management and analysis, survey support, estimating infections averted, and supporting mapping of country-level activities.

U.S. Department of Labor

The U.S. Department of Labor (DoL) implements PEPFAR workplace-targeted projects that focus on the prevention and reduction of HIV/AIDS-related stigma and discrimination. DoL has programs in over 23 countries and has received PEPFAR funding for projects in Guyana, Haiti, India, Nigeria, and Vietnam. DoL programs that work with the International Labor Organization (ILO) and the Academy for Educational Development (AED) have helped 415 enterprises adopt policies that promote worker retention and access to treatment. These programs have reached more than 2,500,000 workers now covered under protective HIV/AIDS workplace policies. DoL brings to all these endeavors its unique experience in building strategic alliances with employers, unions, and Ministries of Labor, which are often overlooked and difficult to target.

U.S. Department of Health and Human Services

The U.S. Department of Health and Human Services (HHS) has a long history of HIV/AIDS work within the United States and internationally. Under PEPFAR, HHS implements prevention, treatment, and care programs in developing countries and conducts HIV/AIDS research through these HHS agencies and programs:

- Centers for Disease Control and Prevention (CDC)

- Division of Global HIV and TB (DGHT)

- U.S. Food and Drug Administration (FDA)

- Health Resources and Services Administration (HRSA)

- National Institutes of Health (NIH)

- Office of Global Affairs (OGA)

- Substance Abuse and Mental Health Services Administration (SAMHSA)

- Peace Corps

- Department of the Treasury

Section 3.4

Current Status of Sexually Transmitted Diseases

This section contains text excerpted from "New CDC Analysis Shows Steep and Sustained Increases in STDs in Recent Years," Centers for Disease Control and Prevention (CDC), August 28, 2018.

Recent U.S. Data Reveal Threat to Multiple Populations

Nearly 2.3 million cases of chlamydia, gonorrhea, and syphilis were diagnosed in the United States in 2017, according to preliminary data released by the Centers for Disease Control and Prevention (CDC) at the National STD Prevention Conference in Washington, D.C. This surpassed the previous record set in 2016 by more than 200,000 cases and marked the fourth consecutive year of sharp increases in these sexually transmitted diseases (STDs).

The CDC analysis of STD cases reported for 2013 and preliminary data for 2017 shows steep sustained increases:

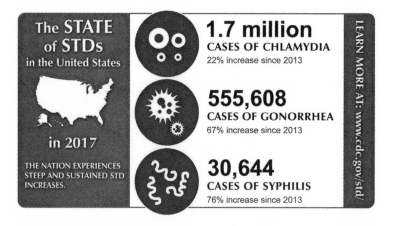

Figure 3.3. *The State of STDs in the United States in 2017* (Source: "The State of STDs Infographic," Centers for Disease Control and Prevention (CDC).)

Chlamydia, gonorrhea, and syphilis are curable with antibiotics, yet most cases go undiagnosed and untreated—which can lead to severe adverse health effects that include infertility, ectopic pregnancy,

44

stillbirth in infants, and increased human immunodeficiency virus (HIV) risk. Prior studies suggest a range of factors may contribute to STD increases, including socioeconomic factors such as poverty, stigma, and discrimination; and drug use.

Continued Concerns about Antibiotic-Resistant Gonorrhea

The threat of untreatable gonorrhea persists in the United States, and reports of antibiotic-resistant gonorrhea abroad have only reinforced those concerns. Over the years, gonorrhea has become resistant to nearly every class of antibiotics used to treat it except ceftriaxone, the only remaining highly effective antibiotic to treat gonorrhea in the United States.

In 2015, the CDC began recommending healthcare providers prescribe a single shot of ceftriaxone accompanied by an oral dose of azithromycin to people diagnosed with gonorrhea. Azithromycin was added to help delay the development of resistance to ceftriaxone.

Emerging resistance to ceftriaxone has not been seen since the dual-therapy approach was implemented, and there has not yet been a confirmed treatment failure in the United States when using this recommended therapy.

The CDC findings released, however, show that emerging resistance to azithromycin is now on the rise in laboratory testing—with the portion of samples that showed emerging resistance to azithromycin increasing from one percent in 2013 to more than four percent in 2017.

The finding adds concerns that azithromycin-resistant genes in some gonorrhea could crossover into strains of gonorrhea with reduced susceptibility to ceftriaxone—and that a strain of gonorrhea may someday surface that does not respond to ceftriaxone.

Chapter 4

Sexually Transmitted Diseases in General Population

Chapter Contents

Section 4.1

Sexually Transmitted Diseases in Women

This section contains text excerpted from the following sources:
Text in this section begins with excerpts from "Stds in Women and
Infants," Centers for Disease Control and Prevention (CDC), July 23,
2018; Text under the heading "How STDs Impact Women Differently
from Men" is excerpted from "How STDs Impact Women Differently
from Men," Centers for Disease Control and Prevention (CDC),
January 2, 2018.

Women and their infants are uniquely vulnerable to the consequences
of sexually transmitted infections (STIs). While individual-level determinants, including high-risk behaviors, contribute to disease transmission and acquisition risk, it is widely accepted that social barriers to
sexually transmitted disease (STD) prevention and control efforts also
contribute to infectious-disease prevalence. A woman's relationship status with her partner, including concurrency of the relationship, may be
an important predictor of her sexual health. In addition to poverty and
lack of access to quality STD services, homelessness or unstable housing
may influence a woman's sexual risk. For some women, maintaining
the relationship with a partner may take a higher priority than STD
risk reduction, affecting her sexual and reproductive health, as well as
the health of her unborn baby. A woman can also be placed at risk for
STIs through her partner's sexual encounter with an infected partner.
Consequently, even a woman who has only one partner may be obliged
to practice safer sex, such as using condoms and/or dental dams.

Chlamydia and gonorrhea disproportionately affect women because
early infection may be asymptomatic and, if untreated, the infection
may ascend to the upper reproductive tract, resulting in pelvic inflammatory disease (PID). Data from studies suggest that as much as
10 percent of untreated chlamydial infections progress to clinically
diagnosed PID and the risk with untreated gonococcal infection may
be even higher. PID is a major concern because it can result in inflammation and damage to the fallopian tubes, elevating the risk of infertility and ectopic pregnancy. Tubal factor infertility ranks among the
most common causes of infertility, accounting for 30 percent of female
infertility in the United States, and much of this damage results from
previous episodes of PID. An important public-health measure for
preventing PID, and ultimately tubal factor infertility, is through the
prevention and control of *Chlamydia trachomatis* and *Neisseria gonorrhoeae*. Strategies to improve the early detection and treatment of

chlamydia and gonorrhea, as demonstrated in randomized controlled trials, has been shown to reduce a woman's risk for PID and ultimately protect the fertility of women.

Human papillomavirus (HPV) infections are highly prevalent in the United States. Although most HPV infections in women appear to be transient and may not result in clinically significant sequelae, high-risk HPV-type infections can cause abnormal changes in the uterine cervical epithelium, which are detected by cytological examination of Papanicolaou (Pap) smears. Persistent high-risk HPV-type infections may lead to cervical cancer precursors, which, if undetected can result in cancer. Other low-risk HPV-type infections can cause genital warts, low-grade Pap smear abnormalities, laryngeal papillomas, and rarely, recurrent respiratory papillomatosis in children born to infected mothers.

Impact on Maternal and Fetal Outcomes

Similar to nonpregnant women, a high proportion of pregnant women with chlamydial and gonococcal infections are asymptomatic. Documented sequelae of untreated infections in pregnancy include premature delivery, premature rupture of the membranes, low birth weight, and stillbirth. Maternal infection can also affect the infant, leading to conjunctivitis infections (termed ophthalmia neonatorum in the first four weeks of life), and, in the case of *C. trachomatis*, pneumonia. Although topical prophylaxis of infants at delivery is effective for the prevention of gonococcal ophthalmia neonatorum, prevention of neonatal pneumonia requires prenatal detection and treatment. The clinical presentation of conjunctivitis can be variable and these infections are especially important to treat promptly, as they can lead to visual impairment.

Syphilis has long been known to be an important risk factor for adverse pregnancy outcomes. The consequences of untreated maternal infection include fetal death, preterm birth, and congenital infection in a proportion of surviving infants, resulting in both physical and mental developmental disabilities. Most cases of congenital syphilis are preventable if women are screened for syphilis and treated early during prenatal care.

Genital infections with herpes simplex virus (HSV) are extremely common, can cause painful outbreaks, and can have serious consequences for pregnant women and their infants. Neonatal herpes can be a severe illness presenting with vesicular lesions on the skin, eye, or mouth, seizures, respiratory collapse, and/or liver failure, following

49

contact with infected cervical or vaginal secretions during delivery. Risk of transmission to the infant is greatest when the mother has a first-episode primary genital infection during pregnancy, especially if she acquires infection towards the end of her pregnancy.

How Sexually Transmitted Diseases Impact Women Differently from Men

STDs remain a major public-health challenge in the United States, especially among women, who disproportionately bear the long-term consequences of STDs. For example, each year untreated STDs cause infertility in at least 20,000 women in the United States, and untreated syphilis in pregnant women results in infant death in up to 30 percent of cases. Testing and treatment are keys to reducing disease and infertility associated with undiagnosed STDs.

- **Women are less likely than men to have symptoms of common STDs such as chlamydia and gonorrhea.** If symptoms do occur, they can go away even though the infection may remain.

- **Women are more likely than men to confuse symptoms of an STD for something else.** Women often have normal discharge or think that burning/itching is related to a yeast infection.

- **Women may not see symptoms as easily as men.** Genital ulcers (such as from herpes or syphilis) can occur in the vagina and may not be easily visible, while men may be more likely to notice sores on their penis.

- **Women typically see their doctor more often than men.** Women should use this time with their doctor as an opportunity to ask for STD testing, and not assume STD testing is part of their annual exam. While the Pap test screens for cervical cancer, it is not a good test for other types of cancer or STDs.

- **A woman's anatomy can place her at a unique risk for STD infection.** The lining of the vagina is thinner and more delicate than the skin on a penis, so it's easier for bacteria and viruses to penetrate. The vagina is a good environment for bacteria to grow.

- **STDs can lead to serious health complications and affect a woman's future reproductive plans.** Untreated STDs can lead to pelvic inflammatory disease (PID), which can result in infertility and ectopic pregnancy.

- **Women who are pregnant can pass STDs to their babies.** Genital herpes, syphilis, and HIV can be passed to babies during pregnancy and at delivery. The harmful effects of STDs in babies may include stillbirth, low birth weight (less than five pounds), brain damage, blindness, and deafness.

- **Human papillomavirus (HPV) is the most common sexually transmitted infection in women and is the main cause of cervical cancer.** While HPV is also very common in men, most do not develop any serious health problems. Women should learn how to protect themselves and their partners from STDs, and where to receive testing and treatment. There are resources available for women to learn how to protect themselves and their partners from STDs, and where to receive testing and treatment.

- **Healthcare providers**—A doctor or physician can provide patient-specific information about STD prevention, protection, and tests.

- **800-232-4636**—Operators can provide information about local STD testing sites and put callers in touch with trained professionals to answer questions about STDs.

- **GetTested.cdc.gov**—This website provides users with locations for HIV, STD, and hepatitis testing, and STD and hepatitis vaccines around the United States.

- **www.cdc.gov/std**—The CDC's website includes comprehensive information about STDs, including fact sheets on STDs and Pregnancy (www.cdc.gov/std/pregnancy) and STDs and Infertility (www.cdc. gov/std/infertility).

Section 4.2

Sexually Transmitted Diseases in Children

This section includes text excerpted from "Special Populations," Centers for Disease Control and Prevention (CDC), June 4, 2015. Reviewed February 2019.

Certain diseases (e.g., gonorrhea, syphilis, and chlamydia), if acquired after the neonatal period, strongly suggest sexual contact. For other diseases (e.g., human papillomavirus (HPV) infections and vaginitis), the association with sexual contact is not as clear.

Sexual Assault and Abuse and Sexually Transmitted Diseases

The identification of sexually transmissible agents in children beyond the neonatal period strongly suggests sexual abuse. Postnatally acquired gonorrhea and syphilis; chlamydia infection; and nontransfusion, nonperinatally acquired human immunodeficiency virus (HIV) are indicative of sexual abuse.

- Chlamydia infection might be indicative of sexual abuse in children ≥3 years of age and among those aged <3 years when infection is not likely perinatally acquired.

- Sexual abuse should be suspected when genital herpes, *T. vaginalis*, or anogenital warts are present.

The general rule that sexually transmissible infections beyond the neonatal period are evidence of sexual abuse has exceptions. For example, genital infection with *T. vaginalis* or rectal or genital infection with *C. trachomatis* (CT) among young children might be the result of perinatally acquired infection and has, in some cases of chlamydia infection, persisted for as long as two to three years, though perinatal CT infection is now uncommon because of prenatal screening and treatment of pregnant women. Genital warts have been diagnosed in children who have been sexually abused, but also in children who have no other evidence of sexual abuse. Bacterial vaginosis (BV) has been diagnosed in children who have been abused, but its presence alone does not prove sexual abuse. Most hepatitis B virus (HBV) infections in children result from household exposure to persons who have chronic HBV infection rather than sexual abuse.

Evaluating Children for Sexually Transmitted Diseases

Evaluations of children for sexual assault or abuse should be conducted in a manner designed to minimize pain and trauma to the child. Examinations and collection of vaginal specimens in prepubertal children can be very uncomfortable and should be performed by an experienced clinician to avoid psychological and physical trauma to the child. The decision to obtain genital or other specimens from a child to evaluate for STDs must be made on an individual basis; however, children who received a diagnosis of one STD should be screened for all STDs. Because STDs are not common in prepubertal children or infants evaluated for abuse, testing all sites for all organisms is not routinely recommended. Factors that make the child considerable for screening for STD include:

- Child has experienced penetration or has evidence of recent or healed penetrative injury to the genitals, anus, or oropharynx.

- Child has been abused by a stranger.

- Child has been abused by a perpetrator known to be infected with an STD or at high risk for STDs (e.g., intravenous drug abusers, men who have sex with men (MSM), persons with multiple sexual partners, and those with a history of STDs).

- Child has a sibling, other relatives, or another person in the household with an STD.

- Child lives in an area with a high rate of STDs in the community.

- Child has signs or symptoms of STDs (e.g., vaginal discharge or pain, genital itching or odor, urinary symptoms, and genital lesions or ulcers).

- Child or parent requests STD testing.

- If a child has symptoms, signs, or evidence of an infection that might be sexually transmitted, the child should be tested for common STDs before the initiation of any treatment that could interfere with the diagnosis of those other STDs. Because of the legal and psychosocial consequences of a false-positive diagnosis, only tests with high specificities should be used. The potential benefit to the child of a reliable STD diagnosis justifies deferring presumptive treatment until specimens for highly specific tests are obtained by providers with experience in the evaluation of sexually abused and assaulted children.

Child-Abuse Survivors Have Higher Risk for Sexually Transmitted Diseases in Adulthood

HIV infection has been reported in children for whom sexual abuse was the only known risk factor. Children might be at higher risk for HIV acquisition than adolescent and adult sexual-assault or sexual-abuse survivors because the sexual abuse of children is frequently associated with multiple episodes of assault and mucosal trauma might be more likely. Serologic testing for HIV infection should be considered for sexually abused children. Although data are insufficient concerning the efficacy of non-occupational post-exposure prophylaxis (nPEP) among children, treatment is well tolerated by infants and children with and without HIV infection, and children have a minimal risk for serious adverse reactions because of the short period recommended for prophylaxis.

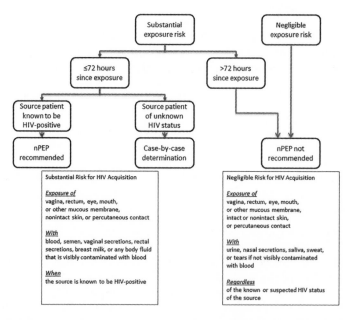

Figure 4.1. *Evaluation and Treatment of Possible Nonoccupational HIV Exposures*

Section 4.3

Sexually Transmitted Diseases in Adolescents and Young Adults

This section includes text excerpted from "Stds in Adolescents and Young Adults," Centers for Disease Control and Prevention (CDC), July 24, 2018.

Incidence and prevalence estimates suggest that young people aged 15 to 24 years acquire half of all new sexually transmitted diseases (STDs) and that one in four sexually active adolescent females has an STD, such as chlamydia or human papillomavirus (HPV).

Compared with older adults, sexually active adolescents aged 15 to 19 years and young adults aged 20 to 24 years are at higher risk of acquiring STDs for a combination of behavioral, biological, and cultural reasons. For some STDs, such as chlamydia, adolescent females may have increased susceptibility to infection because of increased cervical ectopy.

- The higher prevalence of STDs among adolescents may also reflect multiple barriers to accessing quality STD prevention and management services, including inability to pay, lack of transportation, long waiting times, conflict between clinic hours and work and school schedules, embarrassment attached to seeking STD services, method of specimen collection, and concerns about confidentiality (e.g., explanation of benefits for services received mailed to parents or guardians).

- Traditionally, intervention efforts have targeted individual level factors associated with STD risk, which do not address higher level factors (e.g., peer norms and media influences) that may also influence behaviors. Interventions for at-risk adolescents and young adults that address underlying aspects of the social and cultural conditions affecting sexual risk-taking behaviors are needed, as are strategies designed to improve the underlying social conditions themselves.

- In addition, in designing STD programs, consideration should be given to the needs of adolescent and young adult populations, including extended hours, optimizing privacy in waiting rooms, and urine-based specimen collection.

Section 4.4

Sexually Transmitted Diseases in Men

"Sexually Transmitted Diseases in Men,"
© 2019 Omnigraphics. Reviewed February 2019.

List of Sexually Transmitted Diseases in Men

Several types of sexually transmitted diseases (STDs) can affect sexually active men, and some of them are listed below.

Chlamydia

Chlamydia is a bacterial infection that is commonly acquired by sexually active young adults. The causative agent is a bacteria called *"Chlamydia trachomatis."* Many of the infected men and women show no signs or symptoms. However, the most common symptoms for men are urethritis, and an infection of the epididymis and testes. This infection can be cured with the use of antibiotics such as azithromycin. However, re-manifestation of the infection can occur on occasion if the affected sex partners are not treated appropriately.

Gonorrhea

Gonorrhea is a bacterial infection, which may not often show any signs and symptoms; as a result, the individual may remain undiagnosed. Similar to chlamydia, gonorrhea causes urethritis in men, leading to burning or painful urination and discharge from the urethra. This is caused by bacteria called *"Neisseria gonorrhoeae,"* and when symptoms occur, they tend to develop in about four to eight days after contraction. Gonorrhea can cause infection in the rectum and in the throat, in the rare scenario. It is also possible for gonorrhea to spread within the body and cause symptoms such as joint pain, rash, etc. Gonorrhea can be treated with the use of antibiotics such as cefixime (Suprax) and others. Chlamydia and gonorrhea frequently occur together, so in most cases, curative treatment involves a single antibiotic intake that cures both.

Trichomoniasis

The causative is known to be a parasite called *"Trichomonas vaginalis."* Most women and men do not have symptoms, and may not know if they are infected. When it does cause symptoms, it causes symptoms similar to those mentioned with chlamydia and gonorrhea, such as urethritis along with itching, burning, and discharge from the urethra. This can be cured with a single dose of antibiotic regimen; most frequently used antibiotics include metronidazole.

Human Immunodeficiency Virus

The human immunodeficiency virus (HIV) is the most threatening form of a STD. This is caused by the virus, and the infection can occur during sexual contact, by sharing needles, or from an infected pregnant woman to her baby. After some point, the virus causes dysfunction of the immune system, and research suggests that the average time from infection to immune suppression is approximately 10 years. There are no specific symptoms or signals for identifying a case of HIV infection, but on occasion, the individual may develop a fever or flu-like illness two to four weeks after viral contraction. The progression of immunosuppression can lead to complications, such as unusual infections, cancers, and dementia. There are medications available for management of the infection and to delay or prevent progression of the illness, but there is no cure.

Genital Herpes

This is also a viral infection that is caused by herpes simplex viruses (HSV). The symptoms include painful sores with blisters on sexually exposed areas of the body such as the penis, scrotum, buttocks, anus, inside the urethra, and skin of the thighs, etc. They can eventually develop into open ulcers and crust over. Genital herpes can be transmitted with any type of sexual contact. The first outbreak may be more severe than subsequent outbreaks and can sometimes be accompanied by a fever and swollen lymph nodes. HSV type 1 causes cold sores around the mouth, and type 2 causes genital herpes. Like in other STDs, it is possible for an individual to become infected with HSV and have very mild to no symptoms. However, it is possible to transmit the infection even if no symptoms are observed.

Genital Warts

There are different types of human papillomavirus (HPV) that cause different conditions, but HPV infection is a very common STD. Some HPV causes common warts, which are not worrisome, but there are other types of HPV that spread during sexual activity and cause genital warts. Most infected individuals with HPV infection do not develop genital warts or cancers, as the body is often able to clear the infection on its own. Over 75 percent of sexually active people are believed to be infected at some point in their life. Genital warts in men appear as raised bumps that are soft and fleshy in nature, which mostly occurs on the penis or anal area. On occasion, they have a cauliflower-like appearance and can increase in size. Treatments to destroy or remove genital warts are available. Also, vaccines are available for boys and girls that confer immunity to the most common HPV types. Particularly, most of the HPV resolves on its own, and there is no specific cure.

Hepatitis B and C

Inflammation of the liver is called "hepatitis." Hepatitis B (HBV) and hepatitis C (HCV) are two viral diseases that can be transmitted by contact with the blood of an infected individual or by sexual activity.

Often, HBV may not cause symptoms, but symptoms of acute hepatitis can be seen in almost 50 percent of infections. The dangerous part of HBV infection is that around five percent of infected individuals progress to have long-term liver damage or chronic hepatitis B. People with chronic hepatitis B are at an increased risk of liver cancer. There is a very effective vaccine available for hepatitis B prevention. Acute hepatitis can be treated by supportive care and rest, but chronic hepatitis needs interferon or antiviral treatments.

Unlike HBV, HCV is a rare sexually transmitted disease and is usually spread by contact with the blood of an infected person. Individuals infected with HCV show no symptoms, which delays the diagnosis and sometimes leads to a misdiagnosis. The possibility of developing liver damage in people with chronic infection is higher and notably, there is no vaccine available against HCV.

Syphilis

Syphilis is caused by bacteria called *"Treponema pallidum."* In the latent state, it persists and progresses through three phases, if not treated in the initial stage. It manifests initially as a painless ulcer called "chancre" at the site of sexual contact, which develops after 10 to 90 days after infection. It mostly resolves in three to six weeks with antibiotic treatment. If this first stage is untreated, then the individual can develop secondary syphilis as the disease spreads to other organs causing symptoms such as skin rash, swollen lymph nodes, arthritis, kidney disease, or liver problems. Some people may experience latent infection years after this stage, which leads to the development of tertiary syphilis. Tertiary syphilis leads to a brain infection, development of nodules called "gummas," aortic aneurysm, loss of sight, and deafness. Fortunately, syphilis is curable with proper antibiotic treatment.

Zika Virus

The Zika virus is mostly associated with birth defects in babies born to infected mothers. The transmission of the virus occurs among humans through the bite of an infected vector mosquito; however, few studies have found that sexual transmission of the Zika virus is also possible.

What Tests Diagnose Sexually Transmitted Diseases in Men?

Diagnoses are made on the basis of clinical history and physical findings. Identifiable signs and symptoms can occur in herpes and syphilis, but a firm diagnosis is often made after the microbiological culture confirmation of the organism. The tests available to detect STDs in men are performed either by identification of surface proteins of the organism or by the genetic material of the organism and, notably, these methods are more commonly used than the culture.

What Is the Treatment for Sexually Transmitted Diseases in Men?

STDs caused by bacteria are curable with antibiotics. Parasitic infections, such as trichomoniasis, can be cured by effective methods of elimination. Some of the viral STDs may resolve on their own, such as HPV infection, but specifically, there is no treatment for HPV infection. Most genital warts are removed and/or treated by destruction or cryotherapy. HBV and HCV infections may persist and develop into chronic infection. There are antiviral drugs and interferon treatments available for management of these long-term infections, such as HIV and HSV, which can reduce the severity and frequency of outbreaks, but there is no cure.

What Will Be the Consequence If Sexually Transmitted Diseases Are Untreated? Can You Die from a Sexually Transmitted Disease?

There are some STDs that are treatable, but if they are untreated, they can spread throughout the body and cause serious consequences, such as gonorrhea and syphilis. HIV infection leads to immunosuppression, which at a later stage can be accompanied by some rare infections or cancers that can cause death. As mentioned, above treatments are available to postpone the immunosuppressive actions of the virus; however, there is no cure.

Both hepatitis B and C can cause liver damage that on occasion can progress to liver failure. Herpes infection persists throughout life with possible outbreaks, and it has no cure.

Which Specialties of Doctors Treat Sexually Transmitted Diseases in Men?

Infected individuals can consult their primary-care practitioners. Consulting with internists and family practitioners can be beneficial in diagnosing and treating the STD as well.

References

1. Stoppler, Melissa Conrad. "9 Common STDs (Sexually Transmitted Diseases) in Men," MedicineNet, May 6, 2016.

2. "Most Common STDs for Women and Men," WebMD, December 6, 2017.

3. "STD List for Men—STDs Common in Men," The STD Project, May 31, 2012.

Chapter 5

Sexually Transmitted Diseases in Special Populations

Chapter Contents

Section 5.1

Human Immunodeficiency Virus among Pregnant Women

This section includes text excerpted from "HIV among Pregnant Women, Infants, and Children," Centers for Disease Control and Prevention (CDC), March 21, 2018.

Perinatal human immunodeficiency virus (HIV) transmission, also known as mother-to-child transmission, can happen at any time during pregnancy, labor, delivery, and breastfeeding. The Centers for Disease Control and Prevention (CDC) recommends that all women who are pregnant or planning to get pregnant take an HIV test as early as possible before and during every pregnancy. This is because the earlier HIV is diagnosed and treated, the more effective HIV medicine, called antiretroviral treatment (ART), will be at preventing transmission and improving the health outcomes of both mother and child. Advances in HIV research, prevention, and treatment have made it possible for many women living with HIV to give birth without transmitting the virus to their babies.

The annual number of HIV infections through perinatal transmission declined by more than 90 percent since the early 1990s. If a woman takes HIV medicine daily as prescribed throughout pregnancy, labor, and delivery, and gives HIV medicine to her baby for 4 to 6 weeks after delivery, the risk of transmitting HIV to the baby can be as low as 1 percent or less. When the HIV viral load is not adequately reduced, a Cesarean delivery can also help to prevent HIV transmission. After delivery, a mother can prevent transmitting HIV to her baby by not breastfeeding and not pre-chewing her baby's food.

For babies living with HIV, starting treatment early is important because the disease can progress more quickly in children than adults. Providing ART early can help children with perinatal HIV live longer, healthier lives.

Prevention Challenges

Pregnant women with HIV may not know they are infected. The CDC recommends HIV testing for all women as part of routine prenatal care. According to CDC research, more women take the prenatal HIV test if the opt-out approach is used. Opt-out prenatal HIV testing means that a pregnant woman is told she will be given an HIV test as part of routine prenatal care unless she opts out—that is, chooses not to have the test. In some parts of the country where HIV among women is more common, the CDC recommends a second test during the third trimester of pregnancy. In 2016, the American Medical Association (AMA) created a new Common Procedural Terminology (CPT) code that includes HIV testing in the Obstetric Panel. This allows prenatal care providers to order just one panel that includes many standard serologic tests for pregnant women, including HIV.

Women living with HIV may not:

- Know they are pregnant, how to prevent or safely plan a pregnancy, or what they can do to reduce the risk of transmitting HIV to their baby. For women living with HIV, it is important that they visit their healthcare provider regularly.

- Take HIV medicine as directed for their own health and if they want to get pregnant

- Take HIV medicine throughout the pregnancy, labor, and delivery, as prescribed

- Ensure their infant gets HIV medicine after delivery

- Avoid breastfeeding

- Avoid prechewing food for an infant, toddler, or anyone else

To get the full protective benefit of HIV medicine, the mother needs to take it as prescribed—without interruption—throughout pregnancy, labor, and delivery, and provide HIV medicine to her infant. Pregnant women living with HIV may have nausea during pregnancy that can interfere with taking medicines, and new mothers may not be able to see their HIV medical care provider consistently.

Social and economic factors, especially poverty, affect access to all healthcare, and disproportionately affect people living with HIV. Pregnant women living with HIV may face more barriers to accessing medical care if they also use injection drugs; use other substances; or are homeless, incarcerated, mentally ill, or uninsured.

Section 5.2

Sexually Transmitted Diseases in Women Who Have Sex with Women

This section includes text excerpted from "Lesbian and Bisexual Health," Office on Women's Health (OWH), U.S. Department of Health and Human Services (HHS), June 1, 2009. Reviewed February 2019.

What Does It Mean to Be a Lesbian or a Bisexual?

A lesbian is a woman who has sex with another woman, even if it is only sometimes. A lesbian is currently only having sex with a woman, even if she has had sex with men in the past. A bisexual, on the other hand, is a person who is sexually attracted to, or sexually active with, both men and women.

Are Lesbian and Bisexual Women at Risk of Getting Sexually Transmitted Infections?

Women who have sex with women commonly called "WSW" are at risk for STIs. Lesbian and bisexual women can transmit sexually transmitted infections (STIs) to each other through:

- Skin-to-skin contact

- Mucosa contact (e.g., mouth to vagina)

- Vaginal fluids

- Menstrual blood

- Sharing sex toys

Some STIs are more common among lesbians and bisexual women and may be passed easily from woman to woman (such as bacterial vaginosis). Other STIs are much less likely to be passed from woman to woman through sex (such as human immunodeficiency virus (HIV)). When lesbians get these less common STIs, it may be because they also have had sex with men, especially when they were younger. It is also important to remember that some of the less common STIs may not be passed between women during sex, but through sharing needles used to inject drugs. Bisexual women may be more likely to get infected with STIs that are less common for lesbians, since bisexuals are presumably having sex with men and women. Common STIs that can be passed between women include:

Bacterial vaginosis (BV). BV is more common in lesbian and bisexual women than in other women. The reason for this is unknown. BV often occurs in both members of lesbian couples.

The vagina normally has a balance of mostly "good" bacteria and fewer "harmful" bacteria. BV develops when the balance changes. With BV, there is an increase in harmful bacteria and a decrease in good bacteria. Sometimes BV causes no symptoms. But over one-half of women with BV have vaginal itching or discharge with a fishy odor. BV can be treated with antibiotics.

Chlamydia. Chlamydia is caused by bacteria. It is spread through vaginal, oral, or anal sex. It can damage the reproductive organs, such as the uterus, ovaries, and fallopian tubes. The symptoms of chlamydia are often mild—in fact, it's known as a "silent infection." Because the symptoms are mild, you can pass it to someone else without even knowing you have it. Chlamydia can be treated with antibiotics. Infections that are not treated, even if there are no symptoms, can lead to:

- Lower abdominal pain

- Lower back pain

- Nausea

- Fever

- Pain during sex

- Bleeding between periods

Genital herpes. Genital herpes is an STI caused by the herpes simplex viruses type 1 (HSV-1) or type 2 (HSV-2). Most genital herpes is caused by HSV-2. HSV-1 can cause genital herpes. But it more commonly causes infections of the mouth and lips, called "fever blisters or "cold sores." You can spread oral herpes to the genitals through oral sex.

Most people have few or no symptoms from a genital herpes infection. When symptoms do occur, they usually appear as one or more blisters on or around the genitals or rectum. The blisters break, leaving tender sores that may take up to four weeks to heal. Another outbreak can appear weeks or months later. But it almost always is less severe and shorter than the first outbreak. Although the infection can stay in the body forever, the outbreaks tend to become less severe and occur less often over time. You can pass genital herpes to someone else even when you have no symptoms. There is no cure for herpes. Drugs can be used to shorten and prevent outbreaks or reduce the spread of the virus to others

Human papillomavirus (HPV). HPV can cause genital warts. If left untreated, HPV can cause abnormal changes on the cervix that can lead to cancer. Most people don't know they're infected with HPV because they don't have symptoms. Usually, the virus goes away on its own without causing harm. But not always. The Papanicolaou (Pap) test checks for abnormal cell growths caused by HPV that can lead to cancer in women. If you are age 30 or older, your doctor may also do an HPV test with your Pap test. This is a deoxyribonucleic acid (DNA) test that detects most of the high-risk types of HPV. It helps with cervical-cancer screening. If you're younger than 30 years old and have had an abnormal Pap test result, your doctor may give you an HPV test. This test will show if HPV caused the abnormal cells on your cervix.

Both men and women can spread the virus to others whether or not they have any symptoms. Lesbians and bisexual women can transmit HPV through direct genital skin-to-skin contact, touching, or sex toys used with other women. Lesbians who have had sex with men are also at risk of HPV infection. This is why regular Pap tests are just as important for lesbian and bisexual women as they are for heterosexual women.

There is no treatment for HPV, but a healthy immune (body defense) system can usually fight off HPV infection. Two vaccines (Cervarix and Gardasil®) can protect girls and young women against the types of HPV that cause most cervical cancers. The vaccines work best when given before a person's first sexual contact when she could be exposed to HPV. Both vaccines are recommended for 11- and 12-year-old girls. But the vaccines also can be used in girls as young as 9 and in women through age 26 who did not get any or all of the shots when they were younger. These vaccines are given in a series of 3 shots. It is best to use the same vaccine brand for all 3 doses. Ask your doctor which brand vaccine is best for you. Gardasil® also has benefits for men in preventing genital warts and anal cancer caused by HPV. It is approved for use in boys as young as 9 and for young men through age 26. The vaccine does not replace the need to wear condoms or use dental dams to lower your risk of getting other types of HPV and other sexually transmitted infections. If you do get HPV, there are treatments for diseases caused by it. Genital warts can be removed with medicine you apply yourself or treatments performed by your doctor. Cervical and other cancers caused by HPV are most treatable when found early. There are many options for cancer treatment.

Pubic lice. Also known as crabs, pubic lice are small parasites that live in the genital areas and other areas with coarse hair. Pubic lice are spread through direct contact with the genital area. They can also be spread through sheets, towels, or clothes. Pubic lice can be treated with creams or shampoos you can buy at the drugstore.

Trichomoniasis or "Trich." Trichomoniasis is caused by a parasite that can be spread during sex. You can also get trichomoniasis from contact with damp, moist objects, such as towels or wet clothes. Symptoms include:

* Yellow, green, or gray vaginal discharge (often foamy) with a strong odor

* Discomfort during sex and when urinating

* Irritation and itching of the genital area

* Lower abdominal pain (in rare cases)

* Trichomoniasis can be treated with antibiotics.

Less common STIs that may affect lesbians and bisexual women include:

Gonorrhea. Gonorrhea is a common STI but is not commonly passed during woman-to-woman sex. However, it could be, since it does live in vaginal fluid. It is caused by a type of bacteria that can grow in warm, moist areas of the reproductive tract, such as the cervix, uterus, and fallopian tubes. It can grow in the urethra in men and women. It can also grow in the mouth, throat, eyes, and anus. Even when women have symptoms, they are often mild and are sometimes thought to be from a bladder or other vaginal infection.
Symptoms include:

* Pain or burning when urinating

* Yellowish and sometimes bloody vaginal discharge

* Bleeding between menstrual periods

* Gonorrhea can be treated with antibiotics.

Hepatitis B. Hepatitis B is a liver disease caused by a virus. It is spread through bodily fluids, including blood, semen, and vaginal fluid. People can get hepatitis B through sexual contact, by sharing needles with an infected person, or through mother-to-child transmission at birth. Some women have no symptoms if they get infected with the virus.

Women with symptoms may have:

- Mild fever

- Headache and muscle aches

- Tiredness

- Loss of appetite

- Nausea or vomiting

- Diarrhea

- Dark-colored urine and pale bowel movements

- Stomach pain

- Yellow skin and whites of eyes

There is a vaccine that can protect you from hepatitis B.

Human immunodeficiency virus (HIV). HIV is spread through body fluids, such as blood, vaginal fluid, semen, and breast milk. It is primarily spread through sex with men or by sharing needles. Women who have sex with women can spread HIV, but this is rare.

Some women with HIV may have no symptoms for 10 years or more. Women with HIV symptoms may have:

- Extreme fatigue (tiredness)

- Rapid weight loss

- Frequent low-grade fevers and night sweats

- Frequent yeast infections (in the mouth)

- Vaginal yeast infections

- Other STIs

- Pelvic inflammatory disease (PID) (an infection of the uterus, ovaries, or fallopian tubes)

- Menstrual cycle changes

- Red, brown, or purplish blotches on or under the skin or inside the mouth, nose, or eyelids

Acquired immunodeficiency syndrome (AIDS) is the final stage of HIV infection. HIV infection turns to AIDS when you have one or more opportunistic infections, certain cancers, or a very low CD4 cell count.

Syphilis is an STI caused by bacteria. It's passed through direct contact with a syphilis sore during vaginal, anal, or oral sex. Untreated syphilis can infect other parts of the body. It is easily treated with antibiotics. Syphilis is very rare among lesbians. But, you should talk to your doctor if you have any sores that don't heal.

Section 5.3

Sexually Transmitted Diseases in Men Who Have Sex with Men

This section includes text excerpted from "STDs in Men Who Have Sex with Men," Centers for Disease Control and Prevention (CDC), July 24, 2018.

The incidence of many sexually transmitted diseases (STDs) in gay, bisexual, and other men who have sex with men (collectively referred to as MSM)—including primary and secondary syphilis and antimicrobial-resistant gonorrhea—is greater than that reported in women and men who have sex with women only (MSW). In addition to the negative effects of untreated STDs, elevated STD burden is of concern because it may indicate a high risk for subsequent human immunodeficiency virus (HIV) infection. Annual increases in reported STD cases could reflect increased frequency of behaviors that transmit both STDs and HIV (e.g., condomless anal sex), and having an STD increases the risk of acquisition or transmission of HIV.

The relatively high incidence of STD infection among MSM may be related to multiple factors, including individual behaviors and sexual network characteristics. The number of lifetime or recent sex partners, rate of partner exchange, and frequency of condomless sex each influence an individual's probability of exposure to STDs. However, MSM network characteristics, such as a high prevalence of STDs, interconnectedness, and concurrency of sex partners, and possibly limited access to healthcare, also affect the risk of acquiring an STD. Furthermore, experiences of stigma—verbal harassment, discrimination, or physical assault based on attraction to men—are associated with increased sexual-risk behavior among MSM.

For data reported in this section, MSM is defined as men who either reported having one or more male sex partners or who self-reported as gay/homosexual or bisexual. MSW is defined as men who reported having sex with women only or who did not report the sex of their sex partner, but reported that they considered themselves straight/heterosexual.

Chapter 6

Racial Disparities in Sexually Transmitted Disease Rates

Chapter Contents

Section 6.1

Sexually Transmitted Diseases in Racial and Ethnic Minorities

This section includes text excerpted from "STDs in Racial and Ethnic Minorities," Centers for Disease Control and Prevention (CDC), July 24, 2018.

Disparities continue to persist in rates of sexually transmitted diseases (STDs) among some racial minority or Hispanic groups when compared with rates among Whites. This is also true across a wide variety of other health-status indicators, providing evidence that race and Hispanic ethnicity in the United States are population characteristics strongly correlated with other factors affecting overall health statuses, such as income, employment, insurance coverage, and educational attainment.

Access to, and routine use of, quality healthcare—including STD prevention and treatment—is key to reducing STD disparities in the United States. Among all races or ethnic groups in the United States, Hispanics had the lowest rate of health-insurance coverage in 2016 at 84.0 percent (a slight increase from 83.8% in 2015).

Even when healthcare is readily available to racial and ethnic minority populations, fear and distrust of healthcare institutions can negatively affect the healthcare-seeking experience. Social and cultural discrimination, language barriers, provider bias, or the perception that these may exist, likely discourage some people from seeking care. Moreover, the quality of care can differ substantially for minority patients. Broader inequities in social and economic conditions for minority communities are reflected in the profound disparities observed in the incidence of STDs by race and Hispanic ethnicity.

In communities where STD prevalence is higher because of these and other factors, people may experience difficulties reducing their risk for STIs. With each sexual encounter, they face a greater chance of encountering an infected partner than those in lower prevalence settings do, regardless of similar sexual behavior patterns. Acknowledging inequities in STD rates by race and Hispanic ethnicity is a critical first step toward empowering affected groups and the public-health community to collaborate in addressing systemic inequities in the burden of disease—with the ultimate goal of minimizing the health impacts of STDs on individuals and populations.

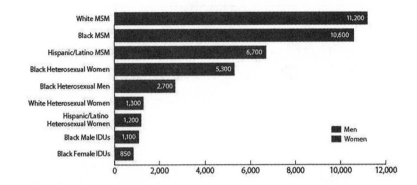

Figure 6.1. *Estimated Numbers of New Human Immunodeficiency Virus Infections in the United States for the Most Affected Subpopulations*

Race and Hispanic ethnicity data:

- **Chlamydia**—27.8 percent of chlamydia case reports were missing race or Hispanic ethnicity data.

- **Gonorrhea**—19.0 percent of gonorrhea case reports were missing information on race or Hispanic ethnicity.

- **Syphilis**—4.2 percent of all primary and secondary syphilis case reports were missing information on race or Hispanic ethnicity.

- **Other STDs**—Data from the National Health and Nutrition Examination Survey (NHANES) indicate the seroprevalence of herpes simplex virus type 2 (HSV-2) in the United States has decreased from 1999 to 2000 to 2015 to 2016 for all race and Hispanic ethnicity groups; however, HSV-2 seroprevalence was highest among non-Hispanic Blacks throughout the entire time period. *Trichomonas vaginalis* prevalence in urine specimens obtained from adult NHANES participants aged 18 to 59 years during 2013 to 2014 indicated a prevalence of 0.5 percent among males and 1.8 percent among females; highest rates were observed among non-Hispanic Black males (4.2%) and females (8.9%). A separate analysis of NHANES data during 2013 to 2016 among men aged 18 to 59 years also found a higher prevalence among non-Hispanic Blacks. An analysis of NHANES data from 2001 to 2004 from cervicovaginal swab specimens also found higher *T. vaginalis* prevalence among non-Hispanic Black females.

Section 6.2

African Americans Disproportionately Affected by Sexually Transmitted Diseases

This section includes text excerpted from "HIV among African Americans," Centers for Disease Control and Prevention (CDC), July 5, 2018.

Blacks/African Americans account for a higher proportion of new human immunodeficiency virus (HIV) diagnoses, those living with HIV, and those who have ever received an acquired immunodeficiency syndrome (AIDS) diagnosis, compared to other races/ethnicities. In 2016, African Americans accounted for 44 percent of HIV diagnoses, though they comprise 12 percent of the U.S. population.

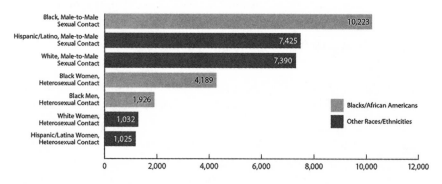

Figure 6.2. *HIV Diagnoses in the United States for the Most-Affected Subpopulations, 2016*

Human Immunodeficiency Virus and Acquired Immunodeficiency Syndrome Diagnoses

In 2016:

- 17,528 African Americans received an HIV diagnosis in the United States (12,890 men and 4,560 women).

- More than half (58% 10,223) of African Americans who received an HIV diagnosis were gay or bisexual men.

- Among African American gay and bisexual men who received an HIV diagnosis, 39 percent (3,993) were young men aged 25 to 34.

• Forty-seven percent (8,501) of those who received an AIDS diagnosis in the United States were African American.

From 2011 to 2015:

• HIV diagnoses decreased 8 percent among African Americans overall.

• HIV diagnoses decreased 16 percent among African American heterosexual men.

• The number of HIV diagnoses among African American women fell 20 percent, though it is still high compared to women of other races/ethnicities. In 2016, 4,560 African American women received an HIV diagnosis, compared with 1,450 White women and 1,168 Hispanic/Latina women.

• HIV diagnoses decreased 39 percent among African Americans who inject drugs.

• HIV diagnoses among African American gay and bisexual men remained stable.

• HIV diagnoses among young African American gay and bisexual men aged 13 to 24 remained stable.

• HIV diagnoses among African American gay and bisexual men aged 25 to 34 increased by 30 percent.

Prevention Challenges

In all communities, lack of awareness of HIV status contributes to HIV risk. People who do not know they have HIV cannot take advantage of HIV care and treatment and may unknowingly pass HIV to others. A number of challenges contribute to the higher rates of HIV infection among African Americans. The greater number of people living with HIV (prevalence) in African American communities and the tendency for African Americans to have sex with partners of the same race/ethnicity mean that African Americans face a greater risk of HIV infection. Some African American communities also experience higher rates of other STDs than other racial/ethnic communities in the United States. Having another STD can significantly increase a person's chance of getting or transmitting HIV.

Stigma, fear, discrimination, and homophobia may place many African Americans at higher risk for HIV. Also, the poverty rate is higher among African Americans than other racial/ethnic groups. The socioeconomic issues associated with poverty—including limited access to high-quality healthcare, housing, and HIV-prevention education—directly and indirectly, increase the risk for HIV infection and affect the health of people living with and at risk for HIV. These factors may explain why African Americans have worse outcomes on the HIV continuum of care, including lower rates of linkage to care and viral suppression.

Section 6.3

Latinxs Bear a Disproportionate Burden

This section includes text excerpted from "HIV among Latinos," Centers for Disease Control and Prevention (CDC), February 2, 2017.

Human immunodeficiency virus (HIV) is a serious health threat to Latinx communities, which bear a disproportionate share of the HIV burden in the United States. Factors driving the HIV epidemic in this population are as diverse as Latinx communities themselves. Prevention efforts led to promising declines in new diagnoses among Latinxs from 2005 to 2010. However, those declines stalled in more recent years, reinforcing the need for expanded access to proven HIV-prevention programs for this important population.

In 2015, approximately 9,290 Latinxs received a diagnosis of HIV infection. Latinxs represent approximately 17 percent of the U.S. population but account for an estimated 21 percent of people living with HIV (263,900 persons in 2013) and an estimated 24 percent of all persons with newly diagnosed infection. Men account for 88 percent of diagnoses among Latinxs. The HIV diagnosis rate among Latinx men is more than three times that among White men. 75 percent of new diagnoses among Latinx men occur among men who have sex with men (MSM). While new HIV diagnoses among MSM overall stabilized between 2010 and 2014, diagnoses among Latinx MSM increased 13 percent during this period. The HIV diagnosis rate among Hispanic women in 2015 was more than three times that of White women. If current rates persist, the Centers for Disease Control and Prevention (CDC) projects that approximately one in 48 Latinx men, one in 227 Latinx women, and one in four Latinx gay and bisexual men will be diagnosed with HIV during their lifetimes. There are substantial regional differences in the HIV burden among Latinxs across the United States. For example, the HIV diagnosis rate is highest among Latinxs in the Northeast. While male-to-male sexual contact is the predominant mode of transmission among all Latinxs newly diagnosed with HIV, Latinxs in the Northeast are more likely than those in other regions to have been infected by intravenous drug use. Latinxs diagnosed with HIV in the South are more likely than those in the Northeast to have been infected through male-to-male sexual contact.

AIDS continues to claim the lives of too many Latinx men and women. Since the beginning of the epidemic, more than 100,000 Latinxs with AIDS have died. HIV treatment helps people with HIV live healthy lives and prevents transmission of the virus to partners. However, too few Latinxs living with HIV receive the care and treatment they need. The CDC estimates that among the roughly 263,900 Latinxs living with HIV in 2013, 85 percent were aware of their status. The CDC study suggests that among Latinxs with diagnosed HIV, 54 percent were virally suppressed (i.e., the virus is under control at a level that helps them stay healthy and reduces the risk of transmission).

Complex Factors Increase Risk

Some of the factors that increase the risk of sexually transmitted diseases (STDs) among Latinxs include:

- **High prevalence of STDs and higher rates of HIV.** Data show that the burden of STDs among Latinxs is high. Because STDs can place individuals at higher risk for HIV infection, high STD prevalence may contribute to higher HIV incidence among Latinx men and women. Additionally, disproportionate rates of HIV among Latinxs and the current high prevalence of HIV in Latinx communities increase the likelihood that Latinxs will encounter HIV-infected sex or drug-injecting partner, placing them at greater risk.

- **Social and economic factors.** The social and economic realities of some Latinxs' lives, including poverty, discrimination, and lack of access to healthcare, can increase HIV risk. Language barriers may also affect the quality of care.

- **Stigma.** The stigma associated with HIV and homosexuality may help to spread HIV in Latinx communities. In some communities, the cultural value of machismo may create a reluctance to acknowledge sensitive, yet risky behaviors, such as male-to-male sexual contact or substance abuse. Fear of disclosing risk behavior or sexual orientation may prevent Latinxs from seeking testing, treatment, and prevention services, and support from friends and family. As a result, too many Latinxs lack critical information about how to prevent infection.

- **Cultural factors.** Latinx culture in the United States is diverse. Research shows that Latinxs born in different countries have different behavioral risk factors for HIV. For example, data suggest that Hispanics born in Puerto Rico are more likely than other Hispanics to contract HIV as a result of injection-drug use or from high-risk heterosexual contact. By contrast, sexual contact with other men is the primary cause of HIV infection among men born in places such as Mexico and the United States.

Chapter 7

Sexually Transmitted Diseases in People in Correctional Facilities

Multiple studies have demonstrated that persons entering correctional facilities have high rates of sexually transmitted diseases (STDs) (including human immunodeficiency virus (HIV)) and viral hepatitis, especially those aged younger than 36 years old. Incarcerated persons are more likely to have low socioeconomic status, live in urban areas, and be ethnic and racial minorities. Risk behaviors for contracting STDs (e.g., having unprotected sex, having multiple sexual partners, using drugs and alcohol, and engaging in commercial, survival, or coerced sex) are common among incarcerated populations. Before incarceration, many have had limited access to medical care.

Although no comprehensive national guidelines regarding STD care and management have been developed for correctional populations, growing evidence demonstrates the utility of expanded STD screening and treatment services in correctional settings. For example, in jurisdictions with comprehensive, targeted jail screening, more chlamydial infections among females (and males if screened) are detected and subsequently treated in the correctional setting than any other single

This chapter includes text excerpted from "Special Populations," Centers for Disease Control and Prevention (CDC), June 4, 2015. Reviewed December 2018.

reporting source and might represent the majority of reported cases in certain jurisdictions.

Both men and women younger than 36 years of age in juvenile and adult detention facilities have been reported to have higher rates of chlamydia and gonorrhea than their nonincarcerated counterparts in the community, and across many studies, rates have been consistently higher among women than men. Syphilis seroprevalence rates, which can indicate previous or current infection, are considerably higher among adult men and women than in adolescents, consistent with the overall national syphilis trends. Detection and treatment of early syphilis in correctional facilities might impact rates of transmission.

In short-term facilities, including jails and juvenile-detention facilities that commonly house entrants for less than one year, up to half of the entrants are released back in the community within 48 hours. As a result, treatment completion rates for those screened for STDs and who receive STD diagnoses in short-term facilities might not be optimal. However, because of the mobility of incarcerated populations in and out of the community, the impact of screening in correctional facilities on the prevalence of infections among detainees and subsequent transmission in the community after release might be considerable. Moreover, treatment completion rates of greater than 95 percent can be achieved by offering screening at or shortly after intake, facilitating earlier receipt of test results; follow-up of untreated persons can be conducted through public-health outreach.

Universal screening for chlamydia and gonorrhea in women younger than 36 years of age entering juvenile and adult correctional facilities has been a long-standing recommendation. However, no such recommendation existed for men until 2006, when the Centers for Disease Control and Prevention (CDC) convened a consultation on male chlamydia screening that resulted in recommendations to screen men younger than thirty years for chlamydia at intake into jails.

Whereas several studies have shown a high prevalence of trichomonas among incarcerated persons, none have demonstrated the impact of trichomonas screening in correctional facilities. Women who report vaginal discharge should be evaluated and treated appropriately.

Chlamydia and Gonorrhea Screening

Women under the age of 36 and men under the age of 30 years in correctional facilities should be screened for chlamydia and gonorrhea. Chlamydia and gonorrhea screening should be conducted at intake.

Syphilis Screening

Universal screening should be conducted on the basis of the local area and institutional prevalence of early (primary, secondary, and early latent) infectious syphilis. Correctional facilities should stay apprised of syphilis prevalence as it changes over time.

Chapter 8

Specific Research Studies on Sexually Transmitted Diseases

Some of the health complications that arise from Sexually Transmitted Diseases (STDs) include pelvic inflammatory disease (PID), infertility, tubal or ectopic pregnancy, cervical cancer, and perinatal or congenital infections in infants born to infected mothers.

Human Immunodeficiency Virus/Acquired Immunodeficiency Syndrome

HIV, or human immunodeficiency virus, is the virus that causes acquired immunodeficiency syndrome (AIDS). HIV attacks the immune system by destroying CD4 positive (CD4+) T cells, a type of white blood cell that is vital to fighting off infection. The destruction of these cells leaves people infected with HIV vulnerable to other infections, diseases, and other complications.

• National Institute of Allergy and Infectious Diseases (NIAID) supports an HIV basic research program that provides valuable scientific information about the basic biology of HIV, the

This chapter contains text excerpted from "Sexually Transmitted Diseases (STD) Disease-Specific Research," National Institute of Allergy and Infectious Diseases (NIAID), October 27, 2016.

immune response to HIV infection, and potential targets for prevention and therapeutic strategies.

Chlamydia

Chlamydia is a common sexually transmitted disease (STD) caused by infection with *Chlamydia trachomatis*. It can cause cervicitis in women and urethritis and proctitis in both men and women. Chlamydial infections in women can lead to serious consequences, including pelvic inflammatory disease (PID), tubal factor infertility (TFI), ectopic pregnancy, and chronic pelvic pain (CPP).

- NIAID and NIAID-supported researchers are studying treatment options for chlamydia infections and developing a vaccine to prevent *Chlamydia trachomatis* infection.

Genital Herpes

Genital herpes is a sexually transmitted disease (STD) caused by the herpes simplex viruses (HSV) type 1 (HSV-1) or type 2 (HSV-2). NIAID supports research on genital herpes and herpes simplex virus (HSV). Studies are currently underway to develop better treatments for the millions of people who suffer from genital herpes. While some scientists are carrying out clinical trials to find the best way to use existing medicines, others are studying the biology of HSV.

- NIAID scientists have identified certain genes and enzymes (proteins) that the virus needs to survive. They are hopeful that drugs aimed at disrupting these viral targets might lead to the design of more effective treatments.

Gonorrhea

Gonorrhea is a sexually transmitted disease (STD) caused by infection with the *Neisseria gonorrhoeae* bacterium. *N. gonorrhoeae* infects the mucous membranes of the reproductive tract, including the cervix, uterus, and fallopian tubes in women, and the urethra in women and men. *N. gonorrhoeae* can also infect the mucous membranes of the mouth, throat, eyes, and rectum.

- NIAID supports a comprehensive, multidisciplinary program of research on *Neissesria gonorrhoeae* (gonococci). Researchers are trying to understand how gonococci infect cells while evading defenses of the human immune system.

Human Papillomavirus and Genital Warts

Human Papillomavirus (HPV) is the most common sexually transmitted infection (STI). HPV is a different virus than HIV and HSV (herpes). HPV is so common that nearly all sexually active men and women get it at some point in their lives. There are many different types of HPV. Some types can cause health problems, including genital warts and cancers. But there are vaccines that can stop these health problems from happening.

- NIAID conducts and supports research to better understand papillomaviruses and the natural history of HPV infection, develop new diagnostics with more accurate and rapid detection of HPV infections, find new treatments, and examine current HPV prevention strategies and the impact of behavior and age on HPV infection.

Pelvic Inflammatory Disease

Pelvic inflammatory disease (PID) is a general term that refers to infection and inflammation of the upper genital tract in women. It can affect the uterus (womb), fallopian tubes (tubes that carry eggs from the ovaries to the uterus), ovaries, and other organs related to reproduction. The scarring that results on these organs can lead to infertility, tubal (ectopic) pregnancy, chronic pelvic pain, abscesses (sores containing pus), and other serious problems. PID is the most common preventable cause of infertility in the United States.

- Scientists supported by NIAID are studying the effects of antibiotics, hormones, and substances that boost the immune system. These studies may lead to insights about how to prevent infertility and other complications of PID.

Syphilis

Syphilis is a sexually transmitted bacterial disease that causes genital ulcers (sores) in its early stages. If untreated, syphilis can also lead to more serious symptoms.

- NIAID-supported researchers are developing new tests that may provide better ways to diagnose syphilis and define the stage of infection. Efforts to develop a diagnostic test that would not require a blood sample are a high priority.

Vaginitis

Vaginitis refers to disorders of the vagina caused by infection, inflammation, or changes in the normal vaginal flora. The three most common diseases diagnosed among women with these symptoms include bacterial vaginosis (40 to 45%), vulvovaginal candidiasis (20 to 25%), and trichomoniasis (15 to 20%). In some cases, there may be more than one disease present. Recurrent vaginitis is also common. Vaginitis is the object of serious studies as scientists try to clarify its role in such conditions as a pelvic inflammatory disease and pregnancy-related complications.

- NIAID-supported research has led to advances in knowledge about the normal microflora of the vagina, reproductive behavior of yeast, and the genetic code of *T. vaginalis*. Other NIAID-funded researchers have sequenced the genome of *T. vaginalis*.

Part Two

Types of Sexually Transmitted Diseases

Chapter 9

Classification of Sexually Transmitted Diseases

Approximately 20 different infections are known to be transmitted through sexual contact. Here are descriptions of some common sexually transmitted infections (STIs).

Chlamydia

- Caused by the bacterium *Chlamydia trachomatis*

- Can be transmitted during vaginal, oral, or anal sexual contact with an infected partner

- Many infected individuals will not experience symptoms, but chlamydia can cause fever, abdominal pain, and unusual discharge from the penis or vagina.

- Can be treated with antibiotics

- If untreated, can cause pelvic inflammatory disease (PID), which can lead to chronic pelvic pain (CPP) and permanent damage to a woman's reproductive organs. This damage may lead to ectopic

This chapter contains text excerpted from "What Are Some Types of and Treatments for Sexually Transmitted Diseases (STDs) or Sexually Transmitted Infections (STIs)?" *Eunice Kennedy Shriver* National Institute of Child Health and Human Development (NICHD), January 31, 2017.

pregnancy (in which the fetus develops outside of the womb, a condition that can be life-threatening) and infertility.

- Can be transmitted to the fetus during pregnancy or to infant during delivery, causing eye infections or pneumonia. Antibiotic ointment is usually applied to a baby's eyes after birth to treat undetected chlamydia.

- Because chlamydia and gonorrhea often occur together, people who have one infection are typically treated for both by their healthcare provider.

- To prevent health complications and sexual transmission, treatment should be provided promptly for all persons testing positive for infection, and recent sexual partners should be treated at the same time to prevent reinfection.

- Infected individuals should follow their healthcare provider's recommendations about how long to abstain from sex after the treatment is completed to avoid passing the infection back and forth.

Gonorrhea

- Caused by the bacterium *Neisseria gonorrhoeae*, which can grow and multiply rapidly in the warm, moist areas of the reproductive tract

- Most common symptoms include discharge from the vagina or penis and painful or difficult urination

- Can be treated with antibiotics

- Like chlamydia, if left untreated, gonorrhea can cause pelvic inflammatory disease, which can lead to chronic pelvic pain and permanent damage to a woman's reproductive organs. This damage may lead to ectopic pregnancy (in which the fetus develops outside of the womb, a condition that can be life-threatening) and infertility.

- In both men and women, gonorrhea can also infect the mouth, throat, eyes, and rectum and can spread to the blood and joints, where it can become a life-threatening illness.

- Can be transmitted to the fetus during pregnancy.

- Because chlamydia and gonorrhea often occur together, people who have one infection are typically treated for both by their healthcare provider.

- People with gonorrhea can more easily contract human immunodeficiency virus (HIV), the virus that causes acquired immunodeficiency syndrome (AIDS). HIV-infected people with gonorrhea are also more likely to transmit the virus to someone else.

Genital Herpes

- Caused by the herpes simplex virus (HSV)

- There are two different strains, or types: HSV type 1 (HSV-1) and type 2 (HSV-2). Both can cause genital herpes, although most cases of genital herpes are caused by HSV-2.

- Symptoms of HSV-1 usually appear as fever blisters or cold sores on the lips, but it can also infect the genital region through oral-genital or genital-genital contact. Symptoms of HSV-2 are typically painful, watery skin blisters on or around the genitals or anus. However, substantial numbers of people who carry these viruses have no or only minimal signs or symptoms.

- Cannot be cured, but can be controlled with medication

- One medication can be taken daily to make it less likely that the infection will pass on to sex partner(s) or to infants during childbirth.

- Periodically, some people will experience outbreaks of symptoms in which new blisters form on the skin in the genital area; at those times, the virus is more likely to be passed on to other people.

- If a pregnant woman has an outbreak when she goes into labor, she may need to have a cesarean section (C-section) to prevent the infant from getting the virus during birth.

- Pregnant women, especially those who acquire genital herpes for the first time during pregnancy, may pass the infection to their newborns, causing life-threatening neonatal HSV, an infection affecting the infant's skin, brain, and other organs.

Human Immunodeficiency Virus/Acquired Immunodeficiency Syndrome

- HIV or human immunodeficiency virus, is the virus that causes AIDS.

- Destroys the body's immune system by killing the blood cells that fight infection. Once HIV destroys a substantial proportion of these cells, the body's ability to fight off and recover from infections is compromised. This advanced stage of HIV infection is known as AIDS.

- People whose HIV infection has progressed to AIDS have a weakened immune system and are very susceptible to opportunistic infections that do not normally make people sick and to certain forms of cancer.

- Transmission of the virus primarily occurs during unprotected sexual activity and by sharing needles used to inject intravenous drugs. HIV can also spread from mother to fetus during pregnancy and from mother to infant during delivery and breastfeeding. However, treatments are available that can virtually eliminate these types of transmission.

- In people who do not have HIV, the infection can be prevented by many tools, including abstaining from sex, limiting the number of sexual partners, never sharing needles, and using condoms and dental dams appropriately. Persons who may be at very high risk of HIV infection may be able to obtain HIV pre-exposure prophylaxis (PrEP), which consists of the HIV medication called Truvada, from their doctor to take every day so they can prevent HIV infection. PrEP will not work if it is not taken consistently. AIDS can be prevented in those with HIV infection by early initiation of antiretroviral therapy.

Human Papillomavirus

- Human papillomavirus (HPV) is the most common STI. More than 40 HPV types exist, and all of them can infect both men and women.

- The types of HPV vary in their ability to cause genital warts; infect other regions of the body, including the mouth and throat; and cause cancers of the cervix, vulva, penis, anus, and mouth.

- Cannot be cured but can be prevented with vaccines and controlled with medications

- Genital warts caused by the virus can be treated.

- Regular screening with a Pap smear test can prevent or detect at an early stage most cases of HPV-caused cervical cancer. (A

Pap smear test involves a healthcare provider taking samples of cells from the cervix during a standard gynecologic exam; these cells are examined under a microscope for signs of developing cancer).

- Two available vaccines protect against most (but not all) HPV types that cause cervical cancer. The Centers for Disease Control and Prevention (CDC) recommends this vaccine for girls and boys starting at 11 or 12 years old.

Syphilis

- Caused by the bacterium *Treponema pallidum*

- Passes from person to person during vaginal, anal, or oral sex through direct contact with syphilis sores

- Syphilis can also be spread from an infected mother to her fetus. In 2001, the number of cases of syphilis was at its lowest in 60 years. But the syphilis rate has increased nearly every year up to 2016, the most recent year for which data are available. Rates have increased among both men and women, but men account for a vast majority of syphilis cases.

- The first sign of syphilis is a chancre, a painless genital sore that most often appears on the penis or in and around the vagina. Chancres typically resolve on their own, but the body does not clear the infection on its own.

- Chancres make a person two to five times more likely to contract an HIV infection. If the person is already infected with HIV, chancres also increase the likelihood that the HIV virus will be passed on to a sexual partner.

- Can be treated with antibiotics:

  - If recognized during the early stages, usually within the first year of infection, syphilis can be treated with a single injection of antibiotic.

  - If not recognized early, or not treated immediately, syphilis may need longer treatment with antibiotics.

- Without treatment:

  - Usually spreads to other organs, including the skin, heart, blood vessels, liver, bones, and joints in secondary syphilis

- Other sores, such as a syphilis rash, can break out in later stages.

- Tertiary syphilis can develop over a period of years and involve the nerves, eyes, and brain, and can potentially cause death.

- Can pass to the fetus during pregnancy and to the infant during delivery.

- Infants who get syphilis infection in the womb may have misshapen bones, very low red blood cell count (called severe anemia), enlarged liver and spleen, jaundice (yellowing of the skin or eyes), nerve problems, blindness or deafness, meningitis, and skin rashes.

- Those being treated for syphilis must avoid sexual contact until the syphilis sores are completely healed to avoid infecting other people.

- Persons with syphilis must notify their sex partners so that they also can be tested and receive treatment if necessary.

- Pregnant women with syphilis, especially untreated syphilis, are at an increased risk of miscarriage and stillbirth.

Bacterial Vaginosis

- Occurs when problematic bacteria that are normally present only in small amounts in the body increase in number. Their levels get so high that they replace normal vaginal bacteria and upset the usual balance.

- More likely if a woman douches frequently or has new or multiple sexual partners

- Most common symptom is a thin, milky discharge that is often described as having a "fishy" odor. However, some women will have no symptoms at all.

- Can be treated with antibiotics, typically metronidazole or clindamycin

- Generally, sexual partners of women with bacterial vaginosis do not need to be treated because treatment of partners has not been shown to reduce the risk of recurrence.

- Treatment is recommended for all pregnant women who show symptoms.

- Increases the risk of getting other STIs even if the woman doesn't have any symptoms

- Associated with preterm labor and birth and having a low-birth-weight baby

- Also associated with pelvic inflammatory disease, an infection of the female reproductive organs, including the uterus and the fallopian tubes (which carry eggs to the uterus), and with infections that commonly occur after surgery

Trichomoniasis

- Caused by the single-celled parasite *Trichomonas vaginalis*

- Common in young, sexually active women but also infects men, though less frequently

- The parasite can be transmitted between men and women as well as between women whenever physical contact occurs between the genital areas.

- Can cause frequent, painful, or "burning" urination in men and women as well as vaginal discharge, genital soreness, redness, or itching in women. However, it may not cause any symptoms.

- Because the infection can occur without symptoms, a person may be unaware of the infection and continue to re-infect a sexual partner who is having recurrent signs of infection.

- Can be treated with a single dose of an antibiotic, usually either metronidazole or tinidazole, taken by mouth

- Because of re-infection, it is important to make sure that the diagnosed individual and all sexual partners are treated at the same time.

- Retesting is recommended for all sexually active women within three months after initial treatment even if they believe their partners were treated.

- Infection during pregnancy is associated with an increased risk of preterm labor or birth and infants with low birth weight.

- Stillbirth and newborn death are more than twice as likely among pregnant women with Trichomonas infection than among uninfected pregnant women.

Viral Hepatitis

Caused by several different viral strains.

- Hepatitis A virus (HAV):

  - Causes a short-term or self-limited liver infection that can be quite serious

  - Does not result in chronic infection

  - Can be transmitted during sexual activity and through oral-anal contact.

  - Vaccination can prevent HAV infection.

  - May cause abdominal pain, nausea, and vomiting

  - Usually, the infection gets better on its own without requiring treatment. In some cases, however, individuals may have such severe nausea and vomiting that they must be admitted to the hospital or may have lasting damage to their livers.

- Hepatitis B virus (HBV):

  - Causes a serious liver infection that can result in both immediate illness and lifelong infection and disease, leading to permanent liver scarring (cirrhosis), cancer, liver failure, and death

  - Can be treated with antiviral medications

  - Vaccination can prevent HBV infection.

  - Spreads through sexual contact, as well as through contact with other bodily fluids, such as blood; through shared contaminated needles used for injecting intravenous drugs; and through tattooing and piercing

  - Pregnant women with HBV can transmit the virus to their infants during delivery, but a series of vaccinations and a shot of hepatitis B immune globulin for the baby beginning at birth can prevent this transmission. Without vaccination, babies born to women with HBV infection can develop chronic infection, which can lead to serious health problems.

  - People with chronic HBV infection will need to see a liver specialist with experience treating individuals with chronic

96

liver disease. These individuals need to take special care not to pass on the virus to their sexual partners, and sexual partners should receive hepatitis B vaccine if they are not already immune.

- Hepatitis C virus (HCV):

  - Serious infection of the liver that can cause an immediate illness but that, in most people, becomes a silent, chronic infection that leads to liver scarring (cirrhosis), cancer, liver failure, and death.

  - Most infected people may not be aware of their infection because they do not develop symptoms.

  - Most commonly transmitted through sharing needles or exposure to infected blood. Less commonly, it can spread through sexual contact or from mother to fetus during pregnancy and delivery.

  - Can be treated. New medications seem to be more effective and have fewer side effects than previous options. The U.S. Food and Drug Administration (FDA) maintains a complete list of approved treatments for Hepatitis C.

Zika

- An infection caused by a virus. In most cases, it is spread by mosquitoes, but Zika virus also can be transmitted sexually.

- Zika is usually mild, with symptoms lasting for several days to a week after being infected.

- Research shows that getting Zika during pregnancy can cause birth defects in the developing fetus. In 2015, Zika virus infection was linked to microcephaly—a condition in which the brain and skull are smaller than normal—in newborns, as well as other birth defects.

- Zika also was linked to problems with the adult nervous system, including Guillain-Barré Syndrome.

- Pregnant women should not travel to areas with Zika. If you must travel to one of these areas, talk to your healthcare provider first and strictly follow steps to prevent mosquito bites during your trip.

- Learn how to protect yourself and your partner from Zika during sex at www.cdc.gov/zika/prevention/protect-yourself-during-sex.html.

- There is currently no specific medication or treatment for Zika infection.

Chapter 10

Chancroid

Chapter Contents

Section 10.1

What Is Chancroid?

This section contains text excerpted from the following sources: Text in this section begins with excerpts from "Chancroid," Genetic and Rare Diseases Information Center (GARD), National Center for Advancing Translational Sciences (NCATS), December 4, 2012. Reviewed February 2019; Text beginning with the heading "Symptoms of Chancroid" is excerpted from "Clinical Presentations and Diagnostic Testing for Specific STDs," Centers for Disease Control and Prevention (CDC), April 6, 2017.

Chancroid is a bacterial infection that is spread through sexual contact. It is caused by the bacteria *Haemophilus ducreyi (H. ducreyi)*. Chancroid is characterized by a small bump on the genital which becomes a painful ulcer. Men may have just one ulcer, but women often develop four or more. About half of the people who are infected with a chancroid will develop enlarged inguinal lymph nodes, the nodes located in the fold between the leg and the lower abdomen. In some cases, the nodes will break through the skin and cause draining abscesses. The swollen lymph nodes and abscesses are often called buboes. Chancroid occurs in Asia, Africa, and the Caribbean, and is an important cofactor of human immunodeficiency virus (HIV) transmission. Chancroid infections can be treated with antibiotics, including azithromycin, ceftriaxone, ciprofloxacin, and erythromycin. Large lymph-node swellings need to be drained, either with a needle or local surgery.

Symptoms of Chancroid

The genital ulcer from chancroid is painful, tender, and nonindurated. Symptoms usually occur four to ten days after exposure. The lesion at the site of infection is, initially, a pustule that breaks down to form a painful, soft, ulcer with a necrotic base and irregular borders. Multiple lesions and inguinal adenopathy often develop. With lymph node involvement, fever, chills, and malaise may also develop. Other symptoms of chancroid include painful urination, vaginal discharge, rectal bleeding, pain with bowel movements, and dyspareunia.

Diagnostic Testing

The combination of a painful genital ulcer and tender suppurative inguinal adenopathy suggests the diagnosis of chancroid. A probable diagnosis of chancroid can be made if:

- One or more painful genital ulcers (regional lymphadenopathy is also typical)

- No evidence of *Treponema pallidum (T. pallidum)* infection by darkfield examination of ulcer exudate or by syphilis serologic testing performed at least seven days after onset of ulcers

- Test for herpes simplex virus (HSV) performed on the ulcer exudate is negative

A definitive diagnosis of chancroid requires the identification of *H. ducreyi* on special culture media. However, culture media for chancroid are not widely available. Nucleic acid amplification tests can be performed in clinical laboratories that have developed their own tests.

Section 10.2

Prevalence and Treatment of Chancroid

This section contains text excerpted from the following sources: Text in this section begins with excerpts from "Other STDs," Centers for Disease Control and Prevention (CDC), July 24, 2018; Text beginning with the heading "Treatment of Chancroid" is excerpted from "Chancroid," Centers for Disease Control and Prevention (CDC), June 4, 2015. Reviewed February 2019.

- Reported cases of chancroid peaked in 1947 and then declined rapidly through 1957, presumably due to the increasing use of antibiotics such as sulfonamides and penicillin, which were introduced in the late 1930s and early 1940s.

- Numerous localized outbreaks, some of which were linked to commercial sex work, were identified during 1981–1990. Chancroid has declined since 1987, and since 2000, the annual number of reported cases has been less than 100.

- From 2008–2017, the number of reported cases has fluctuated, ranging from 28 in 2009 to six in 2014. In 2017, a total of seven cases of chancroid were reported in the United States. Five states reported one or more cases of chancroid in 2017.

Although the overall decline in reported chancroid cases most likely reflects a decline in the incidence of this disease, this should be viewed with caution because *Haemophilus ducreyi* is difficult to culture and no molecular assays have been cleared by the U.S. Food and Drug Administration (FDA) for use in the United States.

Treatment of Chancroid

Successful treatment for chancroid cures the infection, resolves the clinical symptoms, and prevents transmission to others. In advanced cases, scarring can result despite successful therapy.

Recommended Regimens

• Azithromycin 1 g orally in a single dose

• Ceftriaxone 250 mg IM in a single dose

• Ciprofloxacin 500 mg orally twice a day for three days

• Erythromycin base 500 mg orally three times a day for seven days

Azithromycin and ceftriaxone offer the advantage of single-dose therapy. Worldwide, several isolates with intermediate resistance to either ciprofloxacin or erythromycin have been reported. However, because cultures are not routinely performed, data are limited regarding the current prevalence of antimicrobial resistance.

Other Management Considerations

Men who are uncircumcised and patients with human immunodeficiency virus (HIV) infection do not respond as well to treatment as persons who are circumcised or HIV-negative. Patients should be tested for HIV infection at the time chancroid is diagnosed. If the initial test results were negative, a serologic test for syphilis and HIV infection should be performed three months after the diagnosis of chancroid.

Follow-Up

Patients should be re-examined three to seven days after the initiation of therapy. If treatment is successful, ulcers usually improve symptomatically within three days and objectively within seven days after therapy. If no clinical improvement is evident, the clinician must consider whether

- The diagnosis is correct
- The patient is coinfected with another STD
- The patient is infected with HIV
- The treatment was not used as instructed
- The *H. ducreyi* strain causing the infection is resistant to the prescribed antimicrobial

The time required for complete healing depends on the size of the ulcer; large ulcers might require more than two weeks. In addition, healing is slower for some uncircumcised men who have ulcers under the foreskin. Clinical resolution of fluctuant lymphadenopathy is slower than that of ulcers and might require needle aspiration or incision and drainage, despite otherwise successful therapy. Although needle aspiration of buboes is a simpler procedure, incision and drainage might be preferred because of reduced need for subsequent drainage procedures.

Special Considerations

Pregnancy

Data suggest ciprofloxacin presents a low risk to the fetus during pregnancy, with a potential for toxicity during breastfeeding. Alternate drugs should be used during pregnancy and lactation. No adverse effects of chancroid on pregnancy outcome have been reported.

HIV Infection

Persons with HIV infection who have chancroid should be monitored closely because they are more likely to experience treatment failure and to have ulcers that heal slowly. Persons with HIV infection might require repeated or longer courses of therapy, and treatment failures can occur with any regimen. Data are limited concerning the therapeutic efficacy of the recommended single-dose azithromycin and ceftriaxone regimens in persons with HIV infection.

Chapter 11

Chlamydia

Chapter Contents

Section 11.1

What Is Chlamydia?

The text in this section is excerpted from "Chlamydia,"
Office on Women's Health (OWH), U.S. Department of
Health and Human Services (HHS), December 27, 2018.

Chlamydia is a sexually transmitted infection (STI) caused by the
bacteria *Chlamydia trachomatis*. Chlamydia is usually spread through
vaginal, oral, or anal sex. It often has no symptoms. Antibiotics can
treat chlamydia. If left untreated, chlamydia can cause serious health
problems for women, such as difficulty getting pregnant.

Who Gets Chlamydia

Chlamydia is one of the most common STIs for women in the United
States. In 2015, more than one million women in the United States
were diagnosed with chlamydia. It is most common in young women
15 to 24 years old.

How Do You Get Chlamydia?

Chlamydia is spread through:

- Vaginal, oral, or anal sex. Chlamydia can be spread even if
  there are no symptoms. This means you can get chlamydia from
  someone who has no symptoms.

- Genital touching. A man does not need to ejaculate (come) for
  chlamydia to spread. Chlamydia can also be passed between
  women who have sex with women.

- Childbirth from a mother to her baby

What Are the Symptoms of Chlamydia?

Chlamydia is known as a "silent" infection because most women
who have chlamydia do not have symptoms. If you do have symptoms,
you may not notice them until several weeks after you get chlamydia.
Symptoms may include:

- Bleeding between periods

- Burning when urinating

- Fever

- Low back pain

- Lower abdominal pain

- Nausea

- Pain during sex

- Unusual vaginal discharge

If you think you may have chlamydia, you and your sex partner(s) need to see a doctor as soon as possible.

Chlamydia that does not have any symptoms can still lead to future health problems (including not being able to get pregnant). The only way to know if you or a partner has chlamydia is to get tested.

Do I Need to Get Tested for Chlamydia?

- If you are 24 or younger and have sex, you need to get tested for chlamydia. Chlamydia is most common in women between 15 and 24 years old. You need to get tested if you have had any symptoms of chlamydia since your last negative test result or if your sex partner has chlamydia.

- If you are older than 24, you need to get tested if, in the past year or since your last test, you:

  - Had a new sex partner

  - Had your sex partner tell you they have chlamydia

  - Traded sex for money or drugs

  - Have had chlamydia or another STI in the past

  - Did not use condoms and dental dams during sex and are in a relationship that is not monogamous, meaning you or your partner has sex with other people

You also need to be tested if you are pregnant or if you have any symptoms of chlamydia.

How Is Chlamydia Diagnosed?

There are two ways that a doctor or nurse tests for chlamydia:

- **A urine test.** This is the most common. You urinate (pee) into a cup. Your urine is then tested for chlamydia.

107

- **A swab test.** Your doctor uses a cotton swab to take a fluid sample from an infected place (vagina, cervix, rectum, or throat). The fluid is then tested for chlamydia.

A Pap test is not used to detect chlamydia.

Section 11.2

What Is Nongonococcal Urethritis?

This section contains text excerpted from the following sources:
Text in this section begins with excerpts from "Focus on Youth with Impact—An HIV Prevention Program for African American Youth with a Complementary Program for Parents," Centers for Disease Control and Prevention (CDC), 2008. Reviewed February 2019. Text beginning with the heading "Diagnostic Consideration" is excerpted from "Diseases Characterized by Urethritis and Cervicitis," Centers for Disease Control and Prevention (CDC), June 4, 2015. Reviewed February 2019.

Nongonococcal urethritis (NGU) is a treatable bacterial infection of the urethra, often associated with chlamydia. NGU refers to symptoms patients may have when they have an STD.

How Is It Transmitted?

NGU is transmitted through unprotected sex.

What Are the Symptoms in Young Men?

- Pain when urinating
- Painful discharge from the penis

What Are the Symptoms in Young Women?

While men are primarily infected by NGU, women can easily be infected with the main cause of NGU—chlamydia. Symptoms can include:

- Painful urination

- Unusual vaginal discharge

What Are the Health Consequences?

- In young women, it can lead to scarring of the fallopian tubes, which can lead to infertility (the inability to have a baby).

- Complications in young men are rare, but sometimes the infection can spread to the epididymis (a tube that carries sperm from the testes), testicles and prostate causing pain, fever and, rarely, sterility.

- Increases susceptibility to HIV infection

Diagnostic Considerations

NGU is a nonspecific diagnosis that can have many infectious etiologies. NGU is confirmed in symptomatic men when staining of urethral secretions indicates inflammation without gram-negative or purple diplococci. All men who have confirmed NGU should be tested for chlamydia and gonorrhea even if point-of-care tests are negative for evidence of gonococcal infections (GC). Nucleic acid amplification tests (NAATs) for chlamydia and gonorrhea are recommended because of their high sensitivity and specificity; a specific diagnosis can potentially reduce complications, reinfection, and transmission. Testing for T. *vaginalis* should be considered in areas or populations of high prevalence.

How Is It Treated?

NGU can be treated easily and cured with antibiotics.

Presumptive treatment should be initiated at the time of NGU diagnosis. Azithromycin and doxycycline are highly effective for chlamydial urethritis. NGU associated with M. *genitalium* currently responds better to azithromycin than doxycycline, although azithromycin efficacy might be declining.

Recommended Regimens

- Azithromycin 1 g orally in a single dose

- Doxycycline 100 mg orally twice a day for seven days

Alternative Regimens

- Erythromycin base 500 mg orally four times a day for seven days
- Erythromycin ethylsuccinate 800 mg orally four times a day for seven days
- Levofloxacin 500 mg orally once daily for seven days
- Ofloxacin 300 mg orally twice a day for seven days

As a directly observed treatment, single-dose regimens might be associated with higher rates of compliance over other regimens. To maximize compliance with recommended therapies, medications should be dispensed onsite in the clinic, and regardless of the number of doses involved in the regimen, the first should be directly observed.

Other Management Considerations

To minimize transmission and reinfection, patients treated for NGU should be instructed to abstain from sexual intercourse until they and their partner(s) have been adequately treated (i.e., for seven days after single-dose therapy or until completion of a seven-day regimen and symptoms resolved). Patients who receive a diagnosis of NGU should be tested for HIV and syphilis.

Follow-Up

Patients should be provided results of the testing obtained as part of the NGU evaluation, and those with a specific diagnosis of chlamydia, gonorrhea, or trichomonas should be offered partner services and instructed to return three months after treatment for repeat testing because of high rates of reinfection, regardless of whether their sex partners were treated.

If symptoms persist or recur after completion of therapy, patients should be instructed to return for re-evaluation. Symptoms alone, without documentation of signs or laboratory evidence of urethral inflammation, are not a sufficient basis for retreatment. Providers should be alert to the possible diagnosis of chronic prostatitis/chronic pelvic pain syndrome in men experiencing persistent perineal, penile, or pelvic pain or discomfort, voiding symptoms, pain during or after ejaculation, or new-onset premature ejaculation lasting for more than 3 months. Patients with persistent pain should be referred to a urologist.

Management of Sex Partners

All sex partners of patients with NGU within the preceding 60 days should be referred for evaluation, testing, and presumptive treatment with a drug regimen effective against chlamydia. Expedited partner therapy (EPT) is an alternative approach to treating female partners in the absence of signs and symptoms of PID. If N. *gonorrhea* or T. *vaginalis* is documented, all partners should be evaluated and treated according to the management section for their respective pathogen. To avoid reinfection, sex partners should abstain from sexual intercourse until they and their partner(s) are adequately treated.

Persistent and Recurrent Nongonococcal Urethritis

The objective diagnosis of persistent or recurrent NGU should be made before considering additional antimicrobial therapy. In patients who have persistent symptoms after treatment without objective signs of urethral inflammation, the value of extending the duration of anti-microbials has not been demonstrated. Patients who have persistent or recurrent NGU can be retreated with the initial regimen if they did not comply with the treatment regimen or were re-exposed to an untreated sex partner.

- Studies have shown that the most common cause of persistent or recurrent NGU is M. *genitalium*, especially following doxycycline therapy. Azithromycin 1 g orally in a single dose should be administered to men initially treated with doxycycline.

- Certain observational studies have shown that moxifloxacin 400 mg orally once daily for seven days is highly effective against M. *genitalium*. Therefore, patients who fail a regimen of azithromycin should be retreated with moxifloxacin 400 mg orally once daily for seven days. Higher doses of azithromycin have not been found to be effective for M. *genitalium* in cases of azithromycin failure.

- T. *vaginalis* is also known to cause urethritis in men who have sex with women. Although no NAAT for T. *vaginalis* detection in men has been FDA-cleared in the United States, several large reference laboratories have performed the necessary CLIA validation of a urine-based T. *vaginalis* nucleic acid amplification test (NAAT) for men for clinical use.

- Trichomonas NAAT testing is more sensitive than culture. In areas where T. *vaginalis* is prevalent, men who have sex with women and have persistent or recurrent urethritis should be presumptively treated with metronidazole 2 g orally in a single dose or tinidazole 2 g orally in a single dose; their partners should be referred for evaluation and appropriate treatment.

• Persons with persistent or recurrent NGU after presumptive treatment for M. *genitalium* or T. *vaginalis* should be referred to a urologist.

• NGU might facilitate HIV transmission. Persons with NGU and HIV should receive the same treatment regimen as those who are HIV negative.

Section 11.3

Prevalence and Treatment of Chlamydia

This section contains text excerpted from the following sources:
Text under the heading "Chlamydial Infections in Adolescents and Adults" is excerpted from "Chlamydial Infections," Centers for Disease Control and Prevention (CDC), June 4, 2015. Reviewed February 2019; Text under the heading "How Does Chlamydia Affect Pregnancy?" is excerpted from "Chlamydia," Office on Women's Health (OWH), U.S. Department of Health and Human Services (HHS), August 30, 2018.

Chlamydial Infections in Adolescents and Adults

Chlamydial infection is the most frequently reported infectious disease in the United States, and prevalence is highest in people younger than 25 years of age. Several sequelae can result from *Chlamydia trachomatis* (CT) infection in women, the most serious of which include pelvic inflammatory disease (PID), ectopic pregnancy, and infertility. Some women who receive a diagnosis of uncomplicated cervical infection already have subclinical upper-reproductive-tract infection.

Asymptomatic infection is common among both men and women. To detect chlamydial infections, healthcare providers frequently rely on screening tests. Annual screening of all sexually active women younger than 25 is recommended, as is the screening of older women at increased risk for infection (e.g., those who have a new sex partner, more than one sex partner, a sex partner with concurrent partners, or a sex partner who has a sexually transmitted infection. Although CT incidence might be higher in some women older than 25 in some communities, overall the largest burden of infection is among women younger than 25 years of age.

How Does Chlamydia Affect Pregnancy?

For pregnant women, chlamydia may lead to premature birth, or babies born before 37 weeks of pregnancy. Premature birth is the most common cause of infant death and can lead to long-term health and development problems in children.

Babies born to mothers who have chlamydia can get:

* **Infections in their eyes,** called conjunctivitis or pink eye: Signs include discharge from the eyes and swollen eyelids. The signs most often show up within two weeks after birth.

* **Pneumonia:** Signs include congestion, cough, and rapid or labored breathing, although these are not always present. Signs most often show up one to three months after birth.

How Can I Prevent Chlamydia?

The best way to prevent chlamydia or any sexually transmitted infection (STI) is to not have vaginal, oral, or anal sex.

If you do have sex, lower your risk of getting an STI with the following steps:

* **Use condoms and dental dams.** Condoms and dental dams are the best way to prevent STIs when you have sex. Because a man does not need to ejaculate to give or get chlamydia, make sure to put the condom on before the penis touches the vagina, mouth, or anus. Other methods of birth control, such as birth control pills (BCP), shots, implants, or diaphragms, will not protect you from STIs.

* **Get tested.** Be sure you and your partner are tested for STIs. Talk to each other about the test results before you have sex.

* **Be monogamous.** Having sex with just one partner can lower your risk for STIs. After being tested for STIs, be faithful to each other. That means that you have sex only with each other and no one else.

- **Limit your number of sex partners.** Your risk of getting STIs goes up with the number of partners you have.

- **Do not douche.** Douching removes some of the normal bacteria in the vagina that protects you from infection. This may increase your risk of getting STIs.

- **Do not abuse alcohol or drugs.** Drinking too much alcohol or using drugs increases risky behavior and may put you at risk of sexual assault and possible exposure to STIs.

The steps work best when used together. No single step can protect you from every single type of STI.

What Should I Do If I Have Chlamydia?

Chlamydia is easy to treat. But you need to be tested and treated as soon as possible.

If you have chlamydia:

- **See a doctor or nurse as soon as possible.** Antibiotics will treat chlamydia, but they will not fix any permanent damage to your reproductive organs.

- **Take all of your medicine.** Even if symptoms go away, you need to finish all of the antibiotics.

- **Tell your sex partner(s) so they can be tested and treated.** If they are not tested and treated you could get chlamydia again.

- **Avoid sexual contact until you and your partner(s) have been treated and cured.** Even after you finish your antibiotics, you can get chlamydia again if you have sex with someone who has chlamydia.

- **See your doctor or nurse again if you have symptoms that don't go away** within a few days after finishing the antibiotics.

How Is Chlamydia Treated?

- Your doctor or nurse will prescribe antibiotics to treat chlamydia. Antibiotics can cure chlamydia. But they cannot fix any permanent damage done to your body, including scarring of your reproductive organs. For this reason, you should get tested and take the antibiotics as soon as possible.

- For the antibiotics to work, you must finish all of the antibiotics that your doctor gives you, even if the symptoms go away. Do not share your antibiotics for chlamydia with anyone. If symptoms do not go away after treatment, see your doctor or nurse.

- Tell your doctor if you are pregnant. Your doctor can give you antibiotics that are safe to take during pregnancy.

What Can Happen If Chlamydia Is Not Treated?

Untreated chlamydia can cause serious health problems in women, including:

- Pelvic inflammatory disease (PID), an infection of a woman's reproductive organs. PID can lead to chronic pelvic pain, pregnancy problems, and infertility (meaning you can't get pregnant). Untreated chlamydia is a common cause of PID. It affects about 10 percent to 15 percent of women with untreated chlamydia.

- Increased risk of getting human immunodeficiency virus (HIV) (the virus that causes acquired immunodeficiency syndrome (AIDS)) from sexual activity

Chapter 12

Donovanosis (Granuloma Inguinale)

Granuloma inguinale is a genital ulcerative disease caused by the intracellular gram-negative bacterium *Klebsiella granulomatis* (formerly known as *Calymmatobacterium granulomatis*). The disease occurs rarely in the United States, although it is endemic in some tropical and developing areas, including India; Papua, New Guinea; the Caribbean; central Australia; and southern Africa. Clinically, the disease is commonly characterized as painless, slowly progressive ulcerative lesions on the genitals or perineum without regional lymphadenopathy; subcutaneous granulomas (pseudobuboes) also might occur. The lesions are highly vascular (i.e., beefy red appearance) and bleed. Extragenital infection can occur with the extension of infection to the pelvis, or it can disseminate to intra-abdominal organs, bones, or the mouth. The lesions also can develop a secondary bacterial infection and can coexist with other sexually transmitted pathogens.

Diagnostic Considerations

The causative organism of granuloma inguinale is difficult to culture, and diagnosis requires visualization of dark-staining Donovan

This chapter contains text excerpted from "Granuloma Inguinale (Donovanosis)," Centers for Disease Control and Prevention (CDC), June 4, 2015. Reviewed February 2019.

bodies on tissue-crush preparation or biopsy. No U.S. Food and Drug Administration (FDA)-cleared molecular tests for the detection of *K. granulomatis* deoxyribonucleic acid (DNA) exist, but such an assay might be useful when undertaken by laboratories that have conducted a clinical laboratory improvement amendments (CLIA) verification study.

Treatment

Several antimicrobial regimens have been effective, but only a limited number of controlled trials have been published. Treatment has been shown to halt the progression of lesions, and healing typically proceeds inward from the ulcer margins; prolonged therapy is usually required to permit granulation and re-epithelialization of the ulcers. Relapse can occur 6 to 18 months after apparently effective therapy.

Recommended Regimen

Azithromycin 1 g orally once per week or 500 mg daily for at least three weeks and until all lesions have completely healed

Alternative Regimens

- Doxycycline 100 mg orally twice a day for at least three weeks and until all lesions have completely healed, or

- Ciprofloxacin 750 mg orally twice a day for at least three weeks and until all lesions have completely healed, or

- Erythromycin base 500 mg orally four times a day for at least three weeks and until all lesions have completely healed, or

- Trimethoprim-sulfamethoxazole one double-strength (160 mg/800 mg) tablet orally twice a day for at least three weeks and until all lesions have completely healed

The addition of another antibiotic to these regimens can be considered if improvement is not evident within the first few days of therapy. Addition of an aminoglycoside to these regimens is an option (gentamicin 1 mg/kg IV every eight hours).

Follow-Up

Patients should be followed clinically until signs and symptoms resolve.

Special Considerations
Pregnancy

Doxycycline should be avoided in the second and third trimester of pregnancy because of the risk for discoloration of teeth and bones but is compatible with breastfeeding. Data suggest that ciprofloxacin presents a low risk to the fetus during pregnancy. For these reasons, pregnant and lactating women should be treated with a macrolide regimen (erythromycin or azithromycin). The addition of an aminoglycoside (gentamicin 1 mg/kg IV every eight hours) can be considered if improvement is not evident within the first few days of therapy.

Human Immunodeficiency Virus Infection

Persons with both granuloma inguinale and human immunodeficiency virus (HIV) infection should receive the same regimens as those who do not have HIV infection. The addition of an aminoglycoside (gentamicin 1 mg/kg IV every eight hours) can be considered if improvement is not evident within the first few days of therapy.

Chapter 13

Gonorrhea

Chapter Contents

121

Section 13.1

What Is Gonorrhea?

The text in this section is excerpted from "Gonorrhea," Office on Women's Health (OWH), U.S. Department of Health and Human Services (HHS), October 18, 2018.

Gonorrhea is a sexually transmitted infection (STI) that is caused by the bacteria *Neisseria gonorrhoeae*. It is an especially serious problem for women because it can damage the female reproductive organs.

Who Gets Gonorrhea

In 2014, gonorrhea affected more than 162,000 women in the United States. Gonorrhea most often affects women ages 15 to 24. But, gonorrhea is becoming more common in older women too.

How Do You Get Gonorrhea?

Gonorrhea is spread through:

- Vaginal, oral, or anal sex. Gonorrhea can be spread even if there are no symptoms. This means you can get gonorrhea from someone who has no signs or symptoms.

- Genital touching. A man does not need to ejaculate (come) for gonorrhea to spread. Touching infected fluids from the vagina or penis and then touching your eyes can cause an eye infection. Gonorrhea can also be passed between women who have sex with women.

- Childbirth from woman to her baby

What Are the Signs and Symptoms of Gonorrhea?

Most women with gonorrhea do not have any signs or symptoms. If you do get symptoms, they are often mild and can be mistaken for a bladder or vaginal infection. Signs or symptoms of gonorrhea depend on where you are first infected by the gonorrhea bacteria.

Signs and symptoms in the genital area can include:

- Pain or burning when urinating

- More vaginal discharge than usual

- Vaginal discharge that looks different than usual
- Bleeding between periods
- Pain in the pelvis or abdomen

Signs and symptoms in other parts of the body include:

- **Rectum/anus:** Anal itching, pus-like discharge, bright red blood on toilet tissue, or painful bowel movements
- **Eyes:** Pain, itching, sensitivity to light, pus-like discharge
- **Throat:** Sore throat, swollen glands in your neck
- **Joints (such as your knee):** Warmth, redness, swelling or pain while moving

Gonorrhea can cause serious health problems, even if you do not have any signs or symptoms.

How Does Gonorrhea Affect Pregnancy?

For pregnant women, untreated gonorrhea raises the risk of:

- Miscarriage
- Premature birth (babies born before 37 weeks of pregnancy). Premature birth is the most common cause of infant death and can lead to long-term health and developmental problems in children.
- Low birth weight
- Water breaking too early. This can lead to premature birth.

Babies born to infected mothers are at risk for:

- Blindness. Treating the newborn's eyes with medicine right after birth can prevent eye infection. The U.S. Preventive Services Task Force (USPSTF) strongly recommends—and most states require by law—that all babies be treated with medicated eye ointments soon after birth.
- Joint infection
- Life-threatening blood infection

Treatment of gonorrhea as soon as it is found in pregnant women will lower the risk of these problems for both mother and baby. Your baby will get antibiotics if you have gonorrhea or if your baby has a gonorrheal eye infection.

Section 13.2

Diagnosis and Treatment for Gonorrhea

The text in this section is excerpted from the following sources: Text begins with excerpts from "Gonorrhea," Office on Women's Health (OWH), U.S. Department of Health and Human Services (HHS), October 18, 2018; Text under the heading " I Was Treated for Gonorrhea. When Can I Have Sex Again?" is excerpted from "Gonorrhea—CDC Fact Sheet," Centers for Disease Control and Prevention (CDC), January 29, 2014. Reviewed February 2019.

Do I Need to Get Tested for Gonorrhea?

If you are 24 or younger and have sex, you need to get tested for gonorrhea. Gonorrhea is most common in women between ages 15 and 24. You need to get tested if you have had any symptoms of gonorrhea since your last negative test result or if your sex partner has gonorrhea. If you are older than 24, you need to get tested if, in the past year or since your last test, you:

- Had a new sex partner

- Had your sex partner tell you they have gonorrhea

- Have had gonorrhea or another STI in the past

- Traded sex for money or drugs in the past

- Do not use condoms or dental dams during sex and are in a relationship that is not monogamous, meaning you or your partner has sex with other people

- You also need to get tested if you have any symptoms of gonorrhea. Testing is very important because women with untreated gonorrhea can develop serious health problems. If you are tested for gonorrhea, you also need to get tested for other STIs, including chlamydia, syphilis, and HIV.

What Should I Do If I Have Gonorrhea?

Gonorrhea is easy to treat. But you need to get tested and treated as soon as possible.

If you have gonorrhea:

- See a doctor or nurse as soon as possible. Antibiotics will treat gonorrhea, but they will not fix any permanent damage to your reproductive organs.

- Take all of the antibiotics. Even if symptoms go away, you need to finish all of the antibiotics.

- Tell your sex partner(s) so they can be tested and treated. If they are not tested and treated you could get gonorrhea again.

- Avoid sexual contact until you and your partner(s) have been treated and cured. Even after you finish your antibiotics, you can get gonorrhea again if you have sex with someone who has gonorrhea.

- See your doctor or nurse again if you have symptoms that don't go away within a few days after finishing the antibiotics.

How Is Gonorrhea Diagnosed?

There are two ways that a doctor or nurse tests for gonorrhea:

- A urine test. This is the most common. You urinate (pee) into a cup. Your urine is then tested for gonorrhea.

- A swab test. Your doctor or nurse uses a cotton swab to take a fluid sample from an infected place (cervix, rectum, or throat). The fluid is then tested for gonorrhea.

- A Pap test is not used to detect gonorrhea.

How Is Gonorrhea Treated?

Your doctor or nurse will give you antibiotics to treat gonorrhea. The antibiotics are usually a pill you swallow.

Although antibiotics can cure gonorrhea, they cannot fix any permanent damage done to your body. For this reason, it is important to get tested and to take the antibiotics as soon as possible.

For the antibiotics to work, you must finish all of the antibiotics that your doctor gives you, even if the symptoms go away. Do not share your antibiotics for gonorrhea with anyone. If symptoms do not

125

go away after treatment, see your doctor or nurse. It is possible to get gonorrhea again if you have sex with someone who has gonorrhea. Tell your recent sex partner(s) so they can be tested and treated.

What Can Happen If Gonorrhea Is Not Treated?

Gonorrhea that is not treated can cause serious health problems in women:

- Pelvic inflammatory disease (PID), an infection of a woman's reproductive organs. PID can lead to chronic pelvic pain, pregnancy problems, and infertility, meaning you can't get pregnant. Untreated gonorrhea is a common cause of PID.

- Higher risk of getting HIV or spreading HIV.

- Although it does not happen very often, gonorrhea can cause widespread infection in other parts of the body, such as the blood, joints, heart, or brain. This can lead to death.

I Was Treated for Gonorrhea. When Can I Have Sex Again?

You should wait seven days after finishing all medications before having sex. To avoid getting infected with gonorrhea again or spreading gonorrhea to your partner(s), you and your sex partner(s) should avoid having sex until you have each completed treatment. If you've had gonorrhea and took medicine in the past, you can still get infected again if you have unprotected sex with a person who has gonorrhea.

Section 13.3

Antibiotic-Resistant Gonorrhea

The text in this section is excerpted from the following sources: Text beginning with the heading "Antibiotic Resistance (AR) Solutions Initiative" is excerpted from "Antibiotic Resistance (AR) Solutions Initiative," Centers for Disease Control and Prevention (CDC), September 10, 2018; Text under the heading "Combating the Threat of Antibiotic-Resistant Gonorrhea" is excerpted from "Combating the Threat of Antibiotic-Resistant Gonorrhea," Centers for Disease Control and Prevention (CDC), February 21, 2018.

Antibiotic Resistance (AR) Solutions Initiative

Antibiotics have successfully treated gonorrhea for several decades; however, the bacteria has developed resistance to nearly every drug used for treatment.

Drug-resistant gonorrhea is an urgent threat:

• Gonorrhea is a common, sexually transmitted disease. About 820,000 new gonorrheal infections occur each year in the United States, and less than half are detected and reported to the Centers for Disease Control and Prevention (CDC).

• An estimate of 246,000 remains resistant to at least one antibiotic.

Untreated gonorrhea can cause health problems:

• Increases chances of getting or giving HIV, the virus that causes AIDS

• Spreads from mother to baby during childbirth, causing blindness in the baby

• Can cause infertility and ectopic pregnancies

• Spreads to the blood, causing heart and nervous system infections

• Increases healthcare costs

Growing resistance threatens treatment and control:

• Few U.S. labs can test for resistance

• Few healthcare settings have access to these lab tests

- Slow detection of resistance leads to treatment that may not work and delays a rapid response

Action needed:

- Improve monitoring systems to rapidly detect resistant infections

- Rapidly respond to resistant infections to stop the spread

How will the CDC's Solutions Initiative Fight Drug-Resistant Gonorrhea?

Ensure that less than two percent of all gonorrhea infections are resistant to the current treatment.

Rapidly detect resistant gonorrhea:

- Expand the availability of resistance testing

- Reduce time to get test results to providers so that patients can be treated in a timely manner

Ensure effective and timely treatment:

- Use test results to choose correct antibiotics for patients

- Prevent health complications and stop spread with appropriate treatment

Public health action:

- Alert patients and local health departments of a resistant strain quickly

- Identify and contact sexual partners faster to limit the spread of resistant strains

Increase monitoring and awareness:

- Alert healthcare professionals and communities about resistant strains

- Find hot spots

- Predict potential outbreaks

Combating the Threat of Antibiotic-Resistant Gonorrhea

- **Gonococcal Isolate Surveillance Project (GISP)—**
  Established in 1986, the Gonococcal Isolate Surveillance Project

monitors U.S. antibiotic resistance trends in gonorrhea. Through the collaborative effort of selected STD clinics and their local laboratories, regional laboratories, and CDC, GISP's collected data helps ensure gonorrhea receives the right antibiotic treatment. GISP monitors antimicrobial susceptibility of approximately 5,000 male gonococcal urethritis cases seen in 26 STD clinics.

- **Antimicrobial Regional Laboratory Network (ARLN)** — The Antimicrobial Regional Laboratory Network is a network of regional public-health laboratories equipped to respond to emerging health threats and provide cutting-edge antimicrobial resistance laboratory support. Since gonorrhea is an important part of CARB activities, four labs in the ARLN receive funding to build capacity for culture-based antimicrobial-susceptibility testing and genomic sequencing.

- **Strengthening the United States Response to Resistant Gonorrhea (SURRG)** — Strengthening the U.S. Response to Resistant Gonorrhea began in 2016 with three goals:

  - Enhance domestic antibiotic-resistant gonorrhea surveillance and infrastructure.

  - Build capacity for rapid detection and response to resistant gonorrhea through increased culturing and local antibiotic susceptibility testing.

  - Conduct rapid field investigations to stop the spread of resistant infections. The project also aims to gain a better understanding of the epidemiological factors contributing to resistant gonorrhea. Nine jurisdictions collect and analyze data, helping guide national recommendations for the public-health response to resistant gonorrhea.

- **The STD Surveillance Network (SSuN)** — The STD Surveillance Network is a collaborative network of state, county, and/or city health departments funded by the CDC to conduct sentinel and enhanced STD surveillance activities. The purpose of SSuN is to improve the capacity of national, state, and local STD programs to detect, monitor, and respond to trends in STDs through an enhanced collection, reporting, analysis, visualization, and interpretation of disease information.

- **Combating the Threat of Antibiotic-Resistant Gonorrhea Enhanced Gonococcal Isolate Surveillance Project**

(eGISP)—The Enhanced Gonococcal Isolate Surveillance Project strengthens surveillance of resistant gonorrhea and increases state and local capacity to detect and monitor it. In select STD clinics, eGISP not only collects samples from men with gonococcal urethritis but also from women and from extragenital sites. These specimens are sent to regional laboratories for susceptibility testing.

Chapter 14

Herpes Simplex

Chapter Contents

Section 14.1

What Is a Herpes?

The text in this section is excerpted from the following sources: Text beginning with excerpts from "Herpes (HSV) Test," MedlinePlus, National Institutes of Health (NIH), November 2, 2018. Text under the heading "Is Herpes Curable?" is excerpted from "Herpes Can Happen to Anyone—Share Facts, Not Fears," *NIH News in Health,* National Institutes of Health (NIH), June 4, 2018.

Herpes is a skin infection caused by the herpes simplex virus, known as HSV. HSV causes painful blisters or sores in different parts of the body. There are two main types of HSV:

- HSV-1, which usually causes blisters or cold sores around the mouth (oral herpes)

- HSV-2, which usually causes blisters or sores in the genital area (genital herpes)

How Is Herpes Spread?

- HSV-1 is spread through direct contact with sores.

- HSV-2 is usually spread through vaginal, oral, or anal sex.

- Sometimes herpes can be spread even if there are no visible sores.

Are Herpes Infections Recurrent?

Both HSV-1 and HSV-2 are recurring infections. That means after your first outbreak of sores clears up, you may get another outbreak in the future. But the severity and number of outbreaks tend to lessen over time.

What Are the Consequences of Herpes?

- Although oral and genital herpes can be uncomfortable, the viruses usually don't cause any major health problems.

- In rare cases, HSV can infect other parts of the body, including the brain and spinal cord. These infections can be very serious. Herpes can also be dangerous to a newborn baby.

- A mother with herpes can pass the infection to her baby during delivery. A herpes infection can be life-threatening to a baby.

What Is a Herpes Test?

An HSV test looks for the presence of the virus in your body. While there is no cure for herpes, there are medicines that can help manage the condition.

Other names: herpes culture, herpes simplex viral culture, HSV-1 antibodies, HSV-2 antibodies, HSV DNA

What Is It Used For?

An HSV test may be used to:

- Find out whether sores on the mouth or genitals are caused by HSV

- Diagnose an HSV infection in a pregnant woman

- Find out if a newborn is infected with HSV

Why Do I Need an Herpes Simplex Virus Test?

The Centers for Disease Control and Prevention (CDC) does not recommend HSV testing for people without symptoms of HSV, **but you may need an HSV test if**:

- You have symptoms of herpes, such as blisters or sores on the genitals or other parts of the body

- Your sex partner has herpes

- You are pregnant and you or your partner has had a previous herpes infection or symptoms of genital herpes. If you test positive for HSV, your baby may need testing as well.

- HSV-2 may increase your risk of human immunodeficiency virus (HIV) and other sexually transmitted diseases (STDs). You may need a test if you have certain risk factors for STDs.

You may be at higher risk if you:

- Have multiple sex partners

- Are a man who has sex with men

- Have a partner with HIV and/or another STD

In rare cases, HSV can cause encephalitis or meningitis, life-threatening infections of the brain and spinal cord. You may need an HSV test if you have symptoms of a brain or spinal cord disorder. These include:

- Fever

- Stiff neck

- Confusion

- Severe headache

- Sensitivity to light

What Happens during an Herpes Simplex Virus Test

HSV testing is usually done as a swab test, blood test, or lumbar puncture. The type of test you get will depend on your symptoms and health history.

- For a swab test, a healthcare provider will use a swab to collect fluid and cells from a herpes sore.

- For a blood test, a healthcare professional will take a blood sample from a vein in your arm, using a small needle. After the needle is inserted, a small amount of blood will be collected into a test tube or vial. You may feel a little sting when the needle goes in or out. This test usually takes less than five minutes.

- A lumbar puncture, also called a spinal tap, is only done if your provider thinks you may have an infection of the brain or spinal cord.

- During a spinal tap: You will lie on your side or sit on an exam table. A healthcare provider will clean your back and inject an anesthetic into your skin, so you won't feel pain during the procedure. Your provider may put numbing cream on your back before this injection. Once the area on your back is completely numb, your provider will insert a thin, hollow needle between two vertebrae in your lower spine. Vertebrae are the small backbones that make up your spine. Your provider will withdraw a small amount of cerebrospinal fluid for testing. This will take about five minutes. Your provider may ask you to lie on your back for an hour or two after the procedure. This may prevent you from getting a headache afterward.

Will I Need to Do Anything to Prepare for the Test?

You don't need any special preparations for a swab test or a blood test. For a lumbar puncture, you may be asked to empty your bladder and bowels before the test.

Are There Any Risks to the Test?

- There is no known risk to having a swab test.

- There is very little risk to having a blood test. You may have slight pain or bruising at the spot where the needle was put in, but most symptoms go away quickly.

- If you had a lumbar puncture, you may have pain or tenderness in your back where the needle was inserted. You may also get a headache after the procedure.

What Do the Results Mean?

Your HSV test results will be given as negative, also called normal, or positive, also called abnormal.

- **Negative/Normal**—The herpes virus was not found. You may still have an HSV infection if your results were normal. It may mean the sample didn't have enough of the virus to be detected. If you still have symptoms of herpes, you may need to get tested again.

- **Positive/Abnormal**—HSV was found in your sample. It may mean you have an active infection (you currently have sores), or were infected in the past (you have no sores). If you tested positive for HSV, talk to your healthcare provider. While there is no cure for herpes, it hardly ever causes serious health problems. Some people may only have one outbreak of sores their whole lives, while others break out more often. If you want to reduce the severity and number of your outbreaks, your provider may prescribe a medicine that can help.

Is There Anything Else I Need to Know about an Herpes Simplex Virus Test?

- The best way to prevent genital herpes or another STD is to not have sex. If you are sexually active, you can reduce your risk of infection by

- Being in a long-term relationship with one partner who has tested negative for STDs

- Using condoms and dental dams correctly every time you have sex

- If you've been diagnosed with genital herpes, condom and dental dam use can reduce your risk of spreading the infection to others

Is Herpes Curable?

There's no cure for herpes, but antiherpes medicine can speed healing of the sores. If taken every day, this medicine can also lower the risk of future outbreaks.

"It's the first episode that is particularly important to treat," says Dr. Jeffrey I. Cohen, a herpes infection expert at *News in Health*. That's because the first outbreak is often the most severe. In addition to sores, you may have a fever and body aches. Also, the nearby lymph nodes might be swollen and painful.

A doctor may suspect a diagnosis of herpes from looking at a sore, but lab tests on a sample taken from the sore are needed to confirm the diagnosis. A blood test for HSV-1 and HSV-2 is also available to confirm if someone has been infected.

Researchers are working to develop herpes vaccines. "There are two different types of vaccines being developed for herpes virus," Cohen explains. "One is a vaccine that would prevent infection in people who have not been infected with the virus." Cohen's research team at NIH is working on this type of vaccine.

"The other type of vaccine is for people who are already infected," he says. "The idea is that we could boost their immune system so that they have fewer recurrences."

The fact that most people don't know that they're infected makes vaccines especially important. When someone is diagnosed with herpes, they may feel anger, sadness, or shame. They also may fear rejection by romantic partners.

Keep in mind that herpes outbreaks can be managed. People can lower the risk of infecting someone else by avoiding direct contact during an outbreak. For those with genital herpes, using antiherpes medicine every day and condoms during sexual activity also reduces the risk of infection for a romantic partner.

Section 14.2

Genital Herpes in Detail

The text in this section is excerpted from "Genital Herpes,"
Office on Women's Health (OWH), U.S. Department of Health
and Human Services (HHS), August 30, 2018.

What Is Genital Herpes?

Genital herpes is an STI caused by the herpes simplex viruses type
1 (HSV-1) and type 2 (HSV-2). HSV-1 and HSV-2 cause the same symptoms, are both contagious and are treated with the same medicine.
But, they are different in some ways:

- HSV-1 most often causes infections of the mouth and lips, called
  cold sores or "fever blisters." Symptoms are often milder than
  genital herpes, and you may get fewer outbreaks. It can spread
  to the genital area during oral sex and cause genital herpes. If
  HSV-1 spreads to the genital area, it is still HSV-1.

- HSV-2 is the most common cause of genital herpes. It is spread
  through vaginal, oral, or anal sex. HSV-2 can spread to the
  mouth during oral sex. If HSV-2 spreads to the mouth or lips
  during oral sex, it is still HSV-2.

Who Gets Genital Herpes

Genital herpes is more common in women than men. One in five
women ages 14 to 49 has genital herpes, compared with one in 10
men ages 14 to 49. A woman's anatomy (body) puts her more at risk
for genital herpes than men. Small tears in vaginal tissue can make
it easier to get genital herpes.

Genital herpes is also much more common in African-American
women. One in two African American women between the ages of 14
and 49 is infected with HSV-2 that causes genital herpes.

How Do You Get Genital Herpes?

Genital herpes is spread through:

- Vaginal, oral, or anal sex. The herpes virus is usually spread
  through contact with open sores. But you also can get herpes
  from someone without any symptoms or sores.

- Genital touching

- Childbirth from a mother to her baby

- Breastfeeding if a baby touches an open sore

Does a Cold Sore on My Mouth Mean I Have Genital Herpes?

No, a cold sore on your mouth usually means you have herpes simplex virus type 1 (HSV-1). You can get HSV-1 by kissing someone or sharing utensils, towels, razors, or lipstick with someone who has HSV-1.

HSV-1 cannot turn into HSV-2 (the type of genital herpes spread by sexual contact), but you can get a cold sore on your mouth from HSV-2 if you give oral sex to someone with HSV-2.

Cold sores caused by HSV-1 or HSV-2 are contagious. You can spread it to other people or other parts of your body if you touch an open sore and then touch another part of your body. That means if you have a cold sore and give oral sex to someone, that person will get the herpes virus on his or her genitals.

Avoid touching your cold sore as much as possible. If you touch your cold sore, wash your hands right away to avoid spreading the infection to other parts of your body or other people.

What Is the Difference between Genital Herpes and Genital Warts?

Both genital herpes and genital warts are STIs, are spread through skin-to-skin contact, and are caused by a virus. But the viruses that cause genital herpes and genital warts are different:

- Herpes simplex virus (HSV) is the virus that causes genital herpes.

- Human papillomavirus (HPV) is the virus that causes genital warts.

There is no cure for either genital herpes or genital warts. But, different medicines can help manage the symptoms of herpes and treat the complications of HPV infections that can cause genital warts.

What Are the Symptoms of Genital Herpes?

Most people with genital herpes do not know they have it. But, if you get symptoms with the first outbreak of genital herpes, they can be severe. Genital herpes also can be severe and long-lasting in people whose immune systems do not work properly, such as women with HIV.

Within a few days of sexual contact with someone who has the herpes virus, sores (small red bumps that may turn into blisters) may show up where the virus entered your body, such as on your mouth or vagina. Some women might confuse mild sores for insect bites or something else. After a few days, sores become crusted and then heal without scarring. Sometimes, a second set of sores appear soon after the first outbreak, and symptoms can happen again.

The first signs of genital herpes usually show up 2 to 12 days after having sexual contact with someone who has herpes. Symptoms can last from two to four weeks. There are other early symptoms of genital herpes:

- Feeling of pressure in the abdomen

- Flu-like symptoms, including fever

- Itching or burning feeling in the genital or anal area

- Pain in the legs, buttocks, or genital area

- Swollen glands

- Unusual vaginal discharge

If you have any symptoms of genital herpes, see a doctor or nurse.

How Is Genital Herpes Diagnosed?

Often, your doctor can diagnose genital herpes by looking at visible sores. Your doctor or nurse may also use a cotton swab to take a fluid sample from a sore to test in a lab.

Genital herpes can be hard to diagnose, especially between outbreaks. Blood tests that look for antibodies to the herpes virus can help diagnose herpes in women without symptoms or between outbreaks.

A Pap test is not used to detect genital herpes.

How Is Genital Herpes Treated?

Herpes has no cure, but antiviral medicines can prevent or shorten outbreaks during the time you take the medicine. Also, daily suppressive therapy (for example, daily use of antiviral medicine) for herpes can lower your chance of spreading the infection to your partner.

Your doctor will either give you antiviral medicine to take right after getting outbreak symptoms or to take regularly to try to stop outbreaks from happening. Talk to your doctor about treatment options.

During outbreaks, you can take the following steps to speed healing and prevent spreading herpes to other parts of your body or to other people:

- Keep sores clean and dry.
- Try not to touch the sores.
- Wash your hands after any contact with the sores.
- Avoid all sexual contact from the time you first notice symptoms until the sores have healed.

Can Genital Herpes Come Back?

Yes. Genital herpes symptoms can come and go, but the virus stays inside your body even after all signs of the infection have gone away. The virus becomes "active" from time to time, leading to an outbreak. Some people have outbreaks only once or twice. Other people may have four or five outbreaks within a year. Over time, the outbreaks usually happen less often and are less severe.

Experts do not know what causes the virus to become active. Some women say the virus comes back when they are sick, under stress, out in the sun, or during their period.

What Should I Do If I Have Genital Herpes?

If you have genital herpes:

- See a doctor or nurse as soon as possible for testing and treatment.
- Take all of the medicine. Even if symptoms go away, you need to finish all of the antiviral medicine.
- Tell your sex partner(s) so they can be tested and treated if necessary.
- Avoid any sexual contact while you are being treated for genital herpes or while you have an outbreak.

Remember that genital herpes is a lifelong disease. Even though you may not have a genital herpes outbreak for long periods of time, you can still pass the virus to another person at any time. Talk with your doctor or nurse about how to prevent passing the virus to another person.

How Does Genital Herpes Affect Pregnancy?

- If you get genital herpes during pregnancy, you can spread genital herpes to your baby during delivery.

- If you had genital herpes before pregnancy, your baby is still at risk of getting herpes, but the risk is lower.

- Most women with genital herpes have healthy babies. But babies who get herpes from their mother have neonatal herpes. Neonatal herpes is a serious condition that can cause problems in a newborn baby such as brain damage, eye problems, or even death.

Can Pregnant Women Take Genital Herpes Medicine?

Researchers do not know if all antiviral medicines for genital herpes are safe for pregnant women. If you are pregnant, make sure you tell your doctor or nurse that you have genital herpes, even if you are not having an outbreak.

Can I Breastfeed If I Have Genital Herpes?

Yes, you can breastfeed if you have genital herpes, but not if you have herpes sore on one of your breasts. If you have genital herpes, it is possible to spread the infection to any part of your breast, including your nipple and areola.

If you have any genital herpes sores on one or both of your breasts:

- You can keep breastfeeding as long as your baby or pumping equipment does not touch a herpes sore.

- Do not breastfeed from the breast with sores. Herpes is spread through contact with sores and can be dangerous to a newborn baby.

- Pump or hand-express your milk from the breast with sores until the sores heal. Pumping will help keep up your milk supply and prevent your breast from getting overly full and painful. You can store your milk to give to your baby in a bottle for another feeding. But if parts of your pump also touch the sore(s) while pumping, throw the milk away.

Can Genital Herpes Cause Other Problems?

For most women, genital herpes does not usually cause serious health problems.

Women with HIV can have severe herpes outbreaks that are long-lasting. Herpes also may play a role in the spread of HIV. Herpes sores can make it easier for HIV to get into your body. Also, herpes can make people who are HIV-positive more likely to spread the infection to someone else.

How Can I Prevent Genital Herpes?

The best way to prevent genital herpes or any sexually transmitted infection (STI) is to not have vaginal, oral, or anal sex.

If you do have sex, lower your risk of getting an STI with the following steps:

- **Use condoms and dental dams.** Condoms are the best way to prevent STIs when you have sex. Because a man does not need to ejaculate (come) to give or get some STIs, make sure to put the condom on before the penis touches the vagina, mouth, or anus. Other methods of birth control, like birth control pills, shots, implants, or diaphragms, will not protect you from STIs.

- **Get tested.** Be sure you and your partner are tested for STIs. Talk to each other about the test results before you have sex.

- **Be monogamous.** Having sex with just one partner can lower your risk for STIs. After being tested for STIs, be faithful to each other. That means that you have sex only with each other and no one else.

- **Limit your number of sex partners.** Your risk of getting STIs goes up with the number of partners you have.

- **Do not douche.** Douching removes some of the normal bacteria in the vagina that protects you from infection. This may increase your risk of getting STIs.

- **Do not abuse alcohol or drugs.** Drinking too much alcohol or using drugs increases risky behavior and may put you at risk of sexual assault and possible exposure to STIs.

The steps work best when used together. No single step can protect you from every single type of STI.

Can Women Who Have Sex with Women Get Genital Herpes?

Yes. It is possible to get genital herpes or any other STI if you are a woman who has sex only with women.

Talk to your partner about her sexual history before having sex, and ask your doctor or nurse about getting tested if you have signs or symptoms of genital herpes. Use a dental dam during oral sex and avoid sexual activity during an outbreak.

Where Can We Get More Information about Genital Herpes?

You can call the OWH Helpline at 800-994-9662 or contact the following organizations:

- National Center for HIV/AIDS, Viral Hepatitis, STD, and TB Prevention (NCHHSTP), CDC, HHS

- Toll-Free: 800-232-4636

- National Institute of Allergy and Infectious Diseases (NIAID), NIH, HHS

- Toll-Free: 866-284-4107 (Toll-Free TDD: 800-877-8339)

- Herpes Resource Center, ASHA

- Toll-Free: 800-230-6039

Chapter 15

Hepatitis

Chapter Contents

Section 15.1

Viral Hepatitis

This section contains text excerpted from "Viral Hepatitis," Office on Women's Health (OWH), U.S. Department of Health and Human Services (HHS), July 2, 2018.

Hepatitis is an inflammation of the liver. In the United States, viral hepatitis is usually caused by the hepatitis A, B, C, D, and E virus. Different types of hepatitis spread in different ways, including having sex, sharing needles, or eating unclean food. Sometimes, viral hepatitis goes away on its own. In others, the virus is lifelong and can lead to serious health problems. Vaccines can prevent hepatitis A, B, and D, but not C and E. There are medicines to treat and sometimes cure hepatitis B and C.

What Is Viral Hepatitis?

Viral hepatitis is inflammation of the liver caused by the hepatitis virus. Inflammation happens when your immune system senses a danger, such as a virus, and sends white blood cells to surround the area to protect your body. This causes redness, swelling, and sometimes pain. Hepatitis damages the liver and can cause scarring of the liver, called "cirrhosis." Cirrhosis can cause liver cancer, liver failure, and death. Your liver changes the food you eat into energy. It also cleans alcohol and other toxins from your blood, helps your stomach and intestines digest food, and makes proteins that your body needs to control and stop bleeding.

What Are the Different Types of Viral Hepatitis?

The most common types of viral hepatitis in the United States are:

- Hepatitis A

- Hepatitis B

- Hepatitis C

- Hepatitis D

- Hepatitis E

Does Viral Hepatitis Affect Women Differently than Men?

Yes, certain types of viral hepatitis affect women differently than men. Hepatitis A affects women and men in similar ways. Hepatitis B affects women differently than men:

- **Birth control.** Women with severe liver damage may not be able to use birth control. This is because a damaged liver may have problems breaking down estrogen.

- **Pregnancy.** The risk of passing hepatitis B to your baby during pregnancy is high. Hepatitis B raises your risk for pregnancy complications. Talk to your doctor about taking hepatitis B medicine to lower the risk of passing hepatitis B to your baby. Certain hepatitis B medicines are safe to take during pregnancy but are not recommended for everyone.

Hepatitis C affects women differently than men:

- **Younger women.** Research shows that acute (short-term) hepatitis C goes away on its own more often for younger women than men. Also, in women with chronic hepatitis C, liver damage usually happens more slowly than it does for men. Researchers think the hormone estrogen may help protect the liver from damage.

- **Menstrual cycles.** You may miss menstrual periods or have shorter periods. This can happen as a side effect of hepatitis medicines. Since hepatitis C is spread through blood, the risk of passing hepatitis C to a partner is higher during your menstrual period.

- **Birth control.** Women with severe liver damage may not be able to use birth control that contains estrogen. This is because a damaged liver may have problems breaking down estrogen.

- **Pregnancy.** Experts think the risk of passing hepatitis C to your baby during pregnancy is low. But hepatitis C raises your risk for pregnancy complications such as premature birth and gestational diabetes. Some hepatitis C medicines can also cause serious harm to your baby if taken during pregnancy.

- **Menopause.** Liver damage happens more quickly for women after menopause. Hepatitis C medicines also may not work as well for women after menopause as they do for men.

How Do You Get Hepatitis A?

Hepatitis A is found in an infected person's stool (poop). Hepatitis A is spread through:

- Eating or drinking contaminated food or water

  - You can get hepatitis A by eating food prepared by a person with the virus who didn't wash her or his hands after using the bathroom and then touched the food.

  - You can get hepatitis A by eating raw or undercooked shellfish that came from sewage-contaminated water.

- Vaginal, oral, or anal sex. Hepatitis A can be spread even if the infected person has no symptoms.

- Touching unclean diaper-changing areas or toilets. If an infant or toddler had hepatitis A and soiled the changing area, others who come into contact with the stool could become infected.

You are more likely to get hepatitis A if you travel to a developing country with poor sanitation or without access to clean water and have not gotten vaccinated for hepatitis A. Ask your doctor if you need a hepatitis A vaccination.

How Do You Get Hepatitis B?

Hepatitis B is found in an infected person's blood and other body fluids, such as semen and vaginal fluid. Hepatitis B is usually spread through:

- Vaginal, oral, or anal sex. This is the most common way hepatitis B is spread. Hepatitis B can be spread even if the infected person has no symptoms.

- Birth from a mother who has hepatitis B to her child

- Sharing or reusing needles, syringes, and drug-preparation equipment such as cookers and cotton when injecting drugs. Hands or drug-preparation equipment with even a trace amount of blood on them can spread hepatitis B.

- Accidental needle stick or other sharp-instrument injuries (higher risk for healthcare workers)

A less common way to spread hepatitis B is through prechewed food to a baby from a mother who has hepatitis B. However, hepatitis B cannot be spread through breastfeeding.

How Do You Get Hepatitis C?

Hepatitis C is found in an infected person's blood and other body fluids. Hepatitis C is usually spread through:

- Sharing or reusing needles, syringes, and drug preparation equipment such as cookers and cotton when injecting drugs. This is the most common way hepatitis C is spread in the United States. Hands or drug-preparation equipment with even trace amount of blood on them can also spread hepatitis C.

- Accidental needle stick or other sharp-instrument injuries (higher risk for healthcare workers)

Less common ways to spread hepatitis C:

- Vaginal, oral, or anal sex

- Birth to a mother who has hepatitis, though this is rare

- Sharing personal items such as razors and toothbrushes

- Tattoos or body piercings

- Blood transfusions done in the United States before the 1990s (when hepatitis C testing began) or in other parts of the world where hepatitis C testing is less common

How Do You Get Hepatitis D?

The hepatitis D virus is unusual because it can only infect you when you also have a hepatitis B viral infection. In this way, hepatitis D is a double infection. You can protect yourself from hepatitis D by protecting yourself from hepatitis B by getting the hepatitis B vaccine. Hepatitis D spreads the same way that hepatitis B spreads—through contact with an infected person's blood or other body fluids. The hepatitis D virus can cause acute or chronic infection or both:

- **Acute hepatitis D**—This is a short-term infection. The symptoms of acute hepatitis D are the same as the symptoms of any type of hepatitis and are often more severe. Sometimes your body is able to fight off the infection and the virus goes away.

- **Chronic hepatitis D**—This is a long-lasting infection. Chronic hepatitis D occurs when your body is not able to fight off the virus and the virus does not go away. People who have chronic hepatitis B and D develop complications more often and more quickly than people who have chronic hepatitis B alone.

How Do Hepatitis D and Hepatitis B Infections Occur Together?

Hepatitis D and hepatitis B infections may occur together as a coinfection or a superinfection. People can only become infected with hepatitis D when they also have hepatitis B.

Coinfection—A coinfection occurs when you get both hepatitis D and hepatitis B infections at the same time. Coinfections usually cause acute, or short-term, hepatitis D and B infections. Coinfections may cause severe acute hepatitis.

Superinfection—A superinfection occurs if you already have chronic hepatitis B and then become infected with hepatitis D. When you get a superinfection, you may have severe acute hepatitis symptoms.

How Do You Get Hepatitis E?

Hepatitis E is a viral infection that causes liver inflammation and damage. Hepatitis E typically causes acute, or short-term, infection. Some types are spread by drinking contaminated water. These types are more common in developing countries, including parts of Africa, Asia, Central America, and the Middle East. Other types are spread by eating undercooked pork or wild game, such as deer. These types are more common in developed countries, such as the United States, Australia, Japan, and parts of Europe and East Asia.

- **Acute Hepatitis E**—is a short-term infection. In most cases, people's bodies are able to recover and fight off the infection and the virus goes away. People usually get better without treatment after several weeks.

- **Chronic Hepatitis E**—is a long-lasting infection that occurs when your body isn't able to fight off the virus and the virus does not go away. For example, hepatitis E may become chronic in people taking medicines that weaken their immune system after an organ transplant, or in people who have human immunodeficiency virus (HIV) or acquired immunodeficiency syndrome (AIDS).

What Are the Symptoms of Viral Hepatitis?

The symptoms of viral hepatitis are similar for all types of hepatitis. They include:

- Low-grade fever (a temperature between 99.5°F and 101°F)

- Fatigue (tiredness)

- Loss of appetite

- Upset stomach

- Vomiting

- Stomach pain

- Dark urine

- Clay-colored bowel movements

- Joint pain

- Jaundice, which is when the skin and whites of the eyes turn yellow

People who are newly infected are most likely to have one or more of these symptoms, but some people with viral hepatitis do not have any symptoms. Certain blood tests can show if you have hepatitis, even if you do not have symptoms. People with chronic hepatitis B or C often develop symptoms when their liver becomes damaged.

Why Do All Baby Boomers Need to Be Tested for Viral Hepatitis?

The CDC recommends that all Americans born between 1945 and 1965 (called baby boomers) get a one-time test for hepatitis C. This is because three in four adults with hepatitis C are baby boomers, and most baby boomers do not know they have it. It's likely that many baby boomers with hepatitis C were infected many years ago before the blood supply was tested for hepatitis C.

How Is Viral Hepatitis Diagnosed?

Talk to your doctor if you have symptoms of viral hepatitis. Your doctor will:

- Ask questions about your health history

151

- Do a physical exam

- Order blood tests that look for parts of the virus or antibodies that your body makes in response to the virus. Other tests may measure the amount of the virus in your blood.

How Do I Know If I Have Acute or Chronic Viral Hepatitis?

Hepatitis A, B, C, D, and E all start out as an acute (short-term) infection. Some acute infections can develop into lifelong, chronic infections. Your doctor may do a blood test to see if the infection is acute or chronic.

How Is Acute (Short-Term) Viral Hepatitis Treated?

Acute viral hepatitis usually goes away on its own. Hepatitis A causes only acute infection, but hepatitis B, C, D, and E often cause chronic or lifelong infection. If you have acute hepatitis A, B, C, D, or E you may feel sick for a few months before you get better.

- Your doctor may recommend rest and making sure you get enough fluids.

- Avoid alcohol and certain medicines, such as the pain reliever acetaminophen, because they can damage the liver during this time.

- Some people with acute viral hepatitis need to be hospitalized to manage the symptoms.

If you think you have hepatitis, go to the doctor right away.

How Is Chronic (Long-Term) Viral Hepatitis Treated?

If you have chronic viral hepatitis, your treatment depends on the type of hepatitis you have:

- **Hepatitis B.** You will probably meet with your doctor regularly, every 6 to 12 months, to watch for signs of liver disease and liver cancer. If you plan to become pregnant in the future, talk to your doctor first. You may need antiviral medicines to treat hepatitis B, but many people do not need medicine. The U.S. Food and Drug Administration (FDA) has a list of approved medicines to treat hepatitis B.

- **Hepatitis C.** If you have hepatitis C, talk with your doctor about whether you need medicine. Recently approved antiviral medicines treat and may cure hepatitis C in adults. The FDA has a list of approved medicines to treat hepatitis C. If you have health insurance, ask about your copay or coinsurance and which medicines are covered under your plan.

- **Hepatitis D.** Doctors may treat chronic hepatitis D with medicines called interferons, such as peginterferon alfa-2a (Pegasys). Researchers are studying new treatments for hepatitis D. In addition, medicines for hepatitis B may be needed. These are usually medicines taken once daily by mouth. If chronic hepatitis D leads to cirrhosis, you should see a doctor who specializes in liver diseases. Doctors can treat health problems related to cirrhosis with medicines, surgery, and other medical procedures. If you have cirrhosis, you have a greater chance of developing liver cancer. Your doctor may order an ultrasound or another type of imaging test to check for liver cancer. If acute hepatitis D leads to acute liver failure, or if chronic hepatitis D leads to liver failure or liver cancer, you may need a liver transplant.

- **Hepatitis E.** Treatment for acute hepatitis E includes resting, drinking plenty of liquids, and eating healthy foods to help relieve symptoms. Talk with your doctor before taking any prescription or over-the-counter (OTC) medicines, vitamins or other dietary supplements, or complementary or alternative medicines—any of these could damage your liver. You should avoid alcohol until your doctor tells you that you have completely recovered from hepatitis E. See your doctor regularly to make sure your body has fully recovered. Doctors may treat chronic hepatitis E with ribavirin or peginterferon alfa-2a (Pegasys).

What Can Happen If Viral Hepatitis Is Not Treated?

Most people recover from hepatitis A with no treatment or long-lasting health problems.

Chronic hepatitis B, C, D, and E can lead to serious health problems, such as:

- Cirrhosis, or scarring of the liver
- Liver cancer
- Liver failure

People with liver failure may need a liver transplant to survive. In the United States, cirrhosis caused by chronic hepatitis C is currently the most common reason for needing a liver transplant. Viral hepatitis is also the most common cause of liver cancer.

What Should I Do If I Think I Have Been Exposed to Viral Hepatitis?

Call your doctor or your local or state health department if you think you may have been exposed.

- If you may have been exposed to hepatitis A or B, your doctor may recommend getting a vaccine (shot) to keep you from getting the infection.

- The Centers for Disease Control and Prevention (CDC) recommends that people who are exposed to hepatitis C, such as a healthcare worker after an accidental needle stick, get tested for hepatitis C infection. New antiviral medicines for hepatitis C cure most of the people who take them. If you have health insurance, ask about your copay and coinsurance and which medicines are covered under your plan.

How Does Viral Hepatitis Affect Pregnancy?

Hepatitis B and C can cause problems during pregnancy and can be passed to your baby. The risk of passing the virus to your baby is higher with hepatitis B than C.

Research shows that pregnant women with hepatitis B or C may have a higher risk for certain pregnancy complications:

- Gestational diabetes

- Low-birth-weight (LBW) baby (less than 5½ pounds)

- Premature birth (also called preterm birth, or babies born before 37 weeks of pregnancy).

Premature birth is the leading cause of infant death and raises the risk of health and developmental problems at birth and later in life.

Talk to your doctor if you think you may be pregnant or plan to become pregnant. Some antiviral medicines that treat hepatitis C, such as ribavirin, can cause serious birth defects if taken during pregnancy.

I Have Viral Hepatitis and Am Pregnant. Will My Baby Get the Virus?

Maybe. Hepatitis B and C can be passed from a pregnant woman to her baby during childbirth.

- If you have hepatitis B, the risk of passing the infection to your baby is higher. Make sure your baby gets hepatitis B immune globulin (HBIG) and the first shot of the hepatitis B vaccine within 12 hours of birth. Your baby will need two or three more shots of the vaccine over the next 1 to 15 months to help keep them from getting hepatitis B. The timing and the total number of shots will depend on the type of vaccine and your baby's age and weight. All babies should be vaccinated for hepatitis B. Talk to your doctor. One in four people infected at birth will die of hepatitis B-related causes such as liver cancer or liver failure. Your doctor will test your baby after the last shot to make sure he or she is protected from the disease.

- If you have hepatitis C, the risk of passing the virus to your baby is believed to be low, but it is still possible. The only way to know if your baby becomes infected is by doing a test. The CDC recommends testing a child after she or he turns 18 months old. Most infants infected with hepatitis C at birth have no symptoms and do well during childhood.

Can I Breastfeed My Baby If I Have Viral Hepatitis?

- Yes, you can breastfeed your baby if you have viral hepatitis. You cannot pass viral hepatitis through breast milk.

- But, if you have hepatitis C and your nipple or the surrounding skin is cracked or bleeding, stop nursing your baby on that breast until the sores heal. You can pump or hand express your milk from that breast until it heals. Throw any breast milk from that breast away, because it might have been contaminated with hepatitis C from the cracked or bleeding skin.

How Can I Prevent Viral Hepatitis?

You can lower your risk of getting viral hepatitis with the following steps. The steps work best when used together. No single step can protect you from every kind of viral hepatitis. Steps to lower your risk of viral hepatitis:

- Get vaccinated. Getting vaccinated is the best way to prevent hepatitis A and B. There is no vaccine for hepatitis C. The hepatitis A and hepatitis B vaccines are recommended for anyone who wants protection from the viruses and for people with certain risk factors and health problems. Ask your doctor if you need the vaccines.

- Wash your hands after using the bathroom and changing diapers and before preparing or eating food.

- If you have sex, use condoms and dental dams. Condoms lower your risk of getting or passing sexually transmitted infections (STIs), including viral hepatitis. Viral hepatitis can be passed through menstrual blood, vaginal fluid, and semen (cum). Make sure to put the condom on before the penis touches your vagina, mouth, or anus. Other methods of birth control like birth control pills, shots, implants, or diaphragms, will not protect you from viral hepatitis.

- Limit your number of sex partners. Your risk of getting viral hepatitis goes up with the number of lifetime sex partners you have.

- If you use needles or syringes for any reason, do not share them with others.

- Do not share personal items that could have blood on them, such as razors, nail clippers, toothbrushes, or glucose monitors.

- Do not get tattoos or body piercings from an unlicensed person or facility.

- Wear protective gloves if you have to touch another person's blood.

- If you are a healthcare or public-safety worker, get vaccinated for hepatitis A and B, and always follow recommended standard precautions and infection-control principles, including safe injection practices.

Do I Need the Viral Hepatitis Vaccines?

Maybe. Hepatitis A and B vaccines can protect you from getting infected. Talk to your doctor or nurse about getting the recommended vaccines.

There is no vaccine available for hepatitis C and D, but you can take other steps to lower your risk. The hepatitis B vaccine can prevent hepatitis D by preventing hepatitis B. No vaccine for hepatitis E is available in the United States, but vaccines have been developed and are used in China.

How Long Do the Vaccines Protect You?

During your lifetime, you need:

- One series of the hepatitis A vaccine (two shots given at least six months apart)

- One series of the hepatitis B vaccine (three or four shots given over a 6-month period)

Most people don't need a booster dose of either vaccine. But if you have had dialysis, a medical procedure to clean your blood, or have a weakened immune system, your doctor might recommend additional doses of the hepatitis B vaccine.

How Can I Get Free or Low-Cost Hepatitis A and B Vaccines?

Hepatitis A and hepatitis B vaccines are covered under most insurance plans.

- If you have insurance, check with your insurance provider to find out what's included in your plan.

- Medicare Part B covers hepatitis B vaccines for people at risk.

- If you have Medicaid, the benefits covered are different in each state.

Section 15.2

Hepatitis and HIV Coinfection

This section contains text excerpted from the following sources:
Text beginning with the heading "Coinfection with HIV and Viral
Hepatitis" is excerpted from "Coinfection with HIV and Viral
Hepatitis," Centers for Disease Control and Prevention (CDC),
February 7, 2018. Text beginning with the heading "Human
Immunodeficiency Virus and Hepatitis B" is excerpted from "HIV and
Hepatitis B," AIDS*info*, U.S. Department of Health and
Human Services (HHS), June 25, 2018.

Coinfection with Human Immunodeficiency Virus and Viral Hepatitis

An estimated 1.2 million persons are living with human immunodeficiency virus (HIV) in the United States. HIV coinfection more than triples the risk for liver disease, liver failure, and liver-related death from HCV. Because viral hepatitis infection is often serious in people living with HIV and may lead to liver damage more quickly, the Centers for Disease Control and Prevention (CDC) recommends all persons at risk for HIV be vaccinated against hepatitis B virus (HBV) and be tested for HBV and hepatitis C virus (HCV) infection. December 1st has been designated World AIDS Day, creating an opportunity not only for raising awareness about HIV infection, but educating health professionals and the general public worldwide about the overwhelming burden of HIV and viral hepatitis coinfection, and the importance of testing, care, and treatment.

What Is the Connection between Human Immunodeficiency Virus and Hepatitis B Virus?

Both HIV and HBV spread from person to person in semen, blood, or other body fluids. For this reason, the main risk factors for HIV and HBV are the same: having sex without a condom/dental damn and injection drug use.

According to the CDC, approximately 10 percent of people with HIV in the United States also have HBV. Infection with both HIV and HBV is called HIV/HBV coinfection.

Chronic HBV advances faster to cirrhosis, end-stage liver disease, and liver cancer in people with HIV/HBV coinfection than in people with only HBV infection. But chronic HBV doesn't appear to cause HIV to advance faster in people with "HIV/HBV coinfection."

Should People with Human Immunodeficiency Virus Get Tested for Hepatitis B Virus?

The CDC recommends that all people with HIV get tested for HBV. Testing can detect HBV infection even when a person has no symptoms of the infection. There are several HBV blood tests. Results of different tests have different meanings. For example, a positive hepatitis B surface antigen (HBsAg) test result shows that a person has acute or chronic HBV and can spread the virus to others.

What Is the Connection between Human Immunodeficiency Virus and Hepatitis C Virus?

Because both HIV and HCV can spread in blood, a major risk factor for both HIV and HCV infection is injection drug use. Sharing needles or other drug injection equipment increases the risk of contact with HIV- or HCV-infected blood.

According to the CDC, approximately 25 percent of people with HIV in the United States also have HCV. Among people with HIV who inject drugs, about 50 to 90 percent also have HCV. Infection with both HIV and HCV is called "HIV/HCV coinfection."

In people with HIV/HCV coinfection, HIV may cause chronic HCV to advance faster. Whether HCV causes HIV to advance faster is unclear.

Should People with Human Immunodeficiency Virus Get Tested for Hepatitis C Virus?

Every person who has HIV should get tested for HCV. Usually, a person will first get an HCV antibody test. This test checks for HCV antibodies in the blood. HCV antibodies are disease-fighting proteins that the body produces in response to HCV infection.

A positive result on an HCV antibody test means that the person has been exposed to HCV at some point in their life. However, a positive antibody test does not necessarily mean the person has HCV. For this reason, a positive result on an HCV antibody test must be confirmed by a second, follow-up test. The follow-up test checks to see if HCV is present in the person's blood. A positive result on this test confirms that a person has HCV.

Chapter 16

Human Immunodeficiency Virus and Acquired Immunodeficiency Syndrome

Chapter Contents

Section 16.1

An Overview of Human Immunodeficiency Virus and Acquired Immunodeficiency Syndrome

This section includes text excerpted from "HIV Overview—HIV/AIDS: The Basics," AIDS*info*, U.S. Department of Health and Human Services (HHS), November 6, 2018.

What Is Human Immunodeficiency Virus/Acquired Immunodeficiency Syndrome?

"HIV" stands for human immunodeficiency virus, which is the virus that causes HIV infection. The abbreviation "HIV" can refer to the virus or to HIV infection.

AIDS stands for acquired immunodeficiency syndrome. AIDS is the most advanced stage of HIV infection.

HIV attacks and destroys the infection-fighting CD4 cells of the immune system. The loss of CD4 cells makes it difficult for the body to fight infections and certain cancers. Without treatment, HIV can gradually destroy the immune system and advance to AIDS.

How Is Human Immunodeficiency Virus Spread?

HIV is spread through contact with certain body fluids from a person with HIV. These body fluids include:

- Blood
- Semen
- Preseminal fluid
- Vaginal fluids
- Rectal fluids
- Breast milk

The spread of HIV from person to person is called "HIV transmission." The spread of HIV from a woman with HIV to her child during pregnancy, childbirth, or breastfeeding is called "mother-to-child transmission" of HIV.

In the United States, HIV is spread mainly by:

- Having anal or vaginal sex with someone who has HIV without using a condom or taking medicines to prevent or treat HIV

- Sharing injection drug equipment ("works"), such as needles, with someone who has HIV

To reduce your risk of HIV infection, use condoms and dental dams correctly every time you have sex, limit your number of sexual partners, and never share injection-drug equipment. Also, talk to your healthcare provider about pre-exposure prophylaxis (PrEP). PrEP is an HIV prevention option for people who don't have HIV but who are at high risk of becoming infected with HIV. PrEP involves taking a specific HIV medicine every day.

Mother-to-child transmission is the most common way that children get HIV. HIV medicines, given to women with HIV during pregnancy and childbirth and to their babies after birth, reduce the risk of mother-to-child transmission of HIV.

You can't get HIV by shaking hands or hugging a person who has HIV. You also can't get HIV from contact with objects such as dishes, toilet seats, or doorknobs used by a person with HIV. HIV is not spread through the air or in water or by mosquitoes, ticks, or other blood-sucking insects.

What Are the Symptoms of Human Immunodeficiency Virus / Acquired Immunodeficiency Syndrome?

Within two to four weeks after infection with HIV, some people may have flu-like symptoms, such as fever, chills, or rash. The symptoms may last for a few days to several weeks.

After this earliest stage of HIV infection, HIV continues to multiply but at very low levels. More severe symptoms of HIV infection, such as signs of opportunistic infections, generally don't appear for many years. (Opportunistic infections are infections and infection-related cancers that occur more frequently or are more severe in people with weakened immune systems than in people with healthy immune systems.)

Without treatment with HIV medicines, HIV infection usually advances to AIDS in 10 years or longer, though it may advance faster in some people.

HIV transmission is possible at any stage of HIV infection—even if a person with HIV has no symptoms of HIV.

How Is Acquired Immunodeficiency Syndrome Diagnosed?

Symptoms such as fever, weakness, and weight loss may be a sign that a person's HIV has advanced to AIDS. However, a diagnosis of AIDS is based on the following criteria:

- A drop in CD4 count to less than 200 cells/mm3. A CD4 count measures the number of CD4 cells in a sample of blood. Or

- The presence of certain opportunistic infections

Although an AIDS diagnosis indicates severe damage to the immune system, HIV medicines can still help people at this stage of HIV infection.

What Is the Treatment for Human Immunodeficiency Virus?

Antiretroviral therapy (ART) is the use of HIV medicines to treat HIV infection. People on ART take a combination of HIV medicines (called an "HIV regimen") every day. (HIV medicines are often called "antiretrovirals" or "ARTs").

ART is recommended for everyone who has HIV. ART prevents HIV from multiplying and reduces the amount of HIV in the body (also called the "viral load"). Having less HIV in the body protects the immune system and prevents HIV infection from advancing to AIDS. ART can't cure HIV, but HIV medicines help people with HIV live longer, healthier lives.

ART also reduces the risk of HIV transmission. A main goal of ART is to reduce a person's viral load to an undetectable level. An undetectable viral load means that the level of HIV in the blood is too low to be detected by a viral-load test. People with HIV who maintain an undetectable viral load have effectively no risk of transmitting HIV to their HIV-negative partner through sex.

Section 16.2

The Human Immunodeficiency Virus Life Cycle

This section includes text excerpted from "HIV Overview—The HIV Life Cycle" AIDS*info*, U.S. Department of Health and Human Services (HHS), July 27, 2018.

What Is the Human Immunodeficiency Virus Life Cycle?

Human immunodeficiency virus (HIV) attacks and destroys the CD4 cells of the immune system. CD4 cells are a type of white blood cell that plays a major role in protecting the body from infection. HIV uses the machinery of the CD4 cells to multiply (make copies of itself) and spread throughout the body. This process, which is carried out in seven steps or stages, is called the "HIV life cycle."

What Are the Seven Stages of the Human Immunodeficiency Virus Life Cycle?

The seven stages of the HIV life cycle are:

1. Binding
2. Fusion
3. Reverse transcription
4. Integration
5. Replication
6. Assembly
7. Budding

What Is the Connection between the Human Immunodeficiency Virus Life Cycle and Human Immunodeficiency Virus Medicines?

Antiretroviral therapy (ART) is the use of HIV medicines to treat HIV infection. People on ART take a combination of HIV medicines (called an "HIV regimen") every day. HIV medicines protect the

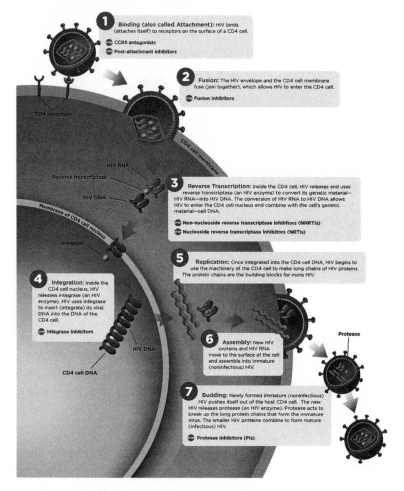

Figure 16.1. *The HIV Life Cycle*

immune system by blocking HIV at different stages of the HIV life cycle.

HIV medicines are grouped into different drug classes according to how they fight HIV. Each class of drugs is designed to target a specific step in the HIV life cycle.

Because an HIV regimen includes HIV medicines from at least two different HIV drug classes, ART is very effective at preventing HIV from multiplying. Having less HIV in the body protects the immune system and prevents HIV from advancing to AIDS. ART also reduces the risk of HIV drug resistance.

ART can't cure HIV, but HIV medicines help people with HIV live longer, healthier lives. HIV medicines also reduce the risk of HIV transmission (the spread of HIV to others).

The Stages of Human Immunodeficiency Virus Infection

Without treatment, HIV infection advances in stages, getting worse over time. HIV gradually destroys the immune system and eventually causes acquired immunodeficiency syndrome (AIDS).

There is no cure for HIV infection, but HIV medicines (called "antiretrovirals" or "ARVs") can slow or prevent HIV from advancing from one stage to the next. HIV medicines help people with HIV live longer, healthier lives. HIV medicines also reduce the risk of HIV transmission (the spread of HIV to others).

There are three stages of HIV infection:

Acute Human Immunodeficiency Virus Infection

Acute HIV infection is the earliest stage of HIV infection, and it generally develops within two to four weeks after infection with HIV. During this time, some people have flu-like symptoms, such as fever, headache, and rash. In the acute stage of infection, HIV multiplies rapidly and spreads throughout the body. The virus attacks and destroys the infection-fighting CD4 cells of the immune system. During the acute HIV infection stage, the level of HIV in the blood is very high, which greatly increases the risk of HIV transmission.

Chronic Human Immunodeficiency Virus Infection

The second stage of HIV infection is chronic HIV infection (also called "asymptomatic HIV infection" or "clinical latency"). During this stage of the disease, HIV continues to multiply in the body but at very low levels. People with chronic HIV infection may not have any HIV-related symptoms, but they can still spread HIV to others. Without treatment with HIV medicines, chronic HIV infection usually advances to AIDS in 10 years or longer, though in some people it may advance faster.

Acquired Immunodeficiency Syndrome

AIDS is the final, most severe stage of HIV infection. Because HIV has severely damaged the immune system, the body can't fight off opportunistic infections. (Opportunistic infections are infections and infection-related cancers that occur more frequently or are more severe in people with weakened immune systems than in people with healthy immune systems.) People with HIV are diagnosed with AIDS if they have a CD4 count of less than 200 cells/mm3 or if they have certain opportunistic infections. Without treatment, people with AIDS typically survive for about three years.

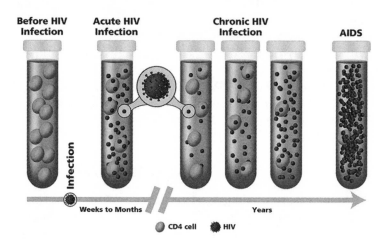

Figure 16.2. *Stages of Human Immunodeficiency Virus Infection—Human Immunodeficiency Virus Progression*

Section 16.3

Symptoms of Human Immunodeficiency Virus

This section includes text excerpted from "Symptoms of HIV," HIV.gov, U.S. Department of Health and Human Services (HHS), May 15, 2017.

The symptoms of human immunodeficiency virus (HIV) vary, depending on the individual and what stage of the disease you are in: the early stage, the clinical latency stage, or acquired immunodeficiency syndrome (AIDS), the late stage of HIV infection. Below are the symptoms that some individuals may experience in these three stages. Not all individuals will experience these symptoms.

Early Stage of Human Immunodeficiency Virus

About 40 to 90 percent of people have flu-like symptoms within two to four weeks after HIV infection. Other people do not feel sick at all during this stage, which is also known as "acute HIV infection." Early infection is defined as HIV infection in the past six months and includes acute infections. Flu-like symptoms can include:

- Fever

- Chills

- Rash

- Night sweats

- Muscle aches

- Sore throat

- Fatigue

- Swollen lymph nodes

- Mouth ulcers

These symptoms can last anywhere from a few days to several weeks. During this time, HIV infection may not show up on some types of HIV tests, but people who have it are highly infectious and can spread the infection to others.

You should not assume you have HIV just because you have any of these symptoms. Each of these symptoms can be caused by other illnesses. And some people who have HIV do not show any symptoms at all for 10 years or more.

However, if you think you may have been exposed to HIV and could be in the early stage of HIV infection, get an HIV test. Most HIV tests detect antibodies (proteins your body makes as a reaction against the presence of HIV), not HIV itself. But it can take a few weeks or longer for your body to produce these antibodies.

Some places use HIV tests that can detect acute and recent infections, but others do not. So be sure to let your testing site know if you think you may have been recently infected with HIV. Tests that can detect acute infection look for HIV Ribonucleic acid (RNA) or p24 antigen. Most doctors and clinics that provide a full range of healthcare services can do this test, but some places that only do HIV testing may not have it. So you may want to contact the site before you go to ask if they can test you for acute HIV infection.

After you get tested, it's important to find out the result of your test. If you are HIV-positive, you should see a doctor and start HIV treatment as soon as possible. You are at high risk of transmitting HIV to others during the early stage of HIV infection, even if you have no symptoms. For this reason, it is very important to take steps to reduce your risk of transmission. If you are HIV-negative, explore HIV-prevention options, such as pre-exposure prophylaxis (PrEP), that can help you stay negative.

Clinical Latency Stage

After the early stage of HIV infection, the disease moves into a stage called the "clinical latency stage" (also called "chronic HIV infection"). During this stage, HIV is still active but reproduces at very low levels. People with chronic HIV infection may not have any HIV-related symptoms or only mild ones.

For people who aren't taking medicine to treat HIV (called "antiretroviral therapy" or "ART"), this period can last a decade or longer, but some may progress through this phase faster. People who are taking medicine to treat HIV, and who take their medications the right way, every day, may be in this stage for several decades because treatment helps keep the virus in check.

It's important to remember that people can still transmit HIV to others during this phase even if they have no symptoms, although people who are on ART and stay virally suppressed (having a very low level of virus in their blood) are much less likely to transmit HIV than those who are not virally suppressed.

Progression to Acquired Immunodeficiency Syndrome

If you have HIV and you are not on ART, eventually the virus will weaken your body's immune system and you will progress to acquired immunodeficiency syndrome (AIDS), the late stage of HIV infection. Symptoms can include:

• Rapid weight loss

• Recurring fever or profuse night sweats

• Extreme and unexplained tiredness

• Prolonged swelling of the lymph glands in the armpits, groin, or neck

• Diarrhea that lasts for more than a week

• Sores of the mouth, anus, or genitals

• Pneumonia

• Red, brown, pink, or purplish blotches on or under the skin or inside the mouth, nose, or eyelids

• Memory loss, depression, and other neurologic disorders

Each of these symptoms can also be related to other illnesses. So the only way to know for sure if you have HIV is to get tested.

Many of the severe symptoms and illnesses of HIV disease come from the opportunistic infections that occur because your body's immune system has been damaged.

Section 16.4

Questions and Answers about Human Immunodeficiency Virus Transmission

This section includes text excerpted from
"HIV/AIDS—HIV Transmission," National Center for Injury
Prevention and Control, Centers for Disease Control and
Prevention (CDC), October 31, 2018.

How Well Does Human Immunodeficiency Virus Survive outside the Body?

HIV does not survive long outside the human body (such as on surfaces), and it cannot reproduce outside a human host. It is not spread by:

- Mosquitoes, ticks, or other insects

- Saliva, tears, or sweat that is not mixed with the blood of an HIV-positive person

- Hugging, shaking hands, sharing toilets, sharing dishes, or closed-mouth or "social" kissing with someone who is HIV-positive

- Other sexual activities that don't involve the exchange of body fluids (for example, touching)

Is There a Connection between Human Immunodeficiency Virus and Other Sexually Transmitted Diseases?

Yes. Having another sexually transmitted disease (STD) can increase the risk of getting or transmitting HIV.

If you have another STD, you are more likely to get or transmit HIV to others. Some of the most common STDs include gonorrhea, chlamydia, syphilis, trichomoniasis, human papillomavirus (HPV), genital herpes, and hepatitis. The only way to know for sure if you have an STD is to get tested. If you are sexually active, you and your partners should get tested for STDs (including HIV if you are HIV-negative) regularly, even if you don't have symptoms.

If you are HIV-negative but have an STD, you are about three times as likely to get HIV if you have unprotected sex with someone who has HIV. There are two ways that having an STD can increase the likelihood of getting HIV. If the STD causes irritation of the skin (for example, from syphilis, herpes, or human papillomavirus), breaks or sores may make it easier for HIV to enter the body during sexual contact. Even STDs that cause no breaks or open sores (for example, chlamydia, gonorrhea, trichomoniasis) can increase your risk by causing inflammation that increases the number of cells that can serve as targets for HIV.

If you are HIV-positive and also have another STD, you are about three times as likely as other people with HIV to transmit HIV through sexual contact. This appears to happen because there is an increased concentration of HIV in the semen and genital fluids of HIV-positive people who also have another STD.

Does My Human Immunodeficiency Virus-Positive Partner's Viral Load Affect My Risk of Getting Human Immunodeficiency Virus?

Yes. As an HIV-positive person's viral load goes down, the chance of transmitting HIV can go down dramatically.

Viral load is the amount of HIV in the blood of someone who has HIV. Taking HIV medicine (called "antiretroviral therapy" or "ART") as prescribed can make the viral load very low—so low that a test can't detect it (called an "undetectable viral load"). People with HIV who take HIV medicine as prescribed and get and keep an undetectable viral load have effectively no risk of transmitting HIV to an HIV-negative partner through sex.

If you are HIV-positive, getting into care and taking HIV medications as prescribed will give you the greatest chance to get and keep an undetectable viral load; live a longer, healthier life; and protect your partners.

If you are HIV-negative and have an HIV-positive partner, encourage your partner to get into care and to take HIV medicine as prescribed.

Treatment is a powerful tool for preventing sexual transmission of HIV. But it works only as long as the HIV-positive partner gets and keeps an undetectable viral load. Here are some things to consider when deciding whether treatment as prevention is right for you and your partner:

- Not everyone taking HIV medicine has an undetectable viral load. Up to one-third of people in HIV care don't keep an undetectable viral load. To stay undetectable, people with HIV must take HIV medicine every day as prescribed.

- Missing some doses can increase the viral load and the risk of transmitting HIV. People who have trouble taking medicine as prescribed can talk with their healthcare provider about the challenges they are facing and develop a plan to ensure they take their medicine every day. They should also consider using other prevention strategies such as condoms.

- We don't know how often people living with HIV need to have their viral load tested if they are using their undetectable viral load status as their only prevention method. But to stay healthy and protect their partners, they need to visit their provider regularly and get a viral load test as recommended.

- Some people who take HIV medicine daily can get an undetectable viral load very quickly, but it can take some people up to six months. The only way to know if you are undetectable is by getting your viral load tested.

- People taking HIV medicine sometimes have small increases or "blips" in their viral load. These blips usually go back down by the next viral load test. But people who experience blips may benefit from using other prevention strategies (condoms) until their viral load is undetectable again.

- HIV medicine does not protect against other STDs.

- Both partners should learn about all their options for preventing HIV, as well as other STDs, so they can make the decisions that are best for them.

Consider other actions to prevent HIV, like using condoms or a negative partner being on Pre-exposure prophylaxis (PrEP), especially if the person with HIV

- Has trouble regularly taking HIV medicine

- Has an increased viral load, or a load of 200 copies/ml of blood or greater

- Hasn't had a recent test (last six months) that shows the viral load is undetectable

- Missed some doses since the last viral load test, or

- Has stopped taking HIV medicine in the past and may choose to do so again

If I Already Have Human Immunodeficiency Virus, Can I Get Another Kind of Human Immunodeficiency Virus

Yes. This is called "HIV superinfection."

HIV superinfection is when a person with HIV gets infected with another strain of the virus. The new strain of HIV can replace the original strain or remain along with the original strain.

The effects of superinfection differ from person to person. Superinfection may cause some people to get sicker faster because they become infected with a new strain of the virus that is resistant to the medicine (antiretroviral therapy or ART) they are taking to treat their original infection.

Research suggests that a hard-to-treat superinfection is rare. Taking medicine to treat HIV (ART) may reduce someone's chance of getting a superinfection.

Can I Get Human Immunodeficiency Virus from Receiving Medical Care?

Although HIV transmission is possible in healthcare settings, it is extremely rare.

Careful practice of infection control, including universal precautions (using protective practices and personal protective equipment to prevent HIV and other blood-borne infections), protects patients as well as healthcare providers from possible HIV transmission in medical and dental offices and hospitals.

The risk of getting HIV from receiving blood transfusions, blood products, or organ/tissue transplants that are contaminated with HIV is extremely small because of rigorous testing of the U.S. blood supply and donated organs and tissues.

It is important to know that you cannot get HIV from donating blood. Blood collection procedures are highly regulated and safe.

Section 16.5

AIDS and Opportunistic Infections

This section includes text excerpted from "HIV/AIDS—AIDS and Opportunistic Infections," Centers for Disease Control and Prevention (CDC), July 23, 2018.

How Does a Person Get Diagnosed with Acquired Immunodeficiency Syndrome?

When a person with human immunodeficiency virus (HIV) gets certain infections (called "opportunistic infections," or "OIs") or specific cancers, they will get diagnosed with acquired immunodeficiency syndrome (AIDS) (also known as HIV Stage 3), the most serious stage of HIV infection. AIDS is also diagnosed if a person's CD4 cells fall below a certain level.

What Are Opportunistic Infections?

Opportunistic infections (OIs) are infections that occur more frequently and are more severe in people with weakened immune systems, including people with HIV. OIs are less common now than they were in the early days of HIV because better treatments reduce the amount of HIV in a person's body and keep a person's immune system stronger. However, many people with HIV still develop OIs because they may not know they have HIV, they may not be on treatment, or their treatment may not be keeping their HIV levels low enough for their immune system to fight off infections.

For those reasons, it is important for people with HIV to be familiar with the most common OIs so that they can work with their healthcare provider to prevent them or to obtain treatment for them as early as possible.

What Are the Most Common Opportunistic Infections?

Table 16.1. Common Opportunistic Infections

Candidiasis of bronchi, trachea, esophagus, or lungs	This illness is caused by infection with a common (and usually harmless) type of fungus called *"Candida."* Candidiasis, or infection with *Candida*, can affect the skin, nails, and mucous membranes throughout the body. Persons with HIV infection often have trouble with Candida, especially in the mouth and vagina. However, candidiasis is only considered an OI when it infects the esophagus (swallowing tube) or lower respiratory tract, such as the trachea and bronchi (breathing tube), or deeper lung tissue.
Invasive cervical cancer	This is cancer that starts within the cervix, which is the lower part of the uterus at the top of the vagina, and then spreads (becomes invasive) to other parts of the body. This cancer can be prevented by having your care provider perform regular examinations of the cervix
Coccidioidomycosis	This illness is caused by the fungus *Coccidioides immitis*. It most commonly acquired by inhaling fungal spores, which can lead to pneumonia that is sometimes called desert fever, San Joaquin Valley fever, or valley fever. The disease is especially common in hot, dry regions of the southwestern United States, Central America, and South America.
Cryptococcosis	This illness is caused by infection with the fungus *Cryptococcus neoformans*. The fungus typically enters the body through the lungs and can cause pneumonia. It can also spread to the brain, causing swelling of the brain. It can infect any part of the body, but (after the brain and lungs) infections of skin, bones, or urinary tract are most common.
Cryptosporidiosis, chronic intestinal (greater than one month's duration)	This diarrheal disease is caused by the protozoan parasite *Cryptosporidium*. Symptoms include abdominal cramps and severe, chronic, watery diarrhea.
Cytomegalovirus diseases (particularly retinitis) (CMV)	This virus can infect multiple parts of the body and cause pneumonia, gastroenteritis (especially abdominal pain caused by infection of the colon), encephalitis (infection) of the brain, and sight-threatening retinitis (infection of the retina at the back of the eye). People with CMV retinitis have difficulty with the vision that worsens over? time. CMV retinitis is a medical emergency because it can cause blindness if not treated promptly.

Table 16.1. Continued

Encephalopathy, HIV-related	This brain disorder is a result of HIV infection. It can occur as part of acute HIV infection or can result from chronic HIV infection. Its exact cause is unknown but it is thought to be related to infection of the brain with HIV and the resulting inflammation.
Herpes simplex (HSV): chronic ulcer(s) (greater than one month's duration); or bronchitis, pneumonitis, or esophagitis	Herpes simplex virus (HSV) is a very common virus that for most people never causes any major problems. HSV is usually acquired sexually or from an infected mother during birth. In most people with healthy immune systems, HSV is usually latent (inactive). However, stress, trauma, other infections, or suppression of the immune system, (such as by HIV), can reactivate the latent virus and symptoms can return. HSV can cause painful cold sores (sometimes called "fever blisters") in or around the mouth or painful ulcers on or around the genitals or anus. In people with severely damaged immune systems, HSV can also cause infection of the bronchus (breathing tube), pneumonia (infection of the lungs), and esophagitis (infection of the esophagus, or swallowing tube).
Histoplasmosis	This illness is caused by the fungus *Histoplasma capsulatum*. Histoplasma most often infects the lungs and produces symptoms that are similar to those of influenza or pneumonia. People with severely damaged immune systems can get a very serious form of the disease called progressive disseminated histoplasmosis. This form of histoplasmosis can last a long time and involves organs other than the lungs.
Isosporiasis, chronic intestinal (greater than one month's duration)	This infection is caused by the parasite *Isospora belli*, which can enter the body through contaminated food or water. Symptoms include diarrhea, fever, headache, abdominal pain, vomiting, and weight loss.
Kaposi's sarcoma (KS)	This cancer, also known as KS, is caused by a virus called "Kaposi's sarcoma herpesvirus" (KSHV) or "human herpesvirus 8" (HHV-8). KS causes small blood vessels, called "capillaries," to grow abnormally. Because capillaries are located throughout the body, KS can occur anywhere. KS appears as firm pink or purple spots on the skin that can be raised or flat. KS can be life-threatening when it affects organs inside the body, such as the lung, lymph nodes, or intestines.

Table 16.1. Continued

Lymphoma, multiple forms	Lymphoma refers to cancer of the lymph nodes and other lymphoid tissues in the body. There are many different kinds of lymphomas. Some types, such as non-Hodgkin lymphoma and Hodgkin lymphoma, are associated with HIV infection.
Tuberculosis (TB)	Tuberculosis (TB) infection is caused by the bacteria Mycobacterium tuberculosis. TB can be spread through the air when a person with active TB coughs, sneezes, or speaks. Breathing in the bacteria can lead to infection in the lungs. Symptoms of TB in the lungs include cough, tiredness, weight loss, fever, and night sweats. Although the disease usually occurs in the lungs, it may also affect other parts of the body, most often the larynx, lymph nodes, brain, kidneys, or bones.
Mycobacterium avium complex (MAC) or *Mycobacterium kansasii*, disseminated or extrapulmonary. Other Mycobacterium, disseminated or extrapulmonary.	MAC is caused by infection with different types of mycobacterium: *Mycobacterium* avium, *Mycobacterium intracellulare*, or *Mycobacterium kansasii*. These mycobacteria live in our environment, including in soil and dust particles. They rarely cause problems for persons with healthy immune systems. In people with severely damaged immune systems, infections with these bacteria spread throughout the body and can be life-threatening.
Pneumocystis carinii pneumonia (PCP)	This lung infection, also called "PCP," is caused by a fungus, which used to be called *"Pneumocystis carinii,"* but now is named *Pneumocystis jirovecii*. PCP occurs in people with weakened immune systems, including people with HIV. The first signs of infection are difficulty breathing, high fever, and dry cough.
Pneumonia, recurrent	Pneumonia is an infection in one or both of the lungs. Many germs, including bacteria, viruses, and fungi can cause pneumonia, with symptoms such as a cough (with mucous), fever, chills, and trouble breathing. In people with immune systems severely damaged by HIV, one of the most common and life-threatening causes of pneumonia is infection with the bacteria *Streptococcus pneumoniae*, also called "Pneumococcus." There are now effective vaccines that can prevent infection with *Streptococcus pneumoniae* and all persons with HIV infection should be vaccinated.

Table 16.1. Continued

Progressive multifocal leukoencephalopathy	This rare brain and spinal cord disease is caused by the JC (John Cunningham) virus. It is seen almost exclusively in persons whose immune systems have been severely damaged by HIV. Symptoms may include loss of muscle control, paralysis, blindness, speech problems, and an altered mental state. This disease often progresses rapidly and may be fatal.
Salmonella septicemia, recurrent	Salmonella is a kind of bacteria that typically enter the body through ingestion of contaminated food or water. Infection with salmonella (called "salmonellosis") can affect anyone and usually causes a self-limited illness with nausea, vomiting, and diarrhea. Salmonella septicemia is a severe form of infection in which the bacteria circulate through the whole body and exceeds the immune system's ability to control it.
Toxoplasmosis of brain	This infection, often called "toxo," is caused by the parasite *Toxoplasma gondii*. The parasite is carried by warm-blooded animals including cats, rodents, and birds and is excreted by these animals in their feces. Humans can become infected with it by inhaling dust or eating food contaminated with the parasite. Toxoplasma can also occur in commercial meats, especially red meats and pork, but rarely poultry. Infection with toxo can occur in the lungs, retina of the eye, heart, pancreas, liver, colon, testes, and brain. Although cats can transmit toxoplasmosis, litter boxes can be changed safely by wearing gloves and washing hands thoroughly with soap and water afterward. All raw red meats that have not been frozen for at least 24 hours should be cooked through to an internal temperature of at least 150°F.
Wasting syndrome due to HIV	Wasting is defined as the involuntary loss of more than 10 percent of one's body weight while having experienced diarrhea or weakness and fever for more than 30 days. Wasting refers to the loss of muscle mass, although part of the weight loss may also be due to loss of fat.

How Do You Prevent Opportunistic Infections?

The best ways to prevent getting an OI are to get into care and to take HIV medications as prescribed. Sometimes, your healthcare provider will also prescribe medications specifically to prevent certain OIs.

In addition to taking HIV medications to keep your immune system strong, there are other steps you can take to prevent getting an OI:

- Prevent exposure to other sexually transmitted infections.

- Don't share drug injection equipment. Blood with hepatitis C in it can remain in syringes and needles after use and the infection can be transmitted to the next user.

- Get vaccinated—your doctor can tell you what vaccines you need. If this information is not provided to you, ask for it.

- Understand what germs you are exposed to (such as tuberculosis or germs found in the stools, saliva, or on the skin of animals) and limit your exposure to them.

- Don't consume certain foods, including undercooked eggs, unpasteurized (raw) milk and cheeses, unpasteurized fruit juices, or raw seed sprouts.

- Don't drink untreated water, such as water directly from lakes or rivers. Tap water in foreign countries is also often not safe. Use bottled water or water filters.

- Ask your doctor to discuss with you the other things you do at work, at home, and on vacation to make sure you aren't exposed to an OI.

If you develop an OI, there are treatments available, such as antibiotics or antifungal drugs

Section 16.6

Testing for Human Immunodeficiency Virus

This section includes text excerpted from "Testing," Centers for Disease Control and Prevention (CDC), December 6, 2015. Reviewed February 2019.

The only way to know for sure whether you have human immunodeficiency virus (HIV) is to get tested. This section answers some of the most common questions related to HIV testing, including the types of tests available, where to get one, and what to expect when you get tested.

Should I Get Tested for Human Immunodeficiency Virus?

The Centers for Disease Control and Prevention (CDC) recommends that everyone between the ages of 13 and 64 gets tested for HIV at least once as part of routine healthcare. About one in eight people in the United States who have HIV don't know they have it.

People with certain risk factors should get tested more often. If you were HIV-negative the last time you were tested and answer yes to any of the following questions, you should get an HIV test because these things increase your chances of getting HIV:

• Are you a man who has had sex with another man?

• Have you had sex—anal or vaginal—with an HIV-positive partner?

• Have you had more than one sex partner since your last HIV test?

• Have you injected drugs and shared needles or works (for example, water or cotton) with others?

• Have you exchanged sex for drugs or money?

• Have you been diagnosed with or sought treatment for another sexually transmitted disease (STD)?

• Have you been diagnosed with or treated for hepatitis or tuberculosis (TB)?

• Have you had sex with someone who could answer yes to any of the above questions or someone whose sexual history you don't know?

You should be tested at least once a year if you keep doing any of these things. Sexually active gay and bisexual men may benefit from more frequent testing (for example, every three to six months).

If you are pregnant, talk to your healthcare provider about getting tested for HIV and other ways to protect you and your child from getting HIV. Also, anyone who has been sexually assaulted should get an HIV test as soon as possible after the assault and should consider post-exposure prophylaxis (PEP), taking antiretroviral medicines after being potentially exposed to HIV to prevent becoming infected.

Before having sex for the first time with a new partner, you and your partner should talk about your sexual and drug-use history, disclose your HIV status, and consider getting tested for HIV and learning the results.

How Can Testing Help Me?

The only way to know for sure whether you have HIV is to get tested.
Knowing your HIV status gives you powerful information to help you take steps to keep you and your partner healthy.

- If you test positive, you can take medicine to treat HIV to stay healthy for many years and greatly reduce the chance of transmitting HIV to your sex partner.

- If you test negative, you have more prevention tools available today to prevent HIV than ever before.

- If you are pregnant, you should be tested for HIV so that you can begin treatment if you are HIV-positive. If an HIV-positive woman is treated for HIV early in her pregnancy, the risk of transmitting HIV to her baby can be very low.

I Don't Believe I Am at High Risk. Why Should I Get Tested?

Some people who test positive for HIV were not aware of their risk. That's why the CDC recommends that everyone between the ages of 13 and 64 gets tested for HIV at least once as part of routine healthcare.

Even if you are in a monogamous relationship (both you and your partner are having sex only with each other), you should find out for sure whether you or your partner has HIV.

I Am Pregnant. Why Should I Get Tested?

All pregnant women should be tested for HIV so that they can begin treatment if they're HIV-positive. If a woman is treated for HIV early in her pregnancy, the risk of transmitting HIV to her baby can be very low. Testing pregnant women for HIV infection and treating those who are infected have led to a big decline in the number of children infected with HIV from their mothers.

The treatment is most effective for preventing HIV transmission to babies when started as early as possible during pregnancy. However, there are still great health benefits to beginning preventive treatment even during labor or shortly after the baby is born.

What Kinds of Tests Are Available, and How Do They Work?

There are three broad types of tests available: antibody tests, combination or fourth-generation tests, and nucleic acid tests (NAT). HIV tests may be performed on blood, oral fluid, or urine.

1. Most HIV tests, including most rapid tests and home tests, are **antibody tests**. Antibodies are produced by your immune system when you're exposed to viruses like HIV or bacteria. HIV antibody tests look for these antibodies to HIV in your blood or oral fluid. In general, antibody tests that use blood can detect HIV slightly sooner after infection than tests done with oral fluid.

   It can take 3 to 12 weeks (21–84 days) for an HIV-positive person's body to make enough antibodies for an antibody test to detect HIV infection. This is called the " window period." Approximately 97 percent of people will develop detectable antibodies during this window period. If you get a negative HIV antibody test result during the window period, you should be re-tested three months after your possible exposure to HIV.

   • With a **rapid antibody screening test**, results are ready in 30 minutes or less.

   • The **OraQuick HIV Test**, which involves taking an oral swab, provides fast results. You have to swab your mouth for an oral fluid sample and use a kit to test it. Results are available in 20 minutes. The manufacturer provides confidential counseling and referral to follow-up testing sites. Because the level of antibody in oral fluid is lower than it is in blood, blood tests find infection sooner after exposure than oral fluid tests. These tests are available for purchase in stores and online. They may be used at home, or they may be used for testing in some community and clinic testing programs.

   • The **Home Access HIV-1 Test System** is a home collection kit, which involves pricking your finger to collect a blood sample, sending the sample by mail to a licensed laboratory, and then calling in for results as early as the next business day. This test is anonymous. The manufacturer provides confidential counseling and referral to treatment.

If you use any type of antibody test and have a positive result, you will need to take a follow-up test to confirm your results. If your first test is a rapid home test and it's positive, you will be sent to a healthcare provider to get follow-up testing. If your first test is done in a testing lab and it's positive, the lab will conduct the follow-up testing, usually on the same blood sample as the first test.

2. **Combination, or fourth-generation, tests** look for both HIV antibodies and antigens. Antigens are foreign substances that cause your immune system to activate. The antigen is part of the virus itself and is present during acute HIV infection (the phase of infection right after people are infected but before they develop antibodies to HIV). If you're infected with HIV, an antigen called "p24" is produced even before antibodies develop. Combination screening tests are now recommended for testing done in labs and are becoming more common in the United States. There is now a rapid combination test available.

It can take two to six weeks (13 to 42 days) for a person's body to make enough antigens and antibodies for a combination, or fourth-generation, test to detect HIV within the window period. If you get a negative combination test result during the window period, you should be retested three months after your possible exposure.

3. **A nucleic acid test** (NAT) looks for HIV in the blood. It looks for the virus and not the antibodies to the virus. The test can give either a positive/negative result or an actual amount of virus present in the blood (known as a viral load test). This test is very expensive and not routinely used for screening individuals unless they recently had a high-risk exposure or a possible exposure with early symptoms of HIV infection.

It can take 7 to 28 days for a NAT to detect HIV. Nucleic acid testing is usually considered accurate during the early stages of infection. However, it is best to get an antibody or combination test at the same time to help the doctor interpret the negative NAT. This is because a small number of people

185

naturally decrease the amount of virus in their blood over time, which can lead to an inaccurate negative NAT result. Taking pre-exposure prophylaxis (PrEP) or post-exposure prophylaxis (PEP) may also reduce the accuracy of NAT if you have HIV.

Talk to your healthcare provider to see what type of HIV test is right for you. After you get tested, it's important for you to find out the result of your test so that you can talk to your healthcare provider about treatment options if you are HIV-positive. If you are HIV-negative, continue to take actions to prevent HIV, such as using condoms the right way every time you have sex and taking medicines to prevent HIV if you are at high risk.

How Soon after an Exposure to HIV Can an HIV Test Detect If I Am Infected?

No HIV test can detect HIV immediately after infection. If you think you've been exposed to HIV, talk to your healthcare provider as soon as possible.

The window period is the time between when a person gets HIV and when a test can accurately detect it. The window period varies from person to person and also depends upon the type of HIV test.

- Most HIV tests are antibody tests. Antibodies are produced by your immune system when you're exposed to viruses such as HIV or bacteria. HIV antibody tests look for these antibodies to HIV in your blood or oral fluid.

- The soonest an antibody test will detect infection is three weeks. Most (approximately 97%), but not all, people will develop detectable antibodies within 3 to 12 weeks (21 to 84 days) of infection.

- Combination, or fourth-generation, tests look for both HIV antibodies and antigens. Antigens are foreign substances that cause your immune system to activate. The antigen is part of the virus itself and is present during acute HIV infection (the phase of infection right after people are infected but before they develop antibodies to HIV).

- Most, but not all people, will make enough antigens and antibodies for fourth-generation, or combination, tests to accurately detect infection two to six weeks (13 to 42 days) after infection.

• A nucleic-acid test (NAT) looks for HIV in the blood. It looks for the virus and not the antibodies to the virus. This test is expensive and not routinely used for screening individuals unless they recently had a high-risk exposure or a possible exposure with early symptoms of HIV infection.

Most, but not all people, will have enough HIV in their blood for a nucleic acid test to detect infection one to four weeks (7 to 28 days) after infection.

Ask your healthcare provider about the window period for the test you are taking. If you are using a home test, you can get that information from the materials included in the test package. If you get an HIV test within three months after a potential HIV exposure and the result is negative, get tested again in three more months to be sure.

If you learned you were HIV-negative the last time you were tested, you can only be sure you are still negative if you haven't had a potential HIV exposure since your last test. If you are sexually active, continue to take actions to prevent HIV, such as using condoms the right way every time you have sex and taking medicines to prevent HIV if you are at high risk.

Where Can I Get Tested?

You can ask your healthcare provider for an HIV test. Many medical clinics, substance abuse programs, community health centers, and hospitals offer them too. You can also find a testing site near you by

• Calling 800-CDC-INFO (800-232-4636)

• Visiting gettested.cdc.gov, or

• Texting your ZIP code to KNOW IT (566948)

You can also buy a home testing kit at a pharmacy or online.

What Should I Expect When I Go in for an HIV Test?

If you take a test in a healthcare setting, when it's time to take the test, a healthcare provider will take your sample (blood or oral fluid), and you may be able to wait for the results if it's a rapid HIV test. If the test comes back negative, and you haven't had an exposure for three months, you can be confident you're not infected with HIV.

If your HIV test result is positive, you may need to get a follow-up test to be sure you have HIV.

Your healthcare provider or counselor may talk with you about your risk factors, answer questions about your general health, and discuss next steps with you, especially if your result is positive.

What Does a Negative Test Result Mean?

A negative result doesn't necessarily mean that you don't have HIV. That's because of the window period—the time between when a person gets HIV and when a test can accurately detect it. The window period varies from person to person and is also different depending upon the type of HIV test.

Ask your healthcare provider about the window period for the test you are taking. If you are using a home test, you can get that information from the materials included in the test's package. If you get an HIV test within three months after a potential HIV exposure and the result is negative, get tested again in three more months to be sure.

If you learned you were HIV-negative the last time you were tested, you can only be sure you are still negative if you haven't had a potential HIV exposure since your last test. If you're sexually active, continue to take actions to prevent HIV, like using condoms the right way every time you have sex and taking medicines to prevent HIV if you are at high risk.

If I Have a Negative Result, Does That Mean That My Partner Is HIV-Negative Also?

No. Your HIV test result reveals only your HIV status.

HIV is not necessarily transmitted every time you have sex. Therefore, taking an HIV test is not a way to find out if your partner is infected.

It's important to be open with your partners and ask them to tell you their HIV status. But keep in mind that your partners may not know or may be wrong about their status, and some may not tell you if they have HIV even if they know they are infected. Consider getting tested together so you can both know your HIV status and take steps to keep yourselves healthy.

What Does a Positive Result Mean?

A follow-up test will be conducted. If the follow-up test is also positive, it means you are HIV-positive.

If you had a rapid screening test, the testing site will arrange a follow-up test to make sure the screening test result was correct. If your blood was tested in a lab, the lab will conduct a follow-up test on the same sample.

It is important that you start medical care and begin HIV treatment as soon as you are diagnosed with HIV. Anti-retroviral therapy—or ART—taking medicines to treat HIV infection is recommended for all people with HIV, regardless of how long they have had the virus or how healthy they are. It slows the progression of HIV and helps protect your immune system. ART can keep you healthy for many years and greatly reduces your chance of transmitting HIV to sex partners if taken the right way, every day.

If you have health insurance, your insurer is required to cover some medicines used to treat HIV. If you do not have health insurance, or you are unable to afford your co-pay or co-insurance amount, you may be eligible for government programs that can help through Medicaid, Medicare, the Ryan White HIV/AIDS Program, and community-health centers. Your healthcare provider or local public-health department can tell you where to get HIV treatment.

To lower your risk of transmitting HIV,

- Take medicines to treat HIV (antiretroviral therapy or ART) the right way every day.

- Use condoms the right way every time you have sex.

- If your partner is HIV-negative, encourage them to talk to their healthcare provider to see if taking daily medicine to prevent HIV (called pre-exposure prophylaxis, or PrEP) is right for them.

- If you think your partner might have been recently exposed to HIV—for example, if the condom breaks during sex and you aren't virally suppressed—they should talk to a healthcare provider right away (within three days) about taking medicines (called post-exposure prophylaxis, or PEP) to prevent getting HIV.

- Get tested and treated for STDs and encourage your partner to do the same.

Receiving a diagnosis of HIV can be a life-changing event. People can feel many emotions—sadness, hopelessness, and even anger. Allied healthcare providers and social service providers, often available at your healthcare provider's office, will have the tools to help you work through the early stages of your diagnosis and begin to manage your HIV.

Talking to others who have HIV may also be helpful. Find a local HIV support group. Learn about how other people living with HIV have handled their diagnosis.

If I Test Positive for HIV, Does That Mean I Have AIDS?

No. Being HIV-positive does not mean you have AIDS. AIDS is the most advanced stage of HIV disease. HIV can lead to AIDS if not treated.

Will Other People Know My Test Result?

If you take an anonymous test, no one but you will know the result. If you take a confidential test, your test result will be part of your medical record, but it is still protected by state and federal privacy laws.

- **Anonymous testing** means that nothing ties your test results to you. When you take an anonymous HIV test, you get a unique identifier that allows you to get your test results.

- **Confidential testing** means that your name and other identifying information will be attached to your test results. The results will go in your medical record and may be shared with your healthcare providers and your health insurance company. Otherwise, the results are protected by state and federal privacy laws, and they can be released only with your permission.

With confidential testing, if you test positive for HIV, the test result and your name will be reported to the state or local health department to help public health officials get better estimates of the rates of HIV in the state. The state health department will then **remove all personal information** about you (name, address, etc.) and share the remaining non-identifying information with the CDC. The CDC does not share this information with anyone else, including insurance companies.

Should I Share My Positive Test Result with Others?

It's important to share your status with your sex partners. Whether you disclose your status to others is your decision.

Partners

It's important to disclose your HIV status to your sex partners even if you're uncomfortable doing it. Communicating with each other about your HIV status means you can take steps to keep both of you healthy. The more practice you have disclosing your HIV status, the easier it will become.

If you are nervous about disclosing your test result, or you have been threatened or injured by your partner, you can ask your doctor or the local health department to tell them that they might have been exposed to HIV. This is called "partner notification services." Health departments do not reveal your name to your partners. They will only tell your partners that they have been exposed to HIV and should get tested.

Many states have laws that require you to tell your sexual partners if you're HIV-positive before you have sex (anal, vaginal, or oral) or tell your drug-using partners before you share drugs or needles to inject drugs. In some states, you can be charged with a crime if you don't tell your partner your HIV status, even if your partner doesn't become infected.

Family and Friends

In most cases, your family and friends will not know your test results or HIV status unless you tell them yourself. While telling your family that you have HIV may seem hard, you should know that disclosure actually has many benefits—studies have shown that people who disclose their HIV status respond better to treatment than those who don't.

If you are under 18, however, some states allow your healthcare provider to tell your parent(s) that you received services for HIV if they think doing so is in your best interest.

Employers

In most cases, your employer will not know your HIV status unless you tell them. But your employer does have a right to ask if you have any health conditions that would affect your ability to do your job or pose a serious risk to others. (An example might be a healthcare professional, like a surgeon, who does procedures where there is a risk of blood or other body fluids being exchanged.)

If you have health insurance through your employer, the insurance company cannot legally tell your employer that you have HIV. But it is possible that your employer could find out if the insurance company provides detailed information to your employer about the benefits it pays or the costs of insurance.

Who Will Pay for My HIV Test?

HIV screening is covered by health insurance without a co-pay, as required by the Affordable Care Act. If you do not have medical insurance, some testing sites may offer free tests.

Who Will Pay for My Treatment If I Am HIV-Positive?

If you have health insurance, your insurer is required to cover some medicines used to treat HIV. If you don't have health insurance, or you're unable to afford your co-pay or co-insurance amount, you may be eligible for government programs that can help through Medicaid, Medicare, the Ryan White HIV/AIDS Program, and community health centers. Your healthcare provider or local public health department can tell you where to get HIV treatment.

Section 16.7

Living with Human Immunodeficiency Virus

This section includes text excerpted from "Living with HIV," Centers for Disease Control and Prevention (CDC), February 23, 2016.

An estimated 1.2 million people are living with HIV in the United States. Thanks to better treatments, people with HIV are now living longer—and with a better quality of life—than ever before. If you are living with HIV, it's important to make choices that keep you healthy and protect others.

Stay Healthy

You should start medical care and begin HIV treatment as soon as you are diagnosed with HIV. Taking medicine to treat HIV, called antiretroviral therapy or ART, is recommended for all people with HIV. Taking medicine to treat HIV slows the progression of HIV and helps protect your immune system. The medicine can keep you healthy for many years and greatly reduces your chance of transmitting HIV to sex partners if taken the right way, every day.

If you are taking medicine to treat HIV, visit your healthcare provider regularly and always take your medicine as directed to keep your viral load (the amount of HIV in the blood and elsewhere in the body) as low as possible.

Do Tell

It is important to disclose your HIV status to your sex and needle-sharing partners even if you are uncomfortable doing it. Communicating with each other about your HIV status allows you and your partner to take steps to keep both of you healthy.

Also, ask your health department about free partner notification services. Health-department staff can help find your sex or needle-sharing partners to let them know they may have been exposed to HIV and provide them with testing, counseling, and referrals for other services. These partner-notification services will not reveal your name unless you want to work with them to tell your partners.

Many states have laws that require you to tell your sexual partners if you are HIV-positive before you have sex (anal, vaginal, or oral) or tell your needle-sharing partners before you share drugs or needles to inject drugs. In some states, you can be charged with a crime if you don't tell your partner your HIV status, even if your partner does not become infected.

Get Support

Receiving a diagnosis of HIV can be a life-changing event. People can feel many emotions—sadness, hopelessness, and even anger. Allied healthcare providers and social-service providers, often available at your healthcare provider's office, will have the tools to help you work through the early stages of your diagnosis and begin to manage your HIV.

Talking to others who have HIV may also be helpful.

Reduce the Risk to Others

HIV is spread through certain body fluids from an HIV-infected person: blood, semen (cum), preseminal fluid (precum), rectal fluids, vaginal fluids, and breast milk. In the United States, HIV is most often transmitted by having anal or vaginal sex with someone who has HIV without using a condom or taking medicines to prevent or treat HIV. In addition, a mother can pass HIV to her baby during pregnancy, during labor, through breastfeeding, or by prechewing her baby's food.

The higher your viral load, the more likely you are to transmit HIV to others. When your viral load is very low (called "viral suppression," with less than 200 copies per milliliter of blood) or undetectable (about 40 copies per milliliter of blood), your chance of transmitting HIV is greatly reduced. However, this is true only if you can stay virally suppressed. One thing that can increase viral load is not taking HIV medicines the right way, every day.

You can also protect your partners by getting tested and treated for other STDs. If you have both HIV and some other STD with sores, like syphilis, your risk of transmitting HIV can be about three times as high as if you did not have any STD with sores.

Taking other actions, like using a condom the right way every time you have sex or having your partners take daily medicine to prevent HIV (called pre-exposure prophylaxis or PrEP) can lower your chances of transmitting HIV even more.

Section 16.8

The Affordable Care Act and People Living with Human Immunodeficiency Virus and Acquired Immunodeficiency Syndrome

This section includes text excerpted from "The Affordable Care Act and HIV/AIDS," U.S. Department of Health and Human Services (HHS), February 4, 2016.

Improving Access to Instant Coverage

The Affordable Care Act (ACA) provides Americans—including those at risk for and living with human immunodeficiency virus (HIV) and acquired immunodeficiency syndrome (AIDS)—better access to healthcare coverage and more health-insurance options.

Coverage for people with preexisting conditions. Thanks to the ACA, no American can ever again be dropped or denied coverage because of a preexisting health condition, such as asthma, cancer, or HIV. Insurers also are prohibited from canceling or rescinding coverage because of mistakes made on an application, and can no longer impose lifetime caps on insurance benefits. These changes are significant because, prior to the ACA, many people living with HIV or other chronic health conditions experienced obstacles in getting health coverage, were dropped from coverage or avoided seeking coverage for fear of being denied. Now they can get covered and get the care they need. The Ryan White Affordable Care Enrollment (ACE) Technical Assistance Center provides tools and resources to support the enrollment of people living with HIV in healthcare coverage.

Broader Medicaid eligibility. Under the ACA, states have the option, which is fully federally funded for the first three years, to expand Medicaid to generally include those with incomes at or below 138 percent of the Federal poverty line, including single adults without children who were previously not generally eligible for Medicaid. Medicaid is the largest payer for HIV care in the United States, and the expansion of Medicaid to low-income childless adults is particularly important for many gay, bisexual, and other men who have sex with men (MSM) who were previously ineligible for Medicaid, and yet remain the population most affected by the HIV epidemic. Further, in states that opt for Medicaid expansion, people living with HIV who meet the income threshold will no longer have to wait for an AIDS diagnosis in order to become eligible for Medicaid. That means they can enroll in life-extending care and treatment before the disease has significantly damaged their immune system.

More affordable coverage. The ACA requires most Americans to have qualifying health insurance. To help people access quality, affordable coverage, the ACA created Health Insurance Marketplaces (sometimes called "exchanges") in every state that helps consumers compare different health plans and determine what savings they may qualify for. The ACA also provides financial assistance for people with low and middle incomes in the form of tax credits that lower the cost of their monthly premiums and lower their out-of-pocket costs. These tax credits depend on a family's household size and income.

Lower prescription drug costs for Medicare recipients. In the past, as many as one in four seniors went without a prescription every year because they could not afford it. The ACA closes, over time, the Medicare Part D prescription drug benefit "donut hole," giving Medicare enrollees living with HIV and AIDS the peace of mind that they will be better able to afford their medications. Beneficiaries receive a 50 percent discount on covered brand-name drugs while they are in the "donut hole," considerable savings for people taking costly HIV/AIDS drugs. And in the years to come, they can expect additional savings on their prescription drugs while they are in the coverage gap until it is closed in 2020. In addition, as a result of the healthcare law, AIDS Drug Assistance Program (ADAP) benefits are now considered as contributions toward Medicare Part D's True Out of Pocket Spending Limit ("TrOOP"). This is a huge relief for ADAP clients who are Medicare Part D enrollees since they will now be able to move through the donut hole more quickly, which was difficult, if not impossible, for ADAP clients to do before this change.

Ensuring Quality Coverage

The Affordable Care Act also helps all Americans, including those at risk for or living with HIV, have access to the best quality coverage and care. This includes:

- **Preventive services.** Under the ACA, most new health insurance plans must cover certain recommended preventive services—including HIV testing for everyone ages 15 to 65, and for people of other ages at increased risk—without additional cost-sharing, such as copays or deductibles. Since one in eight people living with HIV in the United States are unaware of their infection, improving access to HIV testing will help more people learn their status so they can be connected to care and treatment.

- **Comprehensive coverage.** The law establishes a minimum set of benefits (called "essential health benefits") that must be covered under health plans offered in the individual and small group markets, both inside and outside of the Health Insurance Marketplace. These include many health services that are important for people living with HIV/AIDS, including prescription drug services, hospital inpatient care, lab tests, services, and devices to help you manage a chronic disease, and mental-health and substance-use disorder services.

- **Coordinated care for those with chronic health conditions.** The law recognizes the value of patient-centered medical homes as an effective way to strengthen the quality of care, especially for people with complex chronic conditions such as HIV/AIDS. The patient-centered medical home model of care can foster greater patient retention and higher quality HIV care because of its focus on treating the many needs of the patient at once and better coordination across medical specialties and support services. The Ryan White HIV/AIDS Program has been a pioneer in the development of this model in the HIV healthcare system. The ACA also authorized an optional Medicaid State Plan benefit for states to establish Health Homes to coordinate care for Medicaid beneficiaries with certain chronic health conditions. HIV/AIDS is one of the chronic health conditions that states may request approval to cover.

- **Enhancing the capacity of the healthcare delivery system.** The ACA expands the capacity of the healthcare delivery system to better serve all Americans, including those at risk for and living with HIV/AIDS.

- **Expansion of community health centers.** The ACA has made a major investment in expanding the network of community-health centers that provide preventive and primary-care services to more than 20 million Americans every year. These health centers are important partners in implementing the National HIV/AIDS Strategy and expand the opportunities for integrating HIV testing, prevention, care, and treatment services into primary care.

- **Delivering culturally competent care.** The ACA expands initiatives to strengthen cultural-competency training for all healthcare providers and ensure all populations are treated equally. It also bolsters the federal commitment to reducing health disparities. One effort underway to expand the capacity of health centers to deliver culturally competent care to populations heavily impacted by HIV is the National LGBT Health Education Center, funded by HRSA. This center helps healthcare organizations better address the needs of lesbian, gay, bisexual, and transgender individuals, including needs for HIV prevention, testing, and treatment.

- **Increasing the healthcare workforce for underserved communities.** Thanks to the ACA, the National Health Service Corps is providing loans and scholarships to more doctors, nurses, and other healthcare providers. This critical healthcare workforce expansion better serves vulnerable populations. This is in line with a key recommendation of the National HIV/ AIDS Strategy to increase the number and diversity of available providers of clinical care and related services for people living with HIV, many of whom live in underserved communities.

Chapter 17

Human Papillomavirus

Chapter Contents

Section 17.1

What is Human Papillomaviruses?

This section includes text excerpted from "HPV and
Cancer," National Cancer Institute (NCI), February 19, 2015,
Reviewed February 2019.

Human papillomaviruses (HPVs) are a group of more than 200
related viruses. More than 40 HPV types can be easily spread through
direct sexual contact, from the skin and mucous membranes of
infected people to the skin and mucous membranes of their partners. They can be spread by vaginal, anal, and oral sex. Other HPV
types are responsible for nongenital warts, which are not sexually
transmitted.

Sexually transmitted HPV types fall into two categories:

- **Low-risk HPVs,** which do not cause cancer but can
  cause skin warts (technically known as "condylomata
  acuminata") on or around the genitals and anus. For
  example, HPV types 6 and 11 cause 90 percent of all genital
  warts. HPV types 6 and 11 also cause recurrent respiratory
  papillomatosis, a less common disease in which benign tumors
  grow in the air passages leading from the nose and mouth into
  the lungs.

- **High-risk HPVs,** which can cause cancer. About a dozen
  high-risk HPV types have been identified. Two of these, HPV
  types 16 and 18, are responsible for most HPV-caused cancers.

HPV infections are the most common sexually transmitted infections in the United States. About 14 million new genital HPV infections occur each year. In fact, the Centers for Disease Control and
Prevention (CDC) estimates that more than 90 percent and 80 percent,
respectively, of sexually active men and women, will be infected with
at least one type of HPV at some point in their lives.

Most high-risk HPV infections occur without any symptoms, go
away within one to two years, and do not cause cancer. Some HPV
infections, however, can persist for many years. Persistent infections
with high-risk HPV types can lead to cell changes that, if untreated,
may progress to cancer.

How Does High-Risk Human Papillomavirus Cause Cancer?

HPV infects epithelial cells. These cells, which are organized in layers, cover the inside and outside surfaces of the body, including the skin, the throat, the genital tract, and the anus.

Once HPV enters an epithelial cell, the virus begins to make the proteins it encodes. Two of the proteins made by high-risk HPVs (E6 and E7) interfere with cell functions that normally prevent excessive growth, helping the cell to grow in an uncontrolled manner and to avoid cell death.

Many times these infected cells are recognized by the immune system and eliminated. Sometimes, however, these infected cells are not destroyed, and a persistent infection results. As the persistently infected cells continue to grow, they may develop mutations in cellular genes that promote even more abnormal cell growth, leading to the formation of an area of precancerous cells and, ultimately, a cancerous tumor.

Other factors may increase the risk that an infection with a high-risk HPV type will persist and possibly develop into cancer. These include:

- Smoking or chewing tobacco (for increased risk of oropharyngeal cancer)

- Having a weakened immune system

- Having many children (for increased risk of cervical cancer)

- Long-term oral contraceptive use (for increased risk of cervical cancer)

- Poor oral hygiene (for increased risk of oropharyngeal cancer)

- Chronic inflammation

Researchers believe that it can take between 10 and 30 years from the time of an initial HPV infection until a tumor forms. However, even when severely abnormal cells are seen on the cervix (a condition called "cervical intraepithelial neoplasia 3," or "CIN3"), these do not always lead to cancer. The percentage of CIN3 lesions that progress to invasive cervical cancer has been estimated to be 50 percent or less.

Which Cancers Are Caused by Human Papillomavirus?

High-risk HPVs cause several types of cancer.

- **Cervical cancer:** Virtually all cases of cervical cancer are caused by HPV, and just two HPV types, 16 and 18, are responsible for about 70 percent of all cases.

- **Anal cancer:** About 95 percent of anal cancers are caused by HPV. Most of these are caused by HPV type 16.

- **Oropharyngeal cancers (cancers of the middle part of the throat, including the soft palate, the base of the tongue, and the tonsils):** About 70 percent of oropharyngeal cancers are caused by HPV. In the United States, more than half of cancers diagnosed in the oropharynx are linked to HPV type 16.

- **Rarer cancers:** HPV causes about 65 percent of vaginal cancers, 50 percent of vulvar cancers, and 35 percent of penile cancers. Most of these are caused by HPV type 16.

How Is Human Papillomavirus Transmitted?

Anyone who has ever been sexually active (that is, engaged in skin-to-skin sexual conduct, including vaginal, anal, or oral sex) can get HPV. HPV is easily passed between partners through sexual contact. HPV infections are more likely in those who have many sex partners or have sex with someone who has had many partners. Because the infection is so common, most people get HPV infections shortly after becoming sexually active for the first time. A person who has had only one partner can get HPV.

Someone can have an HPV infection even if they have no symptoms and their only sexual contact with an HPV-infected person happened many years ago.

Can Human Papillomavirus Vaccines Prevent Human Papillomavirus Infection?

People who are not sexually active almost never develop genital HPV infections. In addition, HPV vaccination before sexual activity can reduce the risk of infection by the HPV types targeted by the vaccine.

The U.S. Food and Drug Administration (FDA) has approved three vaccines to prevent HPV infection: Gardasil®, Gardasil® 9, and Cervarix®. These vaccines provide strong protection against new HPV infections, but they are not effective at treating established HPV infections or disease caused by HPV.

Correct and consistent condom use is associated with reduced HPV transmission between sexual partners, but less frequent condom use is not. However, because areas not covered by a condom can be infected by the virus, condoms are unlikely to provide complete protection against the infection.

What Is Pap and Human Papillomavirus Testing?

HPV infections can be detected by testing a sample of cells to see if they contain viral deoxyribonucleic acid (DNA) or ribonucleic acid (RNA).

Several HPV tests are currently approved by the FDA for three cervical screening indications: for follow-up testing of women who seem to have abnormal Pap test results, for cervical-cancer screening in combination with a papanicolaou test (Pap) among women over age 30, and for use alone as a first-line primary cervical-cancer screening test for women ages 25 and older.

The most common HPV test detects DNA from several high-risk HPV types in a group, but it cannot identify the specific type(s) that are present. Other tests do tell in addition whether there is DNA or RNA from HPV types 16 and 18, the two types that cause most HPV-associated cancers. These tests can detect HPV infections before abnormal cell changes are evident, and before any treatment for cell changes are needed.

There are no FDA-approved tests to detect HPV infections in men. There are also no currently recommended screening methods similar to a Pap test for detecting cell changes caused by HPV infection in anal, vulvar, vaginal, penile, or oropharyngeal tissues. However, this is an area of ongoing research.

What Are Treatment Options for Human Papillomavirus?

There is currently no medical treatment for persistent HPV infections that are not associated with abnormal cell changes. However, genital warts, benign respiratory-tract tumors, precancerous changes at the cervix, and cancers resulting from HPV infections can be treated.

Methods commonly used to treat precancerous cervical changes include cryosurgery (freezing that destroys tissue), loop electrosurgical excision procedure (LEEP), or the removal of cervical tissue using a hot wire loop), surgical conization (surgery with a scalpel, a laser, or both to remove a cone-shaped piece of tissue from the cervix and cervical canal), and laser vaporization conization (use of a laser to destroy cervical tissue).

Treatments for other types of benign respiratory-tract tumors and precancerous changes caused by HPV (vaginal, vulvar, penile, and anal lesions) and genital warts include topical chemicals or drugs, excisional surgery, cryosurgery, electrosurgery, and laser surgery. Treatment approaches are being tested in clinical trials, including a randomized controlled trial that will determine whether treating anal precancerous lesions will reduce the risk of anal cancer in people who are infected with HIV.

HPV-infected individuals who develop cancer generally receive the same treatment as patients whose tumors do not harbor HPV infections, according to the type and stage of their tumors. However, people who are diagnosed with HPV-positive oropharyngeal cancer may be treated differently than people with oropharyngeal cancers that are HPV-negative. Research has shown that patients with HPV-positive oropharyngeal tumors have a better prognosis and may do just as well on less intense treatment. Ongoing clinical trials are investigating this question.

Section 17.2

Recurrent Respiratory Papillomatosis and Human Papillomaviruses

This section includes text excerpted from "Recurrent Respiratory Papillomatosis or Laryngeal Papillomatosis," National Institute on Deafness and Other Communication Disorders (NIDCD), November 28, 2017.

What Is Recurrent Respiratory Papillomatosis?

Recurrent respiratory papillomatosis (RRP) is a disease in which benign (noncancerous) tumors called papillomas grow in the air passages leading from the nose and mouth into the lungs (respiratory tract). Although the tumors can grow anywhere in the respiratory tract, they most commonly grow in the larynx (voice box)—a condition called "laryngeal papillomatosis." The papillomas may vary in size and grow very quickly. They often grow back after they have been removed.

What Causes Recurrent Respiratory Papillomatosis

RRP is caused by two types of human papillomavirus (HPV): HPV 6 and HPV 11. There are more than 150 types of HPV, and they do not have all the same symptoms.

Most people who encounter HPV never develop a related illness. However, in a small number of people exposed to the HPV 6 or 11 virus, respiratory-tract papillomas and genital warts can form. Although scientists do not fully understand why some people develop the disease and others do not, the virus is thought to be spread through sexual contact or when a mother with genital warts passes the HPV 6 or 11 virus to her baby during childbirth.

Who Is Affected by Recurrent Respiratory Papillomatosis?

RRP may occur in adults (adult-onset RRP) as well as in infants and small children (juvenile-onset RRP) who may have contracted the virus during childbirth. The RRP Foundation estimates that there are roughly 20,000 active cases in the United States. According to the Centers for Disease Control and Prevention (CDC), estimates of the incidence for juvenile-onset RRP are imprecise, but range from two or fewer cases per 100,000 children under age 18. Even less is known about the incidence of the adult form of RRP. Estimates of the incidence for adult-onset RPP range between two to three cases per 100,000 adults in the United States.

What Are the Symptoms of Recurrent Respiratory Papillomatosis?

Normally, the human voice is produced when air from the lungs is pushed through two side-by-side specialized muscles—called "vocal folds"—with enough pressure to cause them to vibrate. Hoarseness, the most common RRP symptom, is caused when RRP papillomas interfere with the normal vibrations of the vocal folds. Eventually, RRP tumors may block the airway passage and cause difficulty breathing.

RRP symptoms tend to be more severe in children than in adults. Because the tumors grow quickly, young children with the disease may

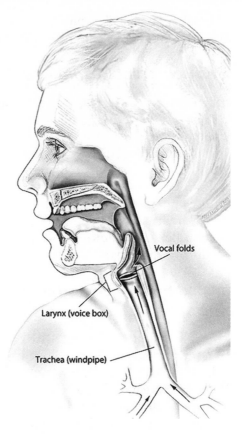

Vocal folds

Larynx (voice box)

Trachea (windpipe)

Figure 17.1. *Parts of the Respiratory Tract Affected by Recurrent Respiratory Papillomatosis*

find it difficult to breathe when sleeping, or they may have difficulty swallowing. Some children experience some relief or remission of the disease when they begin puberty. Both children and adults may experience hoarseness, chronic coughing, or breathing problems. Because of the similarity of the symptoms, RRP is sometimes misdiagnosed as asthma or chronic bronchitis.

How Is Recurrent Respiratory Papillomatosis Diagnosed?

Health professionals use two routine tests for RRP: indirect and direct laryngoscopy. In an indirect laryngoscopy, an otolaryngologist—a doctor who specializes in diseases of the ear, nose, throat, head, and neck—or speech-language pathologist will typically insert a fiber optic telescope, called an "endoscope," into a patient's nose or mouth and then view the larynx on a monitor. Some medical professionals use a video camera attached to this endoscope to view and record the exam. An older, less common method is for the otolaryngologist to place a small mirror in the back of the throat and angle the mirror down toward the larynx to inspect it for papillomas.

A direct laryngoscopy is conducted in the operating room with the use of general anesthesia. This method allows the otolaryngologist to view the vocal folds and other parts of the larynx under high magnification. This procedure is usually used to minimize discomfort, especially with children, or to enable the doctor to biopsy tissue samples from the larynx or other parts of the throat to obtain a diagnosis of RRP.

How Is Recurrent Respiratory Papillomatosis Prevented or Treated?

Vaccination with the HPV vaccine could prevent the development of RRP. The CDC currently recommends that all children receive the HPV vaccine at age 11 or 12. Ask your child's doctor whether the type of HPV vaccine your child will receive will protect against HPV 6 and 11. As more young people receive the vaccine, future research will reveal its effectiveness in preventing HPV-associated diseases such as RRP.

Once RRP develops, there is currently no cure. Surgery is the primary method for removing tumors from the larynx or airway. Because traditional surgery can cause problems due to scarring of the larynx tissue, many surgeons now use laser surgery. Carbon dioxide (CO_2) or potassium titanyl phosphate (KTP) lasers are frequently used for this purpose. Surgeons also commonly use a device called a "microdebrider," which uses suction to hold the tumor in place while a small internal rotary blade removes the growth.

Once the tumors have been removed, they can still return. It is common for patients to require multiple surgeries. With some patients, surgery may be required every few weeks in order to keep the breathing passage open, while others may require surgery only once a year or even less frequently.

In the most extreme cases of aggressive tumor growth, a tracheotomy may be performed. A tracheotomy is a surgical procedure in which an incision is made in the front of the patient's neck and a breathing tube (trach tube) is inserted through an opening, called a stoma, into infection. Having HPV does not mean that a person or his/her partner is having sex outside the relationship.

- Most persons who acquire HPV clear the infection spontaneously and have no associated health problems. When the HPV infection does not clear, genital warts, precancers, and cancers of the cervix, anus, penis, vulva, vagina, head, and neck might develop.

- The types of HPV that cause genital warts are different from the types that can cause cancer.

- Many types of HPV are sexually transmitted through anogenital contact, mainly during vaginal and anal sex. HPV also might be transmitted during genital-to-genital contact without penetration and oral sex. In rare cases, a pregnant woman can transmit HPV to an infant during delivery.

- Having HPV does not make it harder for a woman to get pregnant or carry a pregnancy to term. However, some of the precancers or cancers that HPV can cause, and the treatments needed to treat them, might lower a woman's ability to get pregnant or have an uncomplicated delivery. Treatments are available for the conditions caused by HPV, but not for the virus itself.

- No HPV test can determine which HPV infection will clear and which will progress. However, in certain circumstances, HPV tests can determine whether a woman is at increased risk for cervical cancer. These tests are not for detecting other HPV-related problems, nor are they useful in women less than 25 years of age or men of any age.

and oropharynx. It also protects against the HPV types that cause most genital warts. The HPV vaccine is highly effective in preventing the targeted HPV types, as well as the most common health problems caused by them.

The vaccine is less effective in preventing HPV-related disease in young women who have already been exposed to one or more HPV types. That is because the vaccine prevents HPV before a person is exposed to it. The HPV vaccine does not treat existing HPV infections or HPV-associated diseases.

How Long Does Vaccine Protection Last?

Research suggests that vaccine protection is long-lasting. Current studies have followed vaccinated individuals for ten years, and show that there is no evidence of weakened protection over time.

What Does the Vaccine Not Protect Against?

The vaccine does not protect against all HPV types—so it will not prevent all cases of cervical cancer. Since some cervical cancers will not be prevented by the vaccine, it will be important for women to continue getting screened for cervical cancer. Also, the vaccine does not prevent other sexually transmitted infections (STIs). So it will still be important for sexually active persons to lower their risk for other STIs.

How Safe Is the Human Papillomavirus Vaccine?

The HPV vaccine has been licensed by the U.S. Food and Drug Administration (FDA). The CDC has approved this vaccine as safe and effective. The vaccine was studied in thousands of people around the world, and these studies showed no serious safety concerns. Side effects reported in these studies were mild, including pain where the shot was given, fever, dizziness, and nausea. Vaccine safety continues to be monitored by the CDC and the FDA. More than 60 million doses of HPV vaccine have been distributed in the United States as of March 2014.

Fainting, which can occur after any medical procedure, has also been noted after HPV vaccination. Fainting after any vaccination is more common in adolescents. Because fainting can cause falls and injuries, adolescents and adults should be seated or lying down during HPV vaccination. Sitting or lying down for about 15 minutes after a vaccination can help prevent fainting and injuries.

Why Is the Human Papillomavirus Vaccination Only Recommended for Women through Age 26?

The HPV vaccination is not currently recommended for women older than 26 years. Clinical trials showed that, overall, the HPV vaccination offered women limited or no protection against HPV-related diseases. For women over 26, the best way to prevent cervical cancer is to get routine cervical-cancer screening, as recommended.

What Vaccinated Girls and Women Need to Know: If Vaccinated, Will They Still Need Cervical-Cancer Screening?

Yes, vaccinated women will still need regular cervical-cancer screening because the vaccine protects against most but not all HPV types that cause cervical cancer. Also, women who got the vaccine after becoming sexually active may not get the full benefit of the vaccine if they had already been exposed to HPV.

What about Vaccinating Boys and Men

The HPV vaccine is licensed for use with boys and men. It has been found to be safe and effective for males 9 to 26 years. The Advisory Committee on Immunization Practices (ACIP) recommends routine vaccination of boys aged 11 or 12 years with a series of doses. The vaccination series can be started beginning at 9 years. The vaccination is recommended for males aged 13 through 21 years who have not already been vaccinated or who have not received all recommended doses. The vaccine is most effective when given at younger ages; males aged 22 through 26 years may be vaccinated. The CDC recommends 11- to 12-year-olds get two doses of HPV vaccine to protect against cancers caused by HPV.

Is the Human Papillomavirus Vaccination Covered by Insurance Plans?

Health insurance plans cover the cost of the HPV vaccines. If you don't have insurance, the Vaccines for Children (VFC) program may be able to help.

How Can I Get Help Paying for the Human Papillomavirus Vaccination Vaccine?

The Vaccines for Children (VFC) program helps families of eligible children who might not otherwise have access to vaccines. The program provides vaccines at no cost to doctors who serve eligible children. Children younger than 19 are eligible for VFC vaccines if they are Medicaid-eligible, American Indian, or an Alaska Native, or have no health insurance. "Underinsured" children who have health insurance that does not cover the vaccination can receive VFC vaccines through Federally Qualified Health Centers or Rural Health Centers. Parents of uninsured or underinsured children who receive vaccines at no cost through the VFC Program should check with their healthcare providers about possible administration fees that might apply. These fees help providers cover the costs that result from important services such as storing the vaccines and paying staff members to give vaccines to patients. However, VFC vaccines cannot be denied to an eligible child if a family cannot afford the fee.

Chapter 18

Lymphogranuloma Venereum

Lymphogranuloma venereum (LGV) is caused by *C. trachomatis* serovars L1, L2, or L3. The most common clinical manifestation of LGV among heterosexuals is tender inguinal and/or femoral lymph-adenopathy that is typically unilateral. A self-limited genital ulcer, or papule, sometimes occurs at the site of inoculation. However, by the time patients seek care, the lesions have often disappeared.

Rectal exposure in women or men who have sex with men (MSM) can result in proctocolitis mimicking inflammatory bowel disease, and clinical findings may include mucoid and/or hemorrhagic rectal discharge, anal pain, constipation, fever, and/or tenesmus. Outbreaks of LGV proctocolitis have been reported among MSM.

LGV can be an invasive, systemic infection, and if it is not treated early, LGV proctocolitis can lead to chronic colorectal fistulas and strictures; reactive arthropathy has also been reported. However, reports indicate that rectal LGV can be asymptomatic. Persons with genital and colorectal LGV lesions can also develop a secondary bacterial infection or can be coinfected with other sexually and nonsexually transmitted pathogens.

This chapter includes text excerpted from "Lymphogranuloma Venereum (LGV)," Centers for Disease Control and Prevention (CDC), June 4, 2015. Reviewed February 2019.

Diagnostic Considerations

Diagnosis is based on clinical suspicion, epidemiologic information, and the exclusion of other etiologies for proctocolitis, inguinal lymphadenopathy, or genital or rectal ulcers. Genital lesions, rectal specimens, and lymph-node specimens (i.e., lesion swab or bubo aspirate) can be tested for *C. trachomatis* by culture, direct immunofluorescence, or nucleic-acid detection.

Nucleic-acid amplification tests (NAATs) for *C. trachomatis* perform well on rectal specimens but are not U.S. Food and Drug Administration (FDA) cleared for this purpose. MSM presenting with proctocolitis should be tested for chlamydia; NAAT performed on rectal specimens is the preferred approach to testing.

Additional molecular procedures (e.g., polymerase chain reaction (PCR)-based genotyping) can be used to differentiate LGV from non-LGV *C. trachomatis* in rectal specimens. However, they are not widely available, and results are not available in a timeframe that would influence clinical management.

Treatment

At the time of the initial visit (before diagnostic tests for chlamydia are available), persons with a clinical syndrome consistent with LGV, including proctocolitis or genital-ulcer disease with lymphadenopathy, should be presumptively treated for LGV. As required by state law, these cases should be reported to the state health department.

Treatment cures the infection and prevents ongoing tissue damage, although tissue reaction to the infection can result in scarring. Buboes might require aspiration through intact skin or incision and drainage to prevent the formation of inguinal/femoral ulcerations.

Recommended Regimen

- Doxycycline 100 mg orally twice a day for 21 days

Alternative Regimen

- Erythromycin base 500 mg orally four times a day for 21 days

Although clinical data are lacking, azithromycin 1 g orally once weekly for three weeks is probably effective based on its chlamydial antimicrobial activity. Fluoroquinolone-based treatments also might be effective, but the optimal duration of treatment has not been evaluated.

Follow-Up

Patients should be followed clinically until signs and symptoms resolve.

Management of Sex Partners

Persons who have had sexual contact with a patient who has LGV 60 days before onset of the patient's symptoms should be examined and tested for urethral, cervical, or rectal chlamydial infection, depending on anatomic site of exposure. They should be presumptively treated with a chlamydia regimen (azithromycin 1 g orally single dose or doxycycline 100 mg orally twice a day for seven days).

Special Considerations
Pregnancy

Pregnant and lactating women should be treated with erythromycin. Doxycycline should be avoided in the second and third trimester of pregnancy because of risk for discoloration of teeth and bones, but is compatible with breastfeeding. Azithromycin might prove useful for the treatment of LGV in pregnancy, but no published data are available regarding an effective dose and duration of treatment.

Human Immunodeficiency Virus Infection

Persons with both LGV and HIV infection should receive the same regimens as those who are HIV negative. Prolonged therapy might be required, and delay in resolution of symptoms might occur.

Chapter 19

Syphilis

Syphilis is a sexually transmitted disease (STD) that can have very serious complications when left untreated, but it is simple to cure with the right treatment.

What Is Syphilis?

Syphilis is a sexually transmitted infection (STI) that can cause serious health problems if it is not treated.

How Is Syphilis Spread?

You contract syphilis by direct contact with a syphilis sore during vaginal, anal, or oral sex. The sores are on or around the penis, vagina, anus, or in the rectum, on the lips, or in the mouth. Syphilis can spread from an infected mother to her unborn baby.

What Does Syphilis Look Like?

Syphilis is divided into four stages (primary, secondary, latent, and tertiary), with different signs and symptoms associated with each stage.

- A person with primary syphilis generally has a sore or sores at the original site of infection. These sores usually occur on or

This chapter contains text excerpted from "Syphilis—CDC Fact Sheet," Centers for Disease Control and Prevention (CDC), January 8, 2017.

around the genitals, around the anus, or in the rectum, or in or around the mouth. These sores are usually (but not always) firm, round, and painless.

- Symptoms of secondary syphilis include skin rash, swollen lymph nodes, and fever. The signs and symptoms of primary and secondary syphilis can be mild, and they might not be noticed.

- During the latent stage, there are no signs or symptoms.

- Tertiary syphilis is associated with severe medical problems. A doctor can usually diagnose tertiary syphilis with the help of multiple tests. It can affect the heart, brain, and other organs of the body.

How Can I Reduce My Risk of Getting Syphilis?

The only way to avoid sexually transmitted diseases (STDs) is to not have vaginal, anal, or oral sex.

If you are sexually active, you can do the following things to lower your chances of getting syphilis:

- Be in a long-term mutually monogamous relationship with a partner who has been tested for syphilis and does not have it.

- Use latex condoms or dental dams the right way every time you have sex. Condoms prevent transmission of syphilis by preventing contact with a sore. Sometimes sores occur in areas not covered by a condom or dental dam. Contact with these sores can still transmit syphilis.

Am I at Risk for Syphilis?

Any sexually active person can get syphilis through unprotected vaginal, anal, or oral sex. Have an honest and open talk with your healthcare provider and ask whether you should be tested for syphilis or other STDs.

- All pregnant women should be tested for syphilis at their first prenatal visit.

- You should get tested regularly for syphilis if you are sexually active and

  - Are a man who has sex with men

  - Are living with human immunodeficiency virus (HIV)

  - Or have partner(s) who have tested positive for syphilis

I'm Pregnant. How Does Syphilis Affect My Baby?

If you are pregnant and have syphilis, you can give the infection to your unborn baby. Having syphilis can lead to a low birth weight baby. It can also make it more likely you will deliver your baby too early or stillborn (a baby born dead). To protect your baby, you should be tested for syphilis at least once during your pregnancy. Receive immediate treatment if you test positive.

An infected baby may be born without signs or symptoms of the disease. However, if not treated immediately, the baby may develop serious problems within a few weeks. Untreated babies can have health problems such as cataracts, deafness, or seizures, and can die.

What Are the Signs and Symptoms of Syphilis?

Symptoms of syphilis in adults vary by stage:

Primary Stage

During the first (primary) stage of syphilis, you may notice a single sore or multiple sores. The sore is the location where syphilis entered your body. Sores are usually (but not always) firm, round, and painless. Because the sore is painless, it can easily go unnoticed. The sore usually lasts three to six weeks and heals regardless of whether or not you receive treatment. Even after the sore goes away, you must still receive treatment. This will stop your infection from moving to the secondary stage.

Secondary Stage

During the secondary stage, you may have skin rashes and/or mucous membrane lesions. Mucous membrane lesions are sores in your mouth, vagina, or anus. This stage usually starts with a rash on one or more areas of your body. The rash can show up when your primary sore is healing or several weeks after the sore has healed. The rash can look like rough, red, or reddish brown spots on the palms of your hands and/or the bottoms of your feet. The rash usually won't itch and it is sometimes so faint that you won't notice it. Other symptoms you may have can include fever, swollen lymph glands, sore throat, patchy hair loss, headaches, weight loss, muscle aches, and fatigue (feeling very tired). The symptoms from this stage will go away whether or not you receive treatment. Without the right treatment, your infection will move to the latent and possibly tertiary stages of syphilis.

Latent Stage

The latent stage of syphilis is a period of time when there are no visible signs or symptoms of syphilis. If you do not receive treatment, you can continue to have syphilis in your body for years without any signs or symptoms.

Tertiary Stage

Most people with untreated syphilis do not develop tertiary syphilis. However, when it does happen it can affect many different organ systems. These include the heart and blood vessels, and the brain and nervous system. Tertiary syphilis is very serious and would occur 10 to 30 years after your infection began. In tertiary syphilis, the disease damages your internal organs and can result in death.

Neurosyphilis and Ocular Syphilis

Without treatment, syphilis can spread to the brain and nervous system (neurosyphilis) or to the eye (ocular syphilis). This can happen during any of the stages described above.

Symptoms of neurosyphilis include

- Severe headache

- Difficulty coordinating muscle movements

- Paralysis (not able to move certain parts of your body)

- Numbness

- Dementia (mental disorder)

Symptoms of ocular syphilis include changes in your vision and even blindness.

How Will I or My Doctor Know If I Have Syphilis?

Most of the time, a blood test is used to test for syphilis. Some healthcare providers will diagnose syphilis by testing fluid from a syphilis sore.

Can Syphilis Be Cured?

Yes, syphilis can be cured with the right antibiotics from your healthcare provider. However, treatment might not undo any damage that the infection has already done.

I've Been Treated. Can I Get Syphilis Again?

Having syphilis once does not protect you from getting it again. Even after you've been successfully treated, you can still be re-infected. Only laboratory tests can confirm whether you have syphilis. Follow-up testing by your healthcare provider is recommended to make sure that your treatment was successful.

It may not be obvious that a sex partner has syphilis. This is because syphilis sores can be hidden in the vagina, anus, under the foreskin of the penis, or in the mouth. Unless you know that your sex partner(s) has been tested and treated, you may be at risk of getting syphilis again from an infected sex partner.

Chapter 20

Trichomoniasis

What Is Trichomoniasis?

Trichomoniasis (or "trich") is a very common sexually transmitted disease (STD). It is caused by infection with a protozoan parasite called *Trichomonas vaginalis*. Although symptoms of the disease vary, most people who have the parasite cannot tell they are infected.

How Common Is Trichomoniasis?

Trichomoniasis is the most common curable STD. In the United States, an estimated 3.7 million people have an infection. However, only about 30 percent develop any symptoms of trichomoniasis. Infection is more common in women than in men. Older women are more likely than younger women to have been infected with trichomoniasis.

How Do People Get Trichomoniasis?

The parasite passes from an infected person to an uninfected person during sex. In women, the most commonly infected part of the body is the lower genital tract (vulva, vagina, cervix, or urethra). In men, the most commonly infected body part is the inside of the penis (urethra). During sex, the parasite usually spreads from a

This chapter contains text excerpted from "Trichomoniasis—CDC Fact Sheet," Centers for Disease Control and Prevention (CDC), January 31, 2017.

penis to a vagina, or from a vagina to a penis. It can also spread from a vagina to another vagina. It is not common for the parasite to infect other body parts, like the hands, mouth, or anus. It is unclear why some people with the infection get symptoms while others do not. It probably depends on factors like a person's age and overall health. Infected people without symptoms can still pass the infection on to others.

What Are the Signs and Symptoms of Trichomoniasis?

About 70 percent of infected people do not have any signs or symptoms. When trichomoniasis does cause symptoms, they can range from mild irritation to severe inflammation. Some people with symptoms get them within 5 to 28 days after being infected. Others do not develop symptoms until much later. Symptoms can come and go.

Men with trichomoniasis may notice:

- Itching or irritation inside the penis;

- Burning after urination or ejaculation;

- Discharge from the penis.

Women with trichomoniasis may notice:

- Itching, burning, redness or soreness of the genitals;

- Discomfort with urination;

- A change in their vaginal discharge (i.e., thin discharge or increased volume) that can be clear, white, yellowish, or greenish with an unusual fishy smell.

Having trichomoniasis can make it feel unpleasant to have sex. Without treatment, the infection can last for months or even years.

What Are the Complications of Trichomoniasis?

Trichomoniasis can increase the risk of getting or spreading other sexually transmitted infections (STI). For example, trichomoniasis can cause genital inflammation that makes it easier to get infected with human immunodeficiency virus (HIV) or to pass the HIV virus on to a sex partner.

How Does Trichomoniasis Affect a Pregnant Woman and Her Baby?

Pregnant women with trichomoniasis are more likely to have their babies too early (preterm delivery). Also, babies born to infected mothers are more likely to have a low birth weight (less than 5.5 pounds).

How Is Trichomoniasis Diagnosed?

It is not possible to diagnose trichomoniasis based on symptoms alone. For both men and women, your healthcare provider can examine you and get a laboratory test to diagnose trichomoniasis.

What Is the Treatment for Trichomoniasis?

Trichomoniasis can be treated with medication (either metronidazole or tinidazole). These pills are taken by mouth. It is safe for pregnant women to take this medication. It is not recommended to drink alcohol within 24 hours after taking this medication.

People who have been treated for trichomoniasis can get it again. About one in five people get infected again within three months after receiving treatment. To avoid getting reinfected, make sure that all of your sex partners get treated. Also, wait 7 to 10 days after you and your partner have been treated to have sex again. Get checked again if your symptoms come back.

How Can Trichomoniasis Be Prevented?

The only way to avoid STDs is to not have vaginal, anal, or oral sex. If you are sexually active, you can do the following things to lower your chances of getting trichomoniasis:

- Be in a long-term mutually monogamous relationship with a partner who has been tested and has negative STD test results;

- Use latex condoms the right way every time you have sex. This can lower your chances of getting trichomoniasis. But the parasite can infect areas that are not covered by a condom—so condoms may not fully protect you from getting trichomoniasis.

Another approach is to talk about the potential risk of STDs before you have sex with a new partner. That way you can make informed choices about the level of risk you are comfortable taking with your sex life.

Chapter 21

Infections and Syndromes That Develop after Sexual Contact

Chapter Contents

Section 21.1

Bacterial Vaginosis

This section includes text excerpted from "Bacterial Vaginosis," Office on Women's Health (OWH), U.S. Department of Health and Human Services (HHS), April 24, 2018.

Bacterial vaginosis (BV) is a condition caused by changes in the amount of certain types of bacteria in your vagina. BV is common, and any woman can get it. BV is easily treatable with medicine from your doctor or nurse. If left untreated, it can raise your risk for sexually transmitted infections (STIs) and cause problems during pregnancy.

Who Gets Bacterial Vaginosis?

BV is the most common vaginal condition in women ages 15 to 44. But women of any age can get it, even if they have never had sex. You may be more at risk for BV if you:

- Have a new sex partner

- Have multiple sex partners

- Douche

- Do not use condoms or dental dams

- Are pregnant. BV is common during pregnancy. About one in four pregnant women get BV. The risk for BV is higher for pregnant women because of the hormonal changes that happen during pregnancy.

- Are African American. BV is twice as common in African American women as in White women.

- Have an intrauterine device (IUD), especially if you also have irregular bleeding

What Are the Symptoms of Bacterial Vaginosis?

Many women have no symptoms. If you do have symptoms, they may include:

- Unusual vaginal discharge. The discharge can be white (milky) or gray. It may also be foamy or watery. Some women report a strong fish-like odor, especially after sex.

- Burning when urinating

- Itching around the outside of the vagina

- Vaginal irritation

These symptoms may be similar to vaginal yeast infections and other health problems. Only your doctor or nurse can tell for sure whether you have BV.

What Is the Difference between Bacterial Vaginosis and a Vaginal Yeast Infection?

BV and vaginal yeast infections are both common causes of vaginal discharge. They have similar symptoms, so it can be hard to know if you have BV or a yeast infection. Only your doctor or nurse can tell for sure if you have BV.

With BV, your discharge may be white or gray but may also have a fishy smell. Discharge from a yeast infection may also be white or gray but may look like cottage cheese.

How Is Bacterial Vaginosis Diagnosed?

There are tests to find out if you have BV. Your doctor or nurse takes a sample of vaginal discharge. Your doctor or nurse may then look at the sample under a microscope, use an in-office test, or send the sample to a lab to check for harmful bacteria. Your doctor or nurse may also see signs of BV during an exam.

Before you see a doctor or nurse for a test:

- Don't douche or use vaginal deodorant sprays. They might cover odors that can help your doctor diagnose BV. They can also irritate your vagina.

- Make an appointment for a day when you do not have your period.

How Is Bacterial Vaginosis Treated?

BV is treated with antibiotics. It is also possible to contract BV again. BV and vaginal yeast infections are treated differently. Yeast infections can be treated with over-the-counter (OTC) medicines. But you cannot treat BV with OTC yeast-infection medicine.

Is It Safe to Treat Pregnant Women Who Have Bacterial Vaginosis?

Yes. The medicine used to treat BV is safe for pregnant women. All pregnant women with symptoms of BV should be tested and treated if they have it.

If you have BV, you can be treated safely at any stage of your pregnancy. You will get the same antibiotic given to women who are not pregnant.

What Can Happen If Bacterial Vaginosis Is Not Treated?

If BV is untreated, possible problems may include:

- **Higher risk of getting STIs, including human immunodeficiency virus (HIV).** Having BV can raise your risk of getting HIV, genital herpes, chlamydia, pelvic inflammatory disease (PID), and gonorrhea. Women with HIV who get BV are also more likely to pass HIV to a male sexual partner.

- **Pregnancy problems.** BV can lead to premature birth or a low-birth-weight (LBW) baby (smaller than 5½ pounds at birth). All pregnant women with symptoms of BV should be tested and treated if they have it.

How Can I Lower My Risk of Bacterial Vaginosis?

Researchers do not know exactly how BV spreads. Steps that might lower your risk of BV include:

- **Keeping your vaginal bacteria balanced.** Use warm water only to clean the outside of your vagina. You do not need to use soap. Even mild soap can cause irritate your vagina. Always wipe front to back from your vagina to your anus. Keep the area cool by wearing cotton or cotton-lined underpants.

- **Not douching.** Douching upsets the balance of good and harmful bacteria in your vagina. This may raise your risk of BV. It may also make it easier to get BV again after treatment. Doctors do not recommend douching.

- **Not having sex.** Researchers are still studying how women get BV. You can get BV without having sex, but BV is more common in women who have sex.

- **Limiting your number of sex partners.** Researchers think that your risk of getting BV goes up with the number of partners you have.

How Can I Protect Myself If I Am a Female and My Female Partner Has Bacterial Vaginosis?

If your partner has BV, you might be able to lower your risk by using protection during sex.

- Use a dental dam every time you have sex. A dental dam is a thin piece of latex that is placed over the genitals before oral sex.

- Cover sex toys with condoms before use. Remove the condom and replace it with a new one before sharing the toy with your partner.

Section 21.2

Cytomegalovirus

This section contains text excerpted from the following sources: Text in this section begins with excerpts from "About CMV," Centers for Disease Control and Prevention (CDC), June 6, 2018; Text under the heading "Cytomegalovirus Facts for Pregnant Women and Parents" is excerpted from "CMV Facts for Pregnant Women and Parents," Centers for Disease Control and Prevention (CDC), August 7, 2018; Text beginning with the heading "Babies Born with Cytomegalovirus" is excerpted from "Babies Born with CMV (Congenital CMV Infection)," Centers for Disease Control and Prevention (CDC), June 6, 2018.

Cytomegalovirus (CMV) is a common virus that infects people of all ages. In the United States, nearly one in three children are already infected with CMV by age five. Over half of adults by age 40 have been infected with CMV. Once CMV is in a person's body, it stays there for life and can reactivate. A person can also be re-infected with a different strain (variety) of the virus.

Signs and Symptoms

Most people with CMV infection have no symptoms and aren't aware that they have been infected. In some cases, infection in healthy people can cause mild illness that may include:

- Fever

- Sore throat

- Fatigue

- Swollen glands

Occasionally, CMV can cause mononucleosis or hepatitis (liver problem).

People with weakened immune systems who get CMV can have more serious symptoms affecting the eyes, lungs, liver, esophagus, stomach, and intestines. Babies born with CMV can have brain, liver, spleen, lung, and growth problems. The most common health problem in babies born with congenital CMV infection is hearing loss, which may be detected soon after birth or may develop later in childhood.

Transmission and Prevention

People with CMV may pass the virus in body fluids, such as saliva, urine, blood, tears, semen, and breast milk. CMV is spread from an infected person in the following ways:

- From direct contact with saliva or urine, especially from babies and young children

- Through sexual contact

- From breast milk to nursing infants

- Through transplanted organs and blood transfusions

A woman who is infected with CMV can pass the virus to her developing baby during pregnancy. Women may be able to lessen their risk of getting CMV by reducing contact with saliva and urine from babies and young children. The saliva and urine of children with CMV have high amounts of the virus. A pregnant woman can avoid getting a child's saliva in her mouth by, for example, not sharing food, utensils, or cups with a child. Also, she should wash her hands after changing diapers. These cannot eliminate her risk of getting CMV, but may lessen the chances of getting it.

Cytomegalovirus Facts for Pregnant Women and Parents

For Pregnant Women

- **You Can Pass CMV to Your Baby**—If you are pregnant and have CMV, the virus in your blood can cross through your placenta and infect your developing baby. This is more likely to happen if you have a first-time CMV infection while pregnant, but can also happen if you have a subsequent infection during pregnancy.

- **You Are Not Likely to Be Tested for CMV**—It is not recommended that doctors routinely test pregnant women for CMV infection. This is because laboratory tests cannot predict which developing babies will become infected with CMV or have long-term health problems.

- **You May Be Able to Reduce Your Risk**—You may be able to lessen your risk of getting CMV by reducing contact with saliva and urine from babies and young children. The saliva and urine of children with CMV have high amounts of the virus. You can avoid getting a child's saliva in your mouth by, for example, not sharing food, utensils, or cups with a child. Also, you should wash your hands after changing diapers. These cannot eliminate your risk of getting CMV but may lessen the chances of getting it.

For Parents

About 1 out of every 200 babies is born with congenital CMV. About 1 out of 5 of these babies will have birth defects or other long-term health problems.

- **Babies with Congenital CMV May Show Signs at Birth**—Some signs that a baby might have congenital CMV infection when they are born are:

  - Small head size

  - Seizures

  - Rash

  - Liver, spleen, and lung problems

Tests on a baby's saliva, urine, or blood done within two to three weeks after birth can confirm if the baby has congenital CMV.

- **Early Treatment May Help**—Babies who show signs of congenital CMV at birth may be treated with medicines called antivirals. Antivirals may decrease the severity of health problems and hearing loss but should be used with caution due to side effects.

- **Long-Term Health Problems May Occur**—Babies with signs of congenital CMV at birth are more likely to have long-term health problems, such as:

  - Hearing loss
  - Intellectual disability
  - Vision loss
  - Seizures
  - Lack of coordination or weakness

  Some babies with congenital CMV but without signs of disease at birth may still have or develop hearing loss. Hearing loss may be present at birth or may develop later in babies who passed their newborn hearing test. Sometimes, hearing loss worsens with age.

- **Hearing Checks and Therapies Are Recommended**—Children with congenital CMV should have regular hearing checks. Children with hearing loss should receive services such as speech or occupational therapy (OT). These services help ensure they develop language, social, and communication skills. The earlier your child can get hearing checks and therapies, the more he or she can benefit from them.

Babies Born with Cytomegalovirus

When a baby is born with cytomegalovirus (CMV) infection, it is called congenital CMV. About 1 out of every 200 babies is born with congenital CMV infection. However, only about 1 in 5 babies with congenital CMV infection will be sick from the virus or have long-term health problems.

Transmission

A pregnant woman can pass CMV to her unborn baby. The virus in the woman's blood can cross through the placenta and infect the baby. This can happen when a pregnant woman is infected with CMV for the first time or is infected with CMV again during pregnancy.

240

Signs and Symptoms

Most babies with congenital CMV infection never show signs or have health problems. However, some babies may have health problems that are apparent at birth or develop later during infancy or childhood. In the most severe cases of infection, CMV can cause the death of an unborn baby (pregnancy loss). Some babies with congenital CMV infection have signs at birth. These signs include:

- Rash

- Jaundice (yellowing of the skin or whites of the eyes)

- Microcephaly (small head)

- Intrauterine growth restriction (low weight)

- Hepatosplenomegaly (HSM) (enlarged liver and spleen)

- Seizures

- Retinitis (damaged eye retina)

Some babies with signs of congenital CMV infection at birth may have long-term health problems, such as:

- Hearing loss

- Developmental and motor delay

- Vision loss

- Microcephaly (small head)

- Seizures

Some babies without signs of congenital CMV infection at birth may have hearing loss. Hearing loss may be present at birth or may develop later, even in babies who passed the newborn hearing test.

Diagnosis

Congenital CMV infection can be diagnosed by testing a newborn baby's saliva, urine (preferred specimens), or blood. These specimens must be collected for testing within two to three weeks after the baby is born in order to confirm a diagnosis of congenital CMV infection.

Treatment and Management

For babies with signs of congenital CMV infection at birth, anti-viral medications, primarily valganciclovir, may improve hearing and developmental outcomes. Valganciclovir can have serious side effects and has only been studied in babies with signs of congenital CMV infection. There is limited information on the effectiveness of valganciclovir to treat infants with hearing loss alone. Babies with congenital CMV infection, with or without signs at birth, should have regular hearing checks. Follow-up regularly with your baby's doctor to discuss the care and additional services your child may need.

Section 21.3

Fungal (Yeast) Infection

This section includes text excerpted from "Vaginal Yeast Infections," Office on Women's Health (OWH), U.S. Department of Health and Human Services (HHS), May 23, 2018.

Most women will get a vaginal yeast infection at some point in their life. Symptoms of vaginal yeast infections include burning, itching, and thick, white discharge. Yeast infections are easy to treat, but it is important to see your doctor or nurse if you think you have an infection. Yeast infection symptoms are similar to other vaginal infections and sexually transmitted infections (STIs). If you have a more serious infection and not a yeast infection, it can lead to major health problems.

What Is a Vaginal Yeast Infection?

A vaginal yeast infection is an infection of the vagina that causes itching and burning of the vulva, the area around the vagina. Vaginal yeast infections are caused by an overgrowth of the fungus *Candida*.

Who Gets Vaginal Yeast Infections

Women and girls of all ages can get vaginal yeast infections. Three out of four women will have a yeast infection at some point in their life. Almost half of women have two or more infections.

Vaginal yeast infections are rare before puberty and after menopause.

Are Some Women More at Risk for Yeast Infections?

Yes. Your risk for yeast infections is higher if:

- You are pregnant

- You have diabetes and your blood sugar is not under control

- You use a type of hormonal birth control that has higher doses of estrogen

- You douche or use vaginal sprays

- You recently took antibiotics such as amoxicillin or steroid medicines

- You have a weakened immune system, such as from human immunodeficiency virus (HIV)

What Are the Symptoms of Vaginal Yeast Infections?

The most common symptom of a vaginal yeast infection is extreme itchiness in and around the vagina.

Other signs and symptoms include:

- Burning, redness, and swelling of the vagina and the vulva

- Pain when urinating

- Pain during sex

- Soreness

- A thick, white vaginal discharge that looks like cottage cheese and does not have a bad smell

You may have only a few of these symptoms. They may be mild or severe.

What Causes Yeast Infections

Yeast infections are caused by an overgrowth of the microscopic fungus *Candida*.

Your vagina may have small amounts of yeast at any given time without causing any symptoms. But when too much yeast grows, you can get an infection.

Can I Get a Yeast Infection from Having Sex?

Yes. A yeast infection is not considered a sexually transmitted infection (STI), because you can get a yeast infection without having sex. But you can get a yeast infection from your sexual partner. Condoms and dental dams may help prevent getting or passing yeast infections through vaginal, oral, or anal sex.

How Is a Yeast Infection Diagnosed?

Your doctor will do a pelvic exam to look for swelling and discharge. Your doctor may also use a cotton swab to take a sample of the discharge from your vagina. A lab technician will look at the sample under a microscope to see whether there is an overgrowth of the fungus *Candida* that causes a yeast infection.

How Is a Yeast Infection Treated?

Yeast infections are usually treated with antifungal medicine. See your doctor or nurse and make sure that you have a vaginal yeast infection and not another type of infection.

You can then buy antifungal medicine for yeast infections at a store, without a prescription. Antifungal medicines come in the form of creams, tablets, ointments, or suppositories that you insert into your vagina. You can apply treatment in one dose or daily for up to seven days, depending on the brand you choose.

Your doctor or nurse can also give you a single dose of antifungal medicine taken by mouth, such as fluconazole. If you get more than four vaginal yeast infections a year, or if your yeast infection doesn't go away after using over-the-counter (OTC) treatment, you may need to take regular doses of antifungal medicine for up to six months.

Is It Safe to Use Over-the-Counter Medicines for Yeast Infections?

Yes, but always talk with your doctor or nurse before treating yourself for a vaginal yeast infection. This is because:

- **You may be trying to treat an infection that is not a yeast infection.** Studies show that two out of three women who buy yeast infection medicine don't really have a yeast infection. Instead, they may have an STI or bacterial vaginosis (BV). STIs and BV require different treatments than yeast infections and, if left untreated, can cause serious health problems.

- **Using treatment when you do not actually have a yeast infection can cause your body to become resistant to yeast infection medicine.** This can make actual yeast infections harder to treat in the future.

- **Some yeast infection medicine may weaken condoms and diaphragms, increasing your chance of getting pregnant or an STI when you have sex.** Talk to your doctor or nurse about what is best for you, and always read and follow the directions on the medicine carefully.

How Do I Treat a Yeast Infection If I'm Pregnant?

During pregnancy, it's safe to treat a yeast infection with vaginal creams or suppositories that contain miconazole or clotrimazole.

Do not take the oral fluconazole tablet to treat a yeast infection during pregnancy. It may cause birth defects.

Can I Get a Yeast Infection from Breastfeeding?

Yes. Yeast infections can happen on your nipples or in your breast (commonly called "thrush") from breastfeeding. Yeast thrives on milk and moisture. A yeast infection you get while breastfeeding is different from a vaginal yeast infection. However, it is caused by an overgrowth of the same fungus.

Symptoms of thrush during breastfeeding include:

- Sore nipples that last more than a few days, especially after several weeks of pain-free breastfeeding

- Flaky, shiny, itchy, or cracked nipples

- Deep pink and blistered nipples

- Achy breast

- Shooting pain in the breast during or after feedings

If you have any of these signs or symptoms or think your baby might have thrush in his or her mouth, call your doctor.

If I Have a Yeast Infection, Does My Sexual Partner Need to Be Treated?

Maybe. Yeast infections are not STIs. But it is possible to pass yeast infections to your partner during vaginal, oral, or anal sex.

- **If your partner is a man**, the risk of infection is low. About 15 percent of men get an itchy rash on the penis if they have unprotected sex with a woman who has a yeast infection. If this happens to your partner, he should see a doctor. Men who haven't been circumcised and men with diabetes are at higher risk.

- **If your partner is a woman**, she may be at risk. She should be tested and treated if she has any symptoms.

How Can I Prevent a Yeast Infection?

You can take steps to lower your risk of getting yeast infections:

- Do not douche. Douching removes some of the normal bacteria in the vagina that protects you from infection.

- Do not use scented feminine products, including bubble bath, sprays, pads, and tampons.

- Change tampons, pads, and panty liners often.

- Do not wear tight underwear, pantyhose, pants, or jeans. These can increase body heat and moisture in your genital area.

- Wear underwear with a cotton crotch. Cotton underwear helps keep you dry and doesn't hold in warmth and moisture.

- Change out of wet swimsuits and workout clothes as soon as you can.

- After using the bathroom, always wipe from front to back.

- Avoid hot tubs and very hot baths.

- If you have diabetes, be sure your blood sugar is under control.

Does Yogurt Prevent or Treat Yeast Infections?

Maybe. Studies suggest that eating eight ounces of yogurt with "live cultures" daily or taking *Lactobacillus acidophilus* capsules can help prevent infection.

But, more research still needs to be done to say for sure if yogurt with *Lactobacillus* or other probiotics can prevent or treat vaginal yeast infections. If you think you have a yeast infection, see your doctor or nurse and make sure before taking any OTC medicine.

What Should I Do If I Get Repeated Yeast Infections?

If you get four or more yeast infections in a year, talk to your doctor or nurse.

About 5 percent of women get four or more vaginal yeast infections in one year. This is called recurrent vulvovaginal candidiasis (RVVC). RVVC is more common in women with diabetes or weak immune systems, such as with HIV, but it can also happen in otherwise healthy women.

Doctors most often treat RVVC with antifungal medicine for up to six months. Researchers also are studying the effects of a vaccine to help prevent RVVC.

Section 21.4

Intestinal Parasites

This section includes text excerpted from "Communicable Disease," Centers for Disease Control and Prevention (CDC), June 6, 2016.

Parasitic Infections

Resettling refugees over the age of 1 receive 400 mg of albendazole 48 hours prior to departure for the United States as presumptive treatment for helminthiasis. Approximately 20 percent of new arrivals into Texas between June 2009 and May 2011 had positive O and P stool samples during postarrival screening exams. Of 295 records that specified a parasite, more than 50 percent were positive for *Giardia*, 36 percent for *Dientamoeba*, 20 percent for *Entamoeba*, and 2 percent or less for *Ascaris, Clonorchis*, hookworm, *Schistosoma, Strongyloides*, and *Trichuris*. On serological tests, a more sensitive means of detecting Strongyloides infection, of 272 refugees tested, 20 percent were positive.

Intestinal-Parasitic Infection

There are a number of intestinal parasitic infections that may be encountered in Burmese refugees. These are often parasites found commonly in populations residing in tropical areas, such as *Ascaris, Trichuris*, hookworm, and *Giardia*. This section will discuss specific infections that may be unique to, or of particular concern, in this population.

Strongyloides

Strongyloidiasis is a parasitic nematode infection that is common in Asian refugees and is known to persist for more than 50 years in the human host. The infection is frequently asymptomatic, but may lead to morbidity and, when the infected individual is immunosuppressed, even result in death.

The Centers for Disease Control and Prevention (CDC) recommends that all U.S.-bound Burmese refugees either be presumptively treated for strongyloidiasis overseas or, if they have not been treated overseas, be tested and treated (if positive) after arrival in the United States.

The treatment of choice for *Strongyloides* infection is ivermectin, given once daily for two consecutive days. All resettlement-eligible Burmese refugees, whether they originate in Thailand or in Malaysia, are receiving ivermectin prior to departure for the United States. Ivermectin is thought to be more than 90 percent effective in treating *Strongyloides* infection, although it may not eradicate all infections. If a refugee has persistent symptoms, or persistent eosinophilia (more than 3 months after arrival in the United States), strongyloidiasis should still be considered in the differential diagnosis. In this case, it is reasonable to perform serologic testing and/or repeat presumptive treatment, especially if the patient will be immunosuppressed or placed on corticosteroids.

Cysticercosis

Cysticercosis is an infection with the larval stage of the parasitic cestode (tapeworm) *Taenia solium*. Both pigs and humans may be infected by ingesting eggs. The adult tapeworm resides in the human intestine, where it occasionally may cause mild gastrointestinal symptoms. This is called "taeniasis."

Cysticercosis is usually caused when a human ingests eggs shed in the feces of a human tapeworm carrier (although they may also experience cysticercosis from autoinfection). Cysticercosis occurs when an ingested tapeworm invades the intestinal wall, and migrates into striated muscle, the brain, liver, or other tissues, and develops into cysts. When cysts are found in the central nervous system, the infection is referred to as "neurocysticercosis" (NCC), which, when symptomatic, most commonly presents with seizures. Treatment of NCC is complicated, and consultation with a specialist familiar with this disorder is recommended prior to initiating treatment.

Inadvertent treatment of a person with NCC with certain antiparasitics (e.g., albendazole, praziquantel) may precipitate symptoms such as seizures. Therefore, patients with known NCC or a seizure disorder should not be treated with these medications until a formal neurologic evaluation has been performed.

Although data specific to Burmese refugees are not available, an intestinal infection with the adult tapeworm (taeniasis) is typically seen on stool ova and parasite (O and P) screening in approximately 1 to 2 percent of all refugees following arriving in the United States. It is not possible to distinguish between *T. solium* and other Taenia tapeworms on stool O and P unless a segment of the tapeworm is seen. While routine stool studies of asymptomatic refugees are not indicated,

249

if a family member has a known infection then family members and close contacts should be screened. In addition, diagnostic testing with stool O and Ps should be considered in those with gastrointestinal signs or symptoms, if they report or bring in a segment of a tapeworm passed in their stool (generally about the size of a piece of rice). Use of albendazole or praziquantel should be restricted to those without a history of seizures or known NCC. Assistance with screening, diagnosis, and treatment may be obtained from the CDC's Division of Parasitic and Malaria Diseases (DPDM).

Trematode Infections

Trematode ("fluke") infections occur worldwide, but each infection has a specific geographic distribution. Human infection is largely determined by dietary or environmental exposure in endemic areas. All fluke infections may be persistent and last many years following exposure. Although the most common trematode infection is schistosomiasis, considered the only "blood fluke," Myanmar, areas of Thailand and Malaysia, where refugees from Burma have resided, are not endemic. However, other trematodes that may be encountered in these refugees include: *Paragonimus westermani* (lung fluke), the liver flukes (*Clonorchis sinensis, Fasciola hepatica, Opisthorchis viverrini*) and the intestinal flukes (*Fasciolopsis buski, Heterophyes heterophyes, and Metagonimus yokogawai*). These trematode infections are acquired through ingestion of specific food items. Although Burmese refugees may be exposed to multiple trematode species, the most commonly encountered trematodes in this population are *Paragonimus westermani* and *Clonorchis sinensis*, which are discussed below.

Paragonimiasis

Paragonimus, also known as lung fluke, is acquired from eating raw or undercooked freshwater crab or crayfish, which is a common practice in many Burmese populations (where preparation of these crustaceans involves brining them in vinegar or wine, but not cooking them. This fails to kill the organism). Following consumption of the metacercariae and the development of the adult worm, *Paragonimus* will make its way to the pulmonary system, where it will induce inflammation and generates fibrous cysts containing purulent, bloody fluid and may cause an effusion. The eggs are subsequently released into the environment through expectoration or may be swallowed and passed in the stool. Most infected individuals have no or subtle symptoms. The most common clinical presentation resembles chronic bronchitis or tuberculosis (TB) with a cough, which frequently produces coffee-colored or blood-tinged sputum, chest pain, and/or shortness of breath. The sputum may be peppered with visible clumps of eggs. It commonly causes chest radiograph (CXR) abnormalities such as lobar infiltrates, coin lesions, cavities, calcified nodules, hilar enlargement, and, particularly, pleural thickening and effusions. CXR findings of "ring-shaped opacities" of contiguous cavities, often referred to as a "grape bunch," suggest a central nervous system (CNS) infection, and should be considered in persons with symptoms such as headaches, seizures, visual changes, or other CNS symptoms. *Paragonimus* may also invade the liver, spleen, intestinal wall, peritoneum, and abdominal lymph nodes.

No *Paragonimus* prevalence data are available in Burmese refugees, but there have been many clinical cases diagnosed in refugees following their arrival in the United States. Diagnosis can be challenging, but for patients with pulmonary signs or symptoms, sputum O and Ps examination may be helpful (note: acid-fast bacilli staining for TB will destroy the eggs and sputum O and P should not be stained for acid-fast bacilli). Stool O and P may be diagnostic but has low sensitivity for detecting infection. Serum antibody testing is also available. Generally, when paragonimiasis is suspected, an expert should be consulted.

Clonorchis Sinensis

Clonorchis ("liver fluke") infects the liver, gallbladder, and bile ducts. In addition to humans, the reservoir species include dogs and other fish-eating carnivores. This infection is acquired when a human ingests raw, salted, pickled, smoked, marinated, dried, partially or poorly cooked fish. Most individuals have no or minimal symptoms. The most common finding in refugees is a persistently elevated eosinophil count. Common symptoms include fever, right-upper-quadrant pain, and intermittent biliary colic pain (when the worms obstruct the biliary tract). Chronic infection may result in recurrent pyogenic cholangitis and is associated with cholangiohepatitis. Physicians may confuse the gallstones and cholecystitis (Tip: on ultrasound, the fluke is echogenic and appears dark, compared to a gallstone, which is generally lighter in appearance). Chronic infection with *Clonorchis sinensis* has been associated with biliary cancer, and the International Agency for Research on Cancer (IARC) has classified it as a Group one agent (carcinogenic in humans).

Risk of infection is highly dependent on diet, and the infection has been detected in Burmese refugees—and, in the United States, especially among the Hmong. When this infection suspected, the first diagnostic tests indicated are multiple stool O and Ps and ultrasound of the liver and biliary tract. Diagnosis can be challenging since these tests are not sensitive. Serologic testing is available outside the United States. Generally, when *Clonorchis* infection is suspected, an expert should be consulted.

Malaria

Malaria is prevalent in Myanmar, with the most common species being *Plasmodium falciparum* (which causes acute malaria) and *Plasmodium vivax* (which may cause acute malaria or become dormant in the liver, emerging months, or even years, later, and causing clinical malaria.) In Thai refugee camps along the border of Myanmar, frequent travel between the two countries is common. Although malaria in Thailand is unusual, this cross-border travel and the proximity to Myanmar creates an opportunity for acute clinical cases of malaria in Burmese refugees residing in these camps. There is no sustained malaria transmission in Kuala Lumpur, Malaysia. Refugees originating from Malaysia (Kuala Lumpur) are not at risk of acute malaria. However, most Burmese refugees who have resided in Myanmar have had exposure to areas of *Plasmodium vivax* during their lifetime and may harbor dormant infection. This infection may reactivate following immigration to the United States. At present, the presumptive antimalarial treatment program for refugee populations at high risk of malaria prior to immigration to the United States is only in effect in sub-Saharan Africa. At this time, malaria prevalence rates in Burmese refugees in Thailand are not substantial enough to warrant presumptive treatment in this population. Refugees with *Plasmodium falciparum* infection who are from regions of lower prevalence would be expected to show clinical signs of disease (in highly endemic areas, such as many areas of Africa, *Plasmodium falciparum* malaria parasitemia may be asymptomatic or subclinical). In addition, common medications used to treat acute malaria do not treat the dormant liver phase of *Plasmodium vivax*.

The clinician should be aware that clinical malaria may occur in Burmese refugees, with those originating in Thailand at highest risk. In addition, it should be noted that *Plasmodium vivax* relapse may occur many months, or even years, following migration. Any patient with clinical signs and symptoms of malaria should be tested for infection. The CDC provides clinical consultation support for providers seeking information on the diagnosis and management of malaria.

Section 21.5

Molluscum Contagiosum

This section includes text excerpted from "Molluscum Contagiosum," Centers for Disease Control and Prevention (CDC), May 11, 2015. Reviewed February 2019.

Molluscum contagiosum is an infection caused by a poxvirus (*Molluscum contagiosum* virus (MCV)). The result of the infection is usually a benign, mild skin disease characterized by lesions (growths) that may appear anywhere on the body. Within 6 to 12 months, Molluscum contagiosum typically resolves without scarring but may take as long as four years.

The lesions, known as "Mollusca," are small, raised, and usually white, pink, or flesh-colored with a dimple or pit in the center. They often have a pearly appearance. They're usually smooth and firm. In most people, the lesions range from about the size of a pinhead to as large as a pencil eraser (2 to 5 millimeters in diameter). They may become itchy, sore, red, and/or swollen.

Mollusca may occur anywhere on the body, alone or in groups. The lesions are rarely found on the palms of the hands or the soles of the feet.

Transmission

The virus that causes molluscum spreads from direct person-to-person physical contact and through contaminated fomites. Fomites are inanimate objects that can become contaminated with the virus; in the instance of molluscum contagiosum, this can include linens such as clothing and towels, bathing sponges, pool equipment, and toys. Although the virus might be spread by sharing swimming pools, baths, saunas, or, other wet and warm environments, this has not been proven. Researchers who have investigated this idea think it is more likely the virus is spread by sharing towels and other items around a pool or sauna than through water.

Someone with molluscum can spread it to other parts of their body by touching or scratching a lesion and then touching their body somewhere else. This is called "autoinoculation." Shaving and electrolysis can also spread Mollusca to other parts of the body.

Molluscum can spread from one person to another by sexual contact. Many, but not all, cases of molluscum in adults are caused by sexual contact.

Conflicting reports make it unclear whether the disease may be spread by simple contact with seemingly intact lesions or if the breaking of a lesion and the subsequent transferring of the core material is necessary to spread the virus.

The *molluscum contagiosum* virus remains in the top layer of skin (epidermis) and does not circulate throughout the body; therefore, it cannot spread through coughing or sneezing.

Since the virus lives only in the top layer of skin, once the lesions are gone the virus is gone and you cannot spread it to others. *Molluscum contagiosum* is not like herpes viruses, which can remain dormant ("sleeping") in your body for long periods and then reappear.

Risk Factors
Who Is at Risk for Infection?

Molluscum contagiosum is common enough that you should not be surprised if you see someone with it or if someone in your family becomes infected. Although not limited to children, it is most common in children 1 to 10 years of age.

People at increased risk for getting the disease include:

- People with weakened immune systems (i.e., human immunodeficiency virus (HIV)-infected persons or persons being treated for cancer) are at higher risk for getting molluscum contagiosum. Their growths may look different, be larger, and be more difficult to treat.

- Atopic dermatitis (AD) may also be a risk factor for getting molluscum contagiosum due to frequent breaks in the skin. People with this condition also may be more likely to spread molluscum contagiosum to other parts of their body for the same reason.

- People who live in warm, humid climates where living conditions are crowded

Treatment Options

Because molluscum contagiosum is self-limited in healthy individuals, treatment may be unnecessary. Nonetheless, issues such as lesion visibility, underlying atopic disease, and the desire to prevent transmission may prompt therapy.

Treatment for molluscum is usually recommended if lesions are in the genital area (on or near the penis, vulva, vagina, or anus). If lesions are found in this area it is a good idea to visit your healthcare provider as there is a possibility that you may have another disease spread by sexual contact.

Be aware that some treatments available on the Internet may not be effective and may even be harmful.

Physical Removal

Physical removal of lesions may include cryotherapy (freezing the lesion with liquid nitrogen), curettage (the piercing of the core and scraping of caseous or cheesy material), and laser therapy. These options are rapid and require a trained healthcare provider, may require local anesthesia, and can result in postprocedural pain, irritation, and scarring.

It is not a good idea to try and remove lesions or the fluid inside of lesions yourself. By removing lesions or lesion fluid by yourself you may unintentionally autoinoculate other parts of the body or risk spreading it to others. By scratching or scraping the skin you could cause a bacterial infection.

Oral Therapy

Gradual removal of lesions may be achieved by oral therapy. This technique is often desirable for pediatric patients because it is generally less painful and may be performed by parents at home in a less-threatening environment. Oral cimetidine has been used as an alternative treatment for small children who are either afraid of the pain associated with cryotherapy, curettage, and laser therapy or because the possibility of scarring is to be avoided. While cimetidine is safe, painless, and well tolerated, facial Mollusca does not respond as well as lesions elsewhere on the body.

Topical Therapy

Podophyllotoxin (PPT) cream (0.5%) is reliable as a home therapy for men and some women but is not recommended for pregnant women because of presumed toxicity to the fetus. Each lesion must be treated individually as the therapeutic effect is localized. Other options for topical therapy include iodine and salicylic acid, potassium hydroxide, tretinoin, cantharidin (a blistering agent usually applied in an office setting), and imiquimod (T cell modifier). Imiquimod has not been proven effective for the treatment of molluscum contagiosum in children and is not recommended for children because of possible adverse events. These treatments must be prescribed by a healthcare professional.

Therapy for Immunocompromised Persons

Most therapies are effective in immunocompetent patients; however, patients with human immunodeficiency virus (HIV)/acquired immunodeficiency syndrome (AIDS) or other immunosuppressive conditions often do not respond to traditional treatments. In addition, these treatments are largely ineffective in achieving long-term control in HIV patients.

Low cluster of differentiation 4 (CD4) cell counts have been linked to widespread facial Mollusca, and therefore, have become a marker for severe HIV disease. Thus far, therapies targeted at boosting the immune system have proven the most effective therapy for molluscum contagiosum in immunocompromised persons. In extreme cases, intralesional interferon has been used to treat facial lesions in these patients. However, the severe and unpleasant side effects of interferon, such as influenza-like symptoms, site tenderness, depression, and lethargy, make it a less-than-desirable treatment. Interferon therapy proved most effective in otherwise healthy persons. Radiation therapy is also of little benefit.

Prevention
How Can I Keep It from Spreading?

The best way to avoid getting molluscum is by following good hygiene habits. Remember that the virus lives only in the skin and once the lesions are gone, the virus is gone and you cannot spread the virus to others.

- **Wash Your Hands**—There are ways to prevent the spread of molluscum contagiosum. The best way is to follow good hygiene (cleanliness) habits. Keeping your hands clean is the best way to avoid molluscum infection, as well as many other infections.

Hand washing removes germs that may have been picked up from other people or from surfaces that have germs on them.

- **Don't Scratch or Pick at Molluscum Lesions**—It is important not to touch, pick, or scratch skin that has lesions, that includes not only your own skin but anyone else's. Picking and scratching can spread the virus to other parts of the body and makes it easier to spread the disease to other people too.

- **Keep Molluscum Lesions Covered**—It is important to keep the area with molluscum lesions clean and covered with clothing or a bandage so that others do not touch the lesions and become infected. Do remember to keep the affected skin clean and dry. Any time there is no risk of others coming into contact with your skin, such as at night when you sleep, uncover the lesions to help keep your skin healthy.

Be Careful during Sports Activities

- Do not share towels, clothing, or other personal items.

- People with molluscum should not take part in contact sports such as wrestling, basketball, and football unless all lesions can be covered by clothing or bandages.

- Activities that use shared gear such as helmets, baseball gloves, and balls should also be avoided unless all lesions can be covered.

- Swimming should also be avoided unless all lesions can be covered by watertight bandages. Personal items such as towels, goggles, and swimsuits should not be shared. Other items and equipment such as kickboards and water toys should be used only when all lesions are covered by clothing or watertight bandages.

Other Ways to Avoid Sharing Your Infection

- Do not shave or have electrolysis on areas with lesions.

- Do not share personal items such as unwashed clothes, hair brushes, wrist watches, and bar soap with others.

- If you have lesions on or near the penis, vulva, vagina, or anus, avoid sexual activities until you see a healthcare provider.

Section 21.6

Proctitis, Proctocolitis, and Enteritis

This section includes text excerpted from "Proctitis, Proctocolitis, and Enteritis," Centers for Disease Control and Prevention (CDC), June 4, 2015. Reviewed February 2019.

Sexually Transmitted Gastrointestinal Syndromes

Sexually transmitted gastrointestinal syndromes include proctitis, proctocolitis, and enteritis. Evaluation of these syndromes should include appropriate diagnostic procedures (e.g., anoscopy or sigmoidoscopy, stool examination, and culture).

Proctitis is inflammation of the rectum (i.e., the distal 10 to 12 cm) that can be associated with anorectal pain, tenesmus, or rectal discharge. *N. gonorrhoeae, C. trachomatis* (including Lymphogranuloma venereum (LGV) serovars), *T. pallidum*, and herpes simplex virus (HSV) are the most common sexually transmitted pathogens involved. In persons with human immunodeficiency virus (HIV) infection, herpes proctitis can be especially severe. Proctitis occurs predominantly among persons who participate in receptive anal intercourse.

Proctocolitis is associated with symptoms of proctitis, diarrhea, or abdominal cramps, and inflammation of the colonic mucosa extending to 12 cm above the anus. Fecal leukocytes might be detected on stool examination, depending on the pathogen. Pathogenic organisms include *Campylobacter sp., Shigella sp., Entamoeba histolytica*, and LGV serovars of *C. trachomatis*. CMV or other opportunistic agents can be involved in immunosuppressed HIV-infected patients. Proctocolitis can be acquired through receptive anal intercourse or by oral–anal contact, depending on the pathogen.

Enteritis usually results in diarrhea and abdominal cramping without signs of proctitis or proctocolitis; it occurs among persons whose sexual practices include oral–anal contact. In otherwise healthy persons, *Giardia lamblia* is most frequently implicated. When outbreaks of gastrointestinal illness occur among social or sexual networks of men who have sex with men (MSM), clinicians should consider sexual transmission as a mode of spread and provide counseling accordingly. Among persons with HIV infection, enteritis can be caused by pathogens that may not be sexually transmitted, including cytomegalovirus (CMV), *Mycobacterium avium-intracellulare, Salmonella sp., Campylobacter sp., Shigella sp., Cryptosporidium, Microsporidium*, and

Isospora. Multiple stool examinations might be necessary to detect *Giardia*, and special stool preparations are required to diagnose cryptosporidiosis and microsporidiosis. In addition, enteritis can be directly caused by HIV infection.

Diagnostic Considerations for Acute Proctitis

Persons who present with symptoms of acute proctitis should be examined by anoscopy. A Gram-stained smear of any anorectal exudate from anoscopic or anal examination should be examined for polymorphonuclear leukocytes (PMN). All persons should be evaluated for herpes simplex virus (HSV) (by polymerase chain reaction (PCR) or culture), *N. gonorrhoeae* (nucleic acid amplification testing (NAAT) or culture), *C. trachomatis* (NAAT), and *T. pallidum* (Darkfield if available and serologic testing). If the *C. trachomatis* test is positive on a rectal swab, a molecular test PCR for LGV should be performed, if available, to confirm an LGV diagnosis.

Treatment for Acute Proctitis

Acute proctitis of recent onset among persons who have recently practiced receptive anal intercourse is usually sexually acquired. Presumptive therapy should be initiated while awaiting results of laboratory tests for persons with anorectal exudate detected on examination or polymorphonuclear leukocytes detected on a Gram-stained smear of anorectal exudate or secretions; such therapy also should be initiated when anoscopy or Gram stain is unavailable and the clinical presentation is consistent with acute proctitis in persons reporting receptive anal intercourse.

Recommended Regimen

- Ceftriaxone 250 mg IM in a single dose
- Doxycycline 100 mg orally twice a day for seven days

Bloody discharge, perianal ulcers, or mucosal ulcers among MSM with acute proctitis and either a positive rectal chlamydia NAAT or HIV infection should be offered presumptive treatment for LGV with doxycycline 100 mg twice daily orally for a total of three weeks. If painful perianal ulcers are present or mucosal ulcers are detected on anoscopy, presumptive therapy should also include a regimen for genital herpes.

Other Management Considerations

To minimize transmission and reinfection, men treated for acute proctitis should be instructed to abstain from sexual intercourse until they and their partner(s) have been adequately treated (i.e., until completion of a seven-day regimen and symptoms resolved). All persons with acute proctitis should be tested for HIV and syphilis.

Follow-Up

Follow-up should be based on specific etiology and severity of clinical symptoms. For proctitis associated with gonorrhea or chlamydia, retesting for the respective pathogen should be performed three months after treatment.

Management of Sex Partners

Partners who have had sexual contact with persons treated for gas chromatography (GC), computed tomography (CT), or LGV within the 60 days before the onset of the person's symptoms should be evaluated, tested, and presumptively treated for the respective pathogen. Partners of persons with sexually transmitted enteric infections should be evaluated for any diseases diagnosed in a person with acute proctitis. Sex partners should abstain from sexual intercourse until they and their partner with acute proctitis are adequately treated.

Allergy, Intolerance, and Adverse Reactions

Allergic reactions with third-generation cephalosporins (e.g., ceftriaxone) are uncommon in persons with a history of penicillin allergy. In those persons with a history of an Immunoglobulin E (IgE)-mediated penicillin allergy (e.g., those who have had anaphylaxis, Stevens-Johnson syndrome, or toxic epidermal necrolysis), the use of ceftriaxone is contraindicated.

Human Immunodeficiency Virus Infection

Persons with HIV infection and acute proctitis may present with bloody discharge, painful perianal ulcers, or mucosal ulcers. Presumptive treatment should include a regimen for genital herpes and LGV.

Section 21.7

Pubic Lice

This section includes text excerpted from "Pubic Lice," MedlinePlus,
National Institutes of Health (NIH), April 18, 2018.

Pubic lice (also called "crabs") are tiny insects which usually live
in the pubic or genital area of humans. They are also sometimes
found on other coarse body hair, such as hair on the legs, armpits,
mustache, beard, eyebrows, or eyelashes. Pubic lice on the eyebrows
or eyelashes of children or teens may be a sign of sexual exposure
or abuse.

Pubic lice are parasites, and they need to feed on human blood to
survive. They are one of the three types of lice that live on humans.
The other two types are head lice and body lice. Each type of lice
is different, and getting one type does not mean that you will get
another type.

How Do Pubic Lice Spread and What Are the Symptoms?

- Pubic lice move by crawling because they cannot hop or fly. They
  usually spread through sexual contact. Occasionally, they may
  spread through physical contact with a person who has pubic
  lice, or through contact with clothing, beds, bed linens, or towels
  that were used by a person with pubic lice. You cannot get pubic
  lice from animals.

- The most common symptom of pubic lice is intense itching in the
  genital area. You may also see nits (lice eggs) or crawling lice.

How Do You Know If You Have Pubic Lice?

A diagnosis of pubic lice usually comes from seeing a louse or nit.
But lice and nits can be difficult to find because there may be only a
few present. Also, they often attach themselves to more than one hair,
and they do not crawl as quickly as head and body lice. Sometimes it
takes a magnifying lens to see the lice or nits.

People who have pubic lice should also be checked for other sexually
transmitted diseases (STD), and their sexual partners should also be
checked for pubic lice.

What Are the Treatments for Pubic Lice?

The main treatment for pubic lice is a lice-killing lotion. Options include a lotion that contains permethrin or a mousse containing pyrethrins and piperonyl butoxide (PBO). These products are available over-the-counter (OTC) without a prescription. They are safe and effective when you use them according to the instructions. Usually, one treatment will get rid of the lice. If not, you may need another treatment after 9 to 10 days.

There are other lice-killing medicines that are available with a prescription from your healthcare provider.

You should also wash your clothes, bedding, and towels with hot water, and dry them using the hot cycle of the dryer.

Section 21.8

Scabies

This section includes text excerpted from "Scabies Frequently Asked Questions (FAQs)," Centers for Disease Control and Prevention (CDC), January 10, 2019.

Scabies is an infestation of the skin by the human itch mite (*Sarcoptes scabiei var. hominis*). The microscopic scabies mite burrows into the upper layer of the skin where it lives and lays its eggs. The most common symptoms of scabies are intense itching and a pimple-like skin rash. The scabies mite usually is spread by direct, prolonged, skin-to-skin contact with a person who has scabies.

Scabies is found worldwide and affects people of all races and social classes. Scabies can spread rapidly under crowded conditions where close body and skin contact is frequent. Institutions such as nursing homes, extended-care facilities, and prisons are often sites of scabies outbreaks; child-care facilities also are a common site of scabies infestations.

What Is Crusted (Norwegian) Scabies?

Crusted scabies is a severe form of scabies that can occur in some persons who are immunocompromised (have a weak immune system) and the elderly, disabled, or debilitated. It is also called "Norwegian scabies." Persons with crusted scabies have thick crusts of skin that contain large numbers of scabies mites and eggs. Persons with crusted scabies are very contagious to other persons and can spread the infestation easily both by direct skin-to-skin contact and by contamination of items such as their clothing, bedding, and furniture. Persons with crusted scabies may not show the usual signs and symptoms of scabies, such as the characteristic rash or itching (pruritus). Persons with crusted scabies should receive quick and aggressive medical treatment for their infestation to prevent outbreaks of scabies.

How Soon after Infestation Do Symptoms of Scabies Begin?

If a person has never had scabies before, symptoms may take as long as four to six weeks to begin. It is important to remember that an infested person can spread scabies during this time, even if he or she does not have symptoms yet.

In a person who has had scabies before, symptoms usually appear much sooner (one to four days) after exposure.

What Are the Signs and Symptoms of Scabies Infestation?

The most common signs and symptoms of scabies are intense itchings (pruritus), especially at night, and a pimple-like (papular) itchy rash. The itching and rash each may affect much of the body or be limited to common sites, such as the wrist, elbow, armpit, webbing between the fingers, nipple, penis, waist, belt-line, and buttocks. The rash also can include tiny blisters (vesicles) and scales. Scratching the rash can cause skin sores; sometimes these sores become infected by bacteria.

Tiny burrows sometimes are seen on the skin; these are caused by the female scabies mite tunneling just beneath the surface of the skin. These burrows appear as tiny raised and crooked (serpiginous) grayish-white or skin-colored lines on the skin surface. Because mites are often few in number (only 10 to 15 mites per person), these burrows may be difficult to find. They are found most often in the webbing between the fingers, in the skin folds on the wrist, elbow, or knee, and on the penis, breast, or shoulder blades.

The head, face, neck, palms, and soles often are involved in infants and very young children, but usually not in adults and older children.

Persons with crusted scabies may not show the usual signs and symptoms of scabies, such as the characteristic rash or itching (pruritus).

How Did I Get Scabies?

Scabies usually is spread by direct, prolonged, skin-to-skin contact with a person who has scabies. Contact generally must be prolonged; a quick handshake or hug usually will not spread scabies. Scabies is spread easily to sexual partners and household members. Scabies in adults frequently is contracted through skin-on-skin sexual contact. Scabies sometimes is spread indirectly by sharing articles of clothing, towels, or bedding used by an infested person; however, such indirect spread can occur much more easily when the infested person has crusted scabies.

How Is Scabies Infestation Diagnosed?

Diagnosis of a scabies infestation usually is made based on the customary appearance and distribution of the rash and the presence of burrows. Whenever possible, the diagnosis of scabies should be confirmed by identifying the mite, mite eggs, or mite fecal matter (scybala). This can be done by carefully removing a mite from the end of its burrow using the tip of a needle or by obtaining skin scraping to examine under a microscope for mites, eggs, or mite fecal matter. It is important to remember that a person can still be infested even if mites, eggs, or fecal matter cannot be found; typically fewer than 10 to 15 mites can be present on the entire body of an infested person who is otherwise healthy. However, persons with crusted scabies can be infested with thousands of mites and should be considered highly contagious.

How Long Can Scabies Mites Live?

On a person, scabies mites can live for as long as 1 to 2 months. Off a person, scabies mites usually do not survive more than 48 to 72 hours. Scabies mites will die if exposed to a temperature of 50°C (122°F) for 10 minutes.

Can Scabies Be Treated?

Yes. Products used to treat scabies are called "scabicides" because they kill scabies mites; some also kill eggs. Scabicides to treat human scabies are available only with a prescription; no "over-the-counter (OTC)" (nonprescription) products have been tested and approved for humans.

Always follow carefully the instructions provided by the doctor and pharmacist, as well as those contained in the box or printed on the label. When treating adults and older children, scabicide cream or lotion is applied to all areas of the body from the neck down to the feet and toes; when treating infants and young children, the cream or lotion also is applied to the head and neck. The medication should be left on the body for the recommended time before it is washed off. Clean clothes should be worn after treatment.

In addition to the infested person, treatment also is recommended for household members and sexual contacts, particularly those who have had prolonged skin-to-skin contact with the infested person. All persons should be treated at the same time in order to prevent reinfestation. Retreatment may be necessary if itching continues more than two to four weeks after treatment or if new burrows or rash continue to appear.

Never use a scabicide intended for veterinary or agricultural use to treat humans!

Who Should Be Treated for Scabies?

Anyone who is diagnosed with scabies, as well as her of his sexual partners and other contacts who have had prolonged skin-to-skin contact with the infested person, should be treated. Treatment is recommended for members of the same household as the person with scabies, particularly those persons who have had prolonged skin-to-skin contact with the infested person. All persons should be treated at the same time to prevent reinfestation.

Retreatment may be necessary if itching continues more than two-to-four weeks after treatment or if new burrows or rash continue to appear.

How Soon after Treatment Will I Feel Better?

If itching continues more than two to four weeks after initial treatment or if new burrows or rash continue to appear (if initial treatment includes more than one application or dose, then the two-to-four week time period begins after the last application or dose), retreatment with scabicide may be necessary; seek the advice of a physician.

Did I Get Scabies from My Pet?

No. Animals do not spread human scabies. Pets can become infected with a different kind of scabies mite that does not survive or reproduce on humans but causes mange in animals. If an animal with mange has close contact with a person, the animal mite can get under the person's skin and cause temporary itching and skin irritation. However, the animal mite cannot reproduce on a person and will die on its own in a couple of days. Although the person does not need to be treated, the animal should be treated because mites are harmful to animals and can continue to burrow into the person's skin and cause symptoms until the animal has been treated successfully.

Can Scabies Be Spread by Swimming in a Public Pool?

Scabies is spread by prolonged skin-to-skin contact with a person who has scabies. Scabies sometimes also can be spread by contact with items such as clothing, bedding, or towels that have been used by a person with scabies, but such spread is very uncommon unless the infested person has crusted scabies.

Scabies is very unlikely to be spread by water in a swimming pool. Except for a person with crusted scabies, only about 10 to 15 scabies mites are present on an infested person; it is extremely unlikely that any would emerge from under wet skin.

Although uncommon, scabies can be spread by sharing a towel or item of clothing that has been used by a person with scabies.

How Can I Remove Scabies Mites from My House or Carpet?

Scabies mites do not survive more than two to three days away from human skin. Items such as bedding, clothing, and towels used by a person with scabies can be decontaminated by machine washing in hot water and drying using the hot cycle, or by dry cleaning. Items that cannot be washed or dry cleaned can be decontaminated by removing from any body contact for at least 72 hours.

Because persons with crusted scabies are considered very infectious, careful vacuuming of furniture and carpets in rooms used by these persons is recommended.

Fumigation of living areas is unnecessary.

How Can I Remove Scabies Mites from My Clothes?

Scabies mites do not survive more than two to three days away from human skin. Items such as bedding, clothing, and towels used by a person with scabies can be decontaminated by machine washing in hot water and drying using the hot cycle, or by dry cleaning. Items that cannot be washed or dry cleaned can be decontaminated by removing from any body contact for at least 72 hours.

My Spouse and I Were Diagnosed with Scabies. After Several Treatments, She/he Still Has Symptoms While I Am Cured. Why?

The rash and itching of scabies can persist for several weeks to a month after treatment, even if the treatment was successful and all the mites and eggs have been killed. Your healthcare provider may prescribe additional medication to relieve itching if it is severe. Symptoms that persist for longer than two weeks after treatment can be due to a number of reasons, including:

- Incorrect diagnosis of scabies. Many drug reactions can mimic the symptoms of scabies and cause a skin rash and itching; the diagnosis of scabies should be confirmed by a skin scraping that includes observing the mite, eggs, or mite feces (scybala) under a microscope. If you are sleeping in the same bed with your spouse and have not become reinfested, and you have not retreated yourself for at least 30 days, then it is unlikely that your spouse has scabies.

- Reinfestation with scabies from a family member or other infested person if all patients and their contacts are not treated at the same time; infested persons and their contacts must be treated at the same time to prevent reinfestation.

- Treatment failure caused by resistance to medication, by a faulty application of topical scabicides, or by failure to do a second application when necessary; no new burrows should appear 24 to 48 hours after effective treatment.

- Treatment failure of crusted scabies because of poor penetration of scabicide into thick scaly skin containing large numbers of scabies mites; repeated treatment with a combination of both topical and oral medication may be necessary to treat crusted scabies successfully.

- Reinfestation from items (fomites) such as clothing, bedding, or towels that were not appropriately washed or dry cleaned (this is mainly of concern for items used by persons with crusted scabies); potentially contaminated items (fomites) should be machine washed in hot water and dried using the hot temperature cycle, dry cleaned, or removed from skin contact for at least 72 hours.

- An allergic skin rash (dermatitis); or exposure to household mites that cause symptoms to persist because of cross-reactivity between mite antigens.

If itching continues more than two to four weeks or if new burrows or rash continue to appear, seek the advice of a physician; retreatment with the same or a different scabicide may be necessary.

If I Come in Contact with a Person Who Has Scabies, Should I Treat Myself?

No. If a person thinks he or she might have scabies, that person should contact a doctor. The doctor can examine the person, confirm the diagnosis of scabies, and prescribe an appropriate treatment. Products used to treat scabies in humans are available only with a doctor's prescription.

Sleeping with or having sex with any scabies-infested person presents a high risk of transmission. The longer a person has skin-to-skin exposure, the greater the likelihood for transmission to occur. Although briefly shaking hands with a person who has noncrusted scabies could be considered as presenting a relatively low risk, holding the hand of a person with scabies for five to ten minutes could be considered to present a relatively high risk of transmission. However, transmission can occur even after brief skin-to-skin contact, such as a handshake, with a person who has crusted scabies. In general, a person who has skin-to-skin contact with a person who has crusted scabies would be considered a good candidate for treatment.

To determine when prophylactic treatment should be given to reduce the risk of transmission, early consultation should be sought with a healthcare provider who understands:

- The type of scabies (i.e., noncrusted versus crusted) to which a person has been exposed;

- The degree and duration of skin exposure that a person has had to the infested patient;

- Whether the exposure occurred before or after the patient was treated for scabies; and,

- Whether the exposed person works in an environment where exposure to other people during the asymptomatic incubation period is likely. For example, a nurse or caretaker who works in a nursing home or hospital often would be treated prophylactically to reduce the risk of further scabies transmission in the facility.

Chapter 22

Cervicitis

Inflammation of the cervix is called "cervicitis." Two major diagnostic signs characterize cervicitis:

- A purulent or mucopurulent endocervical exudate visible in the endocervical canal or on an endocervical swab specimen (commonly referred to as mucopurulent cervicitis)

- Sustained endocervical bleeding easily induced by gentle passage of a cotton swab through the cervical os. Either or both signs might be present.

Cervicitis frequently is asymptomatic, but some women complain of an abnormal vaginal discharge and intermenstrual vaginal bleeding (e.g., after sexual intercourse). A finding of leukorrhea (more than 10 white blood cells (WBC) per high-power field on microscopic examination of vaginal fluid) has been associated with chlamydial and gonococcal infection of the cervix. In the absence of the major diagnostic signs of inflammatory vaginitis, leukorrhea might be a sensitive indicator of cervical inflammation with a high negative predictive value (i.e., cervicitis is unlikely in the absence of leucorrhea).

Etiology

When an etiologic organism is isolated in the presence of cervicitis, it is typically *C. trachomatis* or *N. gonorrhoeae*. Cervicitis also

This chapter includes text excerpted from "Diseases Characterized by Urethritis and Cervicitis," Centers for Disease Control and Prevention (CDC), June 4, 2015. Reviewed February 2019.

can accompany trichomoniasis and genital herpes (especially primary HSV-2 infection). However, in most cases of cervicitis, no organism is isolated, especially in women at relatively low risk for recent acquisition of these STDs (e.g., women 30 or more years old). Limited data indicate that infection with *M. genitalium* or bacterial vaginosis (BV) and frequent douching might cause cervicitis. For reasons that are unclear, cervicitis can persist despite repeated courses of antimicrobial therapy. Because most persistent cases of cervicitis are not caused by recurrent or reinfection with *C. trachomatis* or *N. gonorrhoeae*, other factors (e.g., persistent abnormality of vaginal flora, douching [or exposure to other types of chemical irritants], or idiopathic inflammation in the zone of ectopy) might be involved.

Diagnostic Considerations

Because cervicitis might be a sign of upper genital-tract infection (endometritis), women with a new episode of cervicitis should be assessed for signs of pelvic inflammatory disease (PID) and should be tested for *C. trachomatis* and for *N. gonorrhoeae* with nucleic acid amplification testing; such testing can be performed on either vaginal, cervical, or urine samples. Women with cervicitis also should be evaluated for the presence of BV and trichomoniasis, and if these are detected, they should be treated. Because the sensitivity of microscopy to detect T. *vaginalis* is relatively low (approximately 50%), symptomatic women with cervicitis and negative microscopy for trichomonads should receive further testing (i.e., culture, nucleic-acid-amplification testing (NAAT) or other U.S. Food and Drug Administration (FDA)-approved diagnostic test). A finding of greater than 10 WBC per high-power field in vaginal fluid, in the absence of trichomoniasis, might indicate endocervical inflammation caused specifically by *C. trachomatis* or *N. gonorrhoeae*. Although HSV-2 infection has been associated with cervicitis, the utility of specific testing (i.e., PCR, culture or serologic testing) for HSV-2 is unknown. FDA-cleared diagnostic tests for *M. genitalium* are not available.

Treatment

Several factors should affect the decision to provide presumptive therapy for cervicitis. Presumptive treatment with antimicrobials for *C. trachomatis* and *N. gonorrhoeae* should be provided for women at increased risk (e.g., those less than 25 years of age and those with a new sex partner, a sex partner with concurrent partners, or a sex partner who has a sexually transmitted infection), especially if follow up cannot be ensured or if testing with NAAT is not possible. Trichomoniasis and BV should also be treated if detected. For women at lower risk of STDs, deferring treatment until results of diagnostic tests are available is an option. If treatment is deferred and NAATs for *C. trachomatis* and *N. gonorrhoeae* are negative, a follow-up visit to see if the cervicitis has resolved can be considered.

Other Considerations

To minimize transmission and reinfection, women treated for cervicitis should be instructed to abstain from sexual intercourse until they and their partner(s) have been adequately treated (i.e., for seven days after single-dose therapy or until completion of a seven-day regimen) and symptoms have resolved. Women who receive a diagnosis of cervicitis should be tested for human immunodeficiency virus (HIV) and syphilis.

Follow-Up

Women receiving treatment should return to their provider for a follow-up visit, allowing the provider to determine whether cervicitis has resolved. For women who are not treated, a follow-up visit gives providers an opportunity to communicate the results of tests obtained as part of the cervicitis evaluation. Additional follow-up should be conducted as recommended for the infections identified. Women with a specific diagnosis of chlamydia, gonorrhea, or trichomonas should be offered partner services and instructed to return in months after treatment for repeat testing because of high rates of reinfection, regardless of whether their sex partners were treated. If symptoms persist or recur, women should be instructed to return for re-evaluation.

Persistent or Recurrent Cervicitis

Women with persistent or recurrent cervicitis despite having been treated should be reevaluated for possible re-exposure or treatment failure to gonorrhea or chlamydia. If relapse and/or reinfection with a specific STD have been excluded, BV is not present, and sex partners have been evaluated and treated, management options for persistent cervicitis are undefined; in addition, the utility of repeated or prolonged administration of antibiotic therapy for persistent symptomatic cervicitis remains unknown. The etiology of persistent cervicitis, including the potential role of *M. genitalium*, is unclear. *M. genitalium* might be considered for cases of clinically significant cervicitis that persist after azithromycin or doxycycline therapy in which re-exposure to an infected partner or medical nonadherence is unlikely. In settings with validated assays, women with persistent cervicitis could be tested for *M. genitalium* with the decision to treat with moxifloxacin based on results of diagnostic testing. In treated women with persistent symptoms that are clearly attributable to cervicitis, referral to a gynecologic specialist can be considered.

Special Considerations
HIV Infection

Women with cervicitis and HIV infection should receive the same treatment regimen as those who are HIV negative. Cervicitis increases cervical HIV shedding. Treatment of cervicitis in women with HIV infection reduces HIV shedding from the cervix and might reduce HIV transmission to susceptible sex partners.

Pregnancy

Diagnosis and treatment of cervicitis in pregnant women does not differ from that in women that are not pregnant.

Chapter 23

Epididymitis

Acute epididymitis is a clinical syndrome consisting of pain, swelling, and inflammation of the epididymis that lasts six or fewer weeks. Sometimes the testis is also involved—a condition referred to as epididymo-orchitis. A high index of suspicion for spermatic cord (testicular) torsion must be maintained in men who present with a sudden onset of symptoms associated with epididymitis, as this condition is a surgical emergency.

Among sexually active men less than 35 years of age, acute epididymitis is most frequently caused by *C. trachomatis* or *N. gonorrhoeae*. Acute epididymitis caused by sexually transmitted enteric organisms (e.g., *Escherichia coli*) also occurs among men who are the insertive partner during anal intercourse. Sexually transmitted acute epididymitis usually is accompanied by urethritis, which frequently is asymptomatic. Other nonsexually transmitted infectious causes of acute epididymitis (e.g., Fournier's gangrene) are uncommon and should be managed in consultation with a urologist.

In men less than 35 years of age who do not report insertive anal intercourse, sexually transmitted acute epididymitis is less common. In this group, the epididymis usually becomes infected in the setting of bacteriuria secondary to bladder-outlet obstruction (e.g., benign prostatic hyperplasia (BPH)). In older men, nonsexually transmitted acute epididymitis is also associated with prostate biopsy, urinary-tract

---

This chapter includes text excerpted from "Epididymitis," Centers for Disease Control and Prevention (CDC), June 4, 2015. Reviewed February 2019.

instrumentation or surgery, systemic disease, and/or immunosuppression. Chronic epididymitis is characterized by a greater-than-six-week history of symptoms of discomfort and/or pain in the scrotum, testicle, or epididymis.

Chronic infectious epididymitis is most frequently seen in conditions associated with a granulomatous reaction; *Mycobacterium tuberculosis* (TB) is the most common granulomatous disease affecting the epididymis and should be suspected, especially in men with a known history of or recent exposure to tuberculosis (TB). The differential diagnosis of chronic noninfectious epididymitis sometimes termed "orchialgia/epididymalgia" is broad (i.e., trauma, cancer, autoimmune, and idiopathic conditions); men with this diagnosis should be referred to a urologist for clinical management.

Diagnostic Considerations

- Men who have acute epididymitis typically have unilateral testicular pain and tenderness, hydrocele, and palpable swelling of the epididymis. Although inflammation and swelling usually begin in the tail of the epididymis, it can spread to involve the rest of the epididymis and testicle.

- The spermatic cord is usually tender and swollen. Spermatic cord (testicular) torsion, a surgical emergency, should be considered in all cases, but it occurs more frequently among adolescents and in men without evidence of inflammation or infection.

- In men with severe, unilateral pain with sudden onset, those whose test results do not support a diagnosis of urethritis or urinary-tract infection, or men in whom the diagnosis of acute epididymitis is questionable, immediate referral to a urologist for an evaluation of testicular torsion is important because testicular viability might be compromised.

- Bilateral symptoms should raise suspicion of other causes of testicular pain.

Radionuclide scanning of the scrotum is the most accurate method to diagnose epididymitis, but it is not routinely available. Ultrasound should be primarily used for ruling out torsion of the spermatic cord in cases of acute, unilateral, painful scrotum swelling. However, because partial spermatic-cord torsion can mimic epididymitis on scrotal ultrasound when torsion is not ruled out by ultrasound, differentiation between spermatic-cord torsion and epididymitis must be made on the basis of clinical evaluation. Although ultrasound can demonstrate epididymal hyperemia and swelling associated with epididymitis, it provides minimal utility for men with a clinical presentation consistent with epididymitis, because a negative ultrasound does not alter clinical management. Ultrasound should be reserved for men with scrotal pain who cannot receive an accurate diagnosis by history, physical examination, and objective laboratory findings or if torsion of the spermatic cord is suspected.

All suspected cases of acute epididymitis should be evaluated for objective evidence of inflammation by one of the following point-of-care tests.

- Gram or methylene blue or gentian violet (MB/GV) stain of urethral secretions demonstrating two or greater WBC per oil-immersion field. These stains are preferred point-of-care (POC) diagnostic tests for evaluating urethritis because they are highly sensitive and specific for documenting both urethral inflammation and the presence or absence of gonococcal infection. Gonococcal infection is established by documenting the presence of WBC-containing intracellular Gram-negative or purple diplococci in urethral Gram stain or MB/GV smear, respectively.

- Positive leukocyte esterase test on first-void urine.

- Microscopic examination of sediment from a spun first-void urine demonstrating 10 or more WBC per high-power field.

All suspected cases of acute epididymitis should be tested for *C. trachomatis and for N. gonorrhoeae* by nucleic-acid amplification test (NAAT). Urine is the preferred specimen for NAAT testing in men. Urine cultures for chlamydia and gonococcal epididymitis are insensitive and are not recommended. Urine bacterial culture might have a higher yield in men with sexually transmitted enteric infections and in older men with acute epididymitis caused by genitourinary bacteriuria.

Treatment

To prevent complications and transmission of sexually transmitted infections, presumptive therapy is indicated at the time of the visit before all laboratory test results are available. Selection of presumptive therapy is based on risk for chlamydia and gonorrhea and/or enteric organisms. The goals of treatment of acute epididymitis are:

- Microbiologic cure of infection

- Improvement of signs and symptoms

- Prevention of transmission of chlamydia and gonorrhea to others

- A decrease in potential chlamydia/gonorrhea epididymitis complications (e.g., infertility and chronic pain)

Although most men with acute epididymitis can be treated on an outpatient basis, referral to a specialist and hospitalization should be considered when severe pain or fever suggests other diagnoses (e.g., torsion, testicular infarction, abscess, and necrotizing fasciitis) or when men are unable to comply with an antimicrobial regimen. Because high fever is uncommon and indicates a complicated infection, hospitalization for further evaluation is recommended.

Table 23.1. Recommended Regimens

For Acute Epididymitis Most Likely Caused by Sexually Transmitted Chlamydia and Gonorrhea
Ceftriaxone 250 mg IM in a single dose PLUS Doxycycline 100 mg orally twice a day for 10 days
For Acute Epididymitis Most Likely Caused by Sexually-Transmitted Chlamydia and Gonorrhea and Enteric Organisms (Men Who Practice Insertive Anal Sex)
Ceftriaxone 250 mg IM in a single dose PLUS Levofloxacin 500 mg orally once a day for 10 days OR Ofloxacin 300 mg orally twice a day for 10 days
For Acute Epididymitis Most Likely Caused by Enteric Organisms
Levofloxacin 500 mg orally once daily for 10 days OR Ofloxacin 300 mg orally twice a day for 10 days

Therapy including levofloxacin or ofloxacin should be considered if the infection is most likely caused by enteric organisms and gonorrhea has been ruled out by the gram, MB, or GV stain. This includes men who have undergone prostate biopsy, vasectomy, and other urinary-tract instrumentation procedures. As an adjunct to therapy, bed rest, scrotal elevation, and nonsteroidal anti-inflammatory drugs are recommended until fever and local inflammation have subsided. Complete resolution of discomfort might not occur until a few weeks after completion of the antibiotic regimen.

Other Management Considerations

Men who have acute epididymitis confirmed or suspected to be caused by *N. gonorrhoeae or C. trachomatis* should be advised to abstain from sexual intercourse until they and their partners have been adequately treated and symptoms have resolved. All men with acute epididymitis should be tested for other sexually transmitted diseases (STDs), including human immunodeficiency virus (HIV).

Follow-Up

Men should be instructed to return to their healthcare providers if their symptoms fail to improve within 72 hours of the initiation of treatment. Signs and symptoms of epididymitis that do not subside within three days require re-evaluation of the diagnosis and therapy. Men who experience swelling and tenderness that persist after completion of antimicrobial therapy should be evaluated for alternative diagnoses, including tumor, abscess, infarction, testicular cancer, tuberculosis, and fungal epididymitis.

Management of Sex Partners

Men who have acute sexually transmitted epididymitis confirmed or suspected to be caused by *N. gonorrhoeae or C. trachomatis* should be instructed to refer for evaluation, testing, and presumptive treatment all sex partners with whom they have had sexual contact within the 60 days preceding the onset of symptoms. If the last sexual intercourse was more than 60 days before onset of symptoms or diagnosis, the most recent sex partner should be treated. Arrangements should be made to link sexual partners to care. EPT and enhanced referral are effective strategies for treating female sex partners of men who have chlamydia or gonorrhea for whom linkage to care is anticipated to be delayed. Partners should be instructed to abstain from sexual intercourse until they and their sex partners are adequately treated and symptoms have resolved.

Special Considerations
Allergy, Intolerance, and Adverse Reactions

The cross-reactivity between penicillins and cephalosporins is less than 2.5 percent in persons with a history of penicillin allergy. The risk for penicillin cross-reactivity is highest with first-generation cephalosporins, but is negligible between most second-generation (cefoxitin) and all third-generation (ceftriaxone) cephalosporins. Alternative regimens have not been studied; therefore, clinicians should consult infectious-disease specialists if such regimens are required.

Human Immunodeficiency Virus Infection

Men with HIV infection who have uncomplicated acute epididymitis should receive the same treatment regimen as those who are HIV negative. Other etiologic agents have been implicated in acute epididymitis in men with HIV infection, including *cytomegalovirus* (CMV), *salmonella*, toxoplasmosis, *Ureaplasma urealyticum*, *Corynebacterium sp.*, *Mycoplasma sp.*, and *Mima polymorpha*. Fungi and *mycobacteria* also are more likely to cause acute epididymitis in men with HIV infection than in those who are immunocompetent

Chapter 24

Infertility Linked to Sexually Transmitted Disease Infection

"Infertility" is a term that describes when a couple is unable to achieve pregnancy after 1 year of having regular, unprotected sex, or after 6 months if the woman is older than 35 years of age.

The term "infertility" also is used to describe the condition of women who are able to get pregnant but unable to carry a pregnancy to term because of miscarriage (sometimes called clinical "spontaneous abortion"), recurrent pregnancy loss, stillbirth, or other problems.

Recurrent pregnancy loss is considered distinct from infertility. Although there may be some overlap, the causes of pregnancy loss, recurrent pregnancy loss, and stillbirth are often different from the causes of infertility.

This chapter contains text excerpted from the following sources: Text in this chapter begins with excerpts from "About Infertility and Fertility," *Eunice Kennedy Shriver* National Institute of Child Health and Human Development (NICHD), January 31, 2017; Text under the heading "Link between Sexually Transmitted Diseases or Sexually Transmitted Infections (STDs/STIs) and Infertility" is excerpted from "What Is the Link with Infertility?" *Eunice Kennedy Shriver* National Institute of Child Health and Human Development (NICHD), January 31, 2017; Text under the heading "STDs and Infertility" is excerpted from "STDs and Infertility," Centers for Disease Control and Prevention (CDC), October 13, 2013. Reviewed February 2019.

Link between Sexually Transmitted Diseases or Sexually Transmitted Infections and Infertility

In most cases, sexually transmitted diseases (STDs) and sexually transmitted infections (STIs) are linked to infertility primarily when they are left untreated.

For instance, chlamydia and gonorrhea are sexually transmitted bacterial infections that can be cured easily with antibiotics. Left untreated, 10 to 20 percent of chlamydial and gonorrheal infections in women can result in pelvic inflammatory disease (PID)—a condition that can cause long-term complications, such as chronic pelvic pain, ectopic pregnancy (pregnancy outside of the uterus), and infertility.

Additionally, infections with gonorrhea and chlamydia may not cause symptoms and may go unnoticed. These undiagnosed and untreated infections can lead to severe health consequences, especially in women, causing permanent damage to reproductive organs.

The Centers for Disease Control and Prevention (CDC) estimates that these infections cause infertility in at least 24,000 women each year. Although infertility is less common among men, it does occur. More commonly, untreated chlamydia and gonorrhea infections in men may cause epididymitis, a painful infection in the tissue surrounding the testicles, or urethritis, an infection of the urinary canal in the penis, which causes painful urination and fever.

Sexually Transmitted Diseases and Infertility

The CDC Recommends Chlamydia and Gonorrhea Screening of All Sexually Active Women Under 25.
Chlamydia and gonorrhea are important preventable causes of PID and infertility. Untreated, about 10 to 15 percent of women with chlamydia will develop PID. Chlamydia can also cause fallopian-tube infection without any symptoms. PID and "silent" infection in the upper genital tract may cause permanent damage to the fallopian tubes, uterus, and surrounding tissues, which can lead to infertility.

- An estimated 2.86 million cases of chlamydia and 820,000 cases of gonorrhea occur annually in the United States.

- Most women infected with chlamydia or gonorrhea have no symptoms.

The CDC recommends annual chlamydia and gonorrhea screening of all sexually active women younger than 25 years, as well as older women with risk factors such as new or multiple sex partners, or a sex partner who has a sexually transmitted infection.

Chapter 25

Neurosyphilis

Neurosyphilis is a disease of the coverings of the brain, the brain itself, or the spinal cord. It can occur in people with syphilis, especially if they are left untreated. Neurosyphilis is different from syphilis because it affects the nervous system, while syphilis is a sexually transmitted disease with different signs and symptoms. There are five types of neurosyphilis:

• **Asymptomatic neurosyphilis**—means that neurosyphilis is present, but the individual reports no symptoms and does not feel sick.

• **Meningeal neurosyphilis**—can occur between the first few weeks to the first few years of getting syphilis. Individuals with meningeal syphilis can have a headache, stiff neck, nausea, and vomiting. Sometimes there can also be a loss of vision or hearing.

• **Meningovascular neurosyphilis**—causes the same symptoms as meningeal syphilis but affected individuals also have strokes. This form of neurosyphilis can occur within the first few months to several years after infection.

• **General paresis**—can occur between 3 to 30 years after getting syphilis. People with general paresis can have personality or mood changes.

This chapter includes text excerpted from "Neurosyphilis Information Page," National Institute of Neurological Disorders and Stroke (NINDS), July 10, 2018.

• **Tabes dorsalis**—is characterized by pains in the limbs or abdomen, failure of muscle coordination, and bladder disturbances. Other signs include vision loss, loss of reflexes and sense of vibration, poor gait, and impaired balance. Tabes dorsalis can occur anywhere from 5 to 50 years after initial syphilis infection.

General paresis and tabes dorsalis are now less common than the other forms of neurosyphilis because of advances made in prevention, screening, and treatment. People with human immunodeficiency virus (HIV)/acquired immunodeficiency syndrome (AIDS) are at higher risk of having neurosyphilis.

Treatment

Penicillin, an antibiotic, is used to treat syphilis. Individuals with neurosyphilis can be treated with penicillin given by vein or by daily intramuscular injections for 10 to 14 days. If they are treated with daily penicillin injections, individuals must also take probenecid by mouth four times a day. Some medical professionals recommend another antibiotic called "ceftriaxone" for neurosyphilis treatment. This drug is usually given daily by vein, but can also be given by intramuscular injection. Individuals who receive ceftriaxone are also treated for 10 to 14 days. People with HIV/AIDS who get treated for neurosyphilis may have different outcomes than individuals without HIV/AIDS.

Prognosis

Prognosis can change based on the type of neurosyphilis and how early in the course of the disease people with neurosyphilis get diagnosed and treated. Individuals with asymptomatic neurosyphilis or meningeal neurosyphilis usually return to normal health. People with meningovascular syphilis, general paresis, or tabes dorsalis usually do not return to normal health, although they may get much better. Individuals who receive treatment many years after they have been infected have a worse prognosis. Treatment outcome is different for every person.

Chapter 26

Pelvic Inflammatory Disease

What Is Pelvic Inflammatory Disease?

Pelvic inflammatory disease (PID) is an infection of a woman's reproductive organs. The reproductive organs include the uterus (womb), fallopian tubes, ovaries, and cervix. PID can be caused by many different types of bacteria. Usually, PID is caused by bacteria from STIs. Sometimes PID is caused by normal bacteria found in the vagina.

Who Gets Pelvic Inflammatory Disease

PID affects about five percent of women in the United States. Your risk for PID is higher if you:

- Have had an STI

- Have had PID before

- Are younger than 25 and have sex. PID is most common in women 15 to 24 years old.

- Have more than one sex partner or have a partner who has multiple sexual partners

- Douche. Douching can push bacteria into the reproductive organs and cause PID. Douching can also hide the signs of PID.

This chapter includes text excerpted from "Pelvic Inflammatory Disease," Office on Women's Health (OWH), U.S. Department of Health and Human Services (HHS), August 30, 2018.

- Recently had an intrauterine device (IUD) inserted. The risk of PID is higher for the first few weeks only after insertion of an IUD, but PID is rare after that. Getting tested for STIs before the IUD is inserted lowers your risk for PID.

How Do You Get Pelvic Inflammatory Disease?

A woman can get PID if bacteria move up from her vagina or cervix and into her reproductive organs. Many different types of bacteria can cause PID. Most often, PID is caused by infection from two common STIs: gonorrhea and chlamydia. You can also get PID without having an STI. Normal bacteria in the vagina can travel into a woman's reproductive organs and can sometimes cause PID. Sometimes the bacteria travel up to a woman's reproductive organs because of douching. Do not douche. No doctor or nurse recommends douching.

What Are the Signs and Symptoms of Pelvic Inflammatory Disease?

Many women do not know they have PID because they do not have any signs or symptoms. When symptoms do happen, they can be mild or more serious.

Signs and symptoms include:

- Pain in the lower abdomen (this is the most common symptom)

- Fever (100.4°F or higher)

- Vaginal discharge that may smell foul

- Painful sex

- Pain when urinating

- Irregular menstrual periods

- Pain in the upper right abdomen (this is rare)

PID can come on fast, with extreme pain and fever, especially if it is caused by gonorrhea.

How Is Pelvic Inflammatory Disease Diagnosed?

To diagnose PID, doctors usually do a physical exam to check for signs of PID and test for STIs. If you think that you may have PID, see a doctor or nurse as soon as possible.

If you have pain in your lower abdomen, your doctor or nurse will check for:

- Unusual discharge from your vagina or cervix

- An abscess (collection of pus) near your ovaries or fallopian tubes

- Tenderness or pain in your reproductive organs

Your doctor may do tests to find out whether you have PID or a different problem that looks like PID. These can include:

- Tests for STIs, especially gonorrhea and chlamydia. These infections can cause PID.

- A test for a urinary-tract infection or other conditions that can cause pelvic pain

- Ultrasound or another imaging test so your doctor can look at your internal organs for signs of PID

A Pap test is not used to detect PID.

How Is Pelvic Inflammatory Disease Treated?

Your doctor or nurse will give you antibiotics to treat PID. Most of the time, at least two antibiotics that work against many different types of bacteria are used. You must take all of your antibiotics, even if your symptoms go away. This helps to make sure the infection is fully cured. See your doctor or nurse again two to three days after starting the antibiotics to make sure they are working.

Your doctor or nurse may suggest going into the hospital to treat your PID if:

- You are very sick

- You are pregnant

- Your symptoms do not go away after taking the antibiotics or if you cannot swallow pills. If this is the case, you will need IV antibiotics.

- You have an abscess in a fallopian tube or ovary

If you still have symptoms or if the abscess does not go away after treatment, you may need surgery. Problems caused by PID, such as chronic pelvic pain (CPP) and scarring, are often hard to treat. But sometimes they get better after surgery.

What Can Happen If Pelvic Inflammatory Disease Is Not Treated?

Without treatment, PID can lead to serious problems such as infertility, ectopic pregnancy, and chronic pelvic pain (pain that does not go away). If you think you may have PID, see a doctor or nurse as soon as possible.

Antibiotics will treat PID, but they will not fix any permanent damage done to your internal organs.

Can I Get Pregnant If I Have Had Pelvic Inflammatory Disease?

Maybe. Your chances of getting pregnant are lower if you have had PID more than once. When you have PID, bacteria can get into the fallopian tubes or cause inflammation of the fallopian tubes. This can cause scarring in the tissue that makes up your fallopian tubes. Scar tissue can block an egg from your ovary from entering or traveling down the fallopian tube to your uterus (womb). The egg needs to be fertilized by a man's sperm and then attach to your uterus for pregnancy to happen. Even having just a little scar tissue can keep you from getting pregnant without fertility treatment. Scar tissue from PID can also cause a dangerous ectopic pregnancy (a pregnancy outside of the uterus) instead of a normal pregnancy. Ectopic pregnancies are more than six times more common in women who have had PID compared with women who have not had PID. Most of these pregnancies end in miscarriage.

How Can I Prevent Pelvic Inflammatory Disease?

You may not be able to prevent PID. It is not always caused by an STI. Sometimes, normal bacteria in your vagina can travel up to your reproductive organs and cause PID.

But, you can lower your risk of PID by not douching. You can also prevent STIs by not having vaginal, oral, or anal sex.

If you do have sex, lower your risk of getting an STI with the following steps:

- **Use condoms and dental dams.** Condoms are the best way to prevent STIs when you have sex. Because a man does not need to ejaculate (come) to give or get STIs, make sure to put the condom on before the penis touches the vagina, mouth, or anus.

Other methods of birth control, such as birth control pills, shots, implants, or diaphragms, will not protect you from STIs.

- **Get tested.** Be sure you and your partner are tested for STIs. Talk to each other about the test results before you have sex.

- **Be monogamous.** Having sex with just one partner can lower your risk for STIs. After being tested for STIs, be faithful to each other. That means that you have sex only with each other and no one else.

- **Limit your number of sex partners.** Your risk of getting STIs goes up with the number of partners you have.

- **Do not douche.** Douching removes some of the normal bacteria in the vagina that protect you from infection. Douching may also raise your risk for PID by helping bacteria travel to other areas, such as your uterus, ovaries, and fallopian tubes.

- **Do not abuse alcohol or drugs.** Drinking too much alcohol or using drugs increases risky behavior and may put you at risk of sexual assault and possible exposure to STIs.

The steps work best when used together. No single step can protect you from every single type of STI.

Can Women Who Have Sex with Women Get Pelvic Inflammatory Disease?

Yes. It is possible to get PID, or an STI if you are a woman who has sex only with women.

Talk to your partner about her sexual history before having sex, and ask your doctor about getting tested if you have signs or symptoms of PID.

Chapter 27

Pregnancy Complications and Sexually Transmitted Diseases

How Do Sexually Transmitted Diseases and Sexually Transmitted Infections Affect Pregnancy?

Sexually transmitted diseases (STDs) and sexually transmitted infections (STIs) pose special risks for pregnant women and their infants. If a mother has an STD/STI, it is possible for the fetus or newborn to become infected. Some STDs/STIs, including chlamydia, gonorrhea, genital herpes, and cytomegalovirus (CMV) can be passed from mother to infant during delivery when the infant passes through an infected birth canal. A few STDs/STIs, including syphilis, human immunodeficiency virus (HIV) and CMV, can infect a fetus before birth during the pregnancy. It is important for a pregnant woman to be tested for STDs/STIs, including HIV infection and acquired immune

This chapter contains text excerpted from the following sources: Text under the heading "How Do Sexually Transmitted Diseases and Sexually Transmitted Infections Affect Pregnancy?" is excerpted from "How Do Sexually Transmitted Diseases and Sexually Transmitted Infections Affect Pregnancy?" *Eunice Kennedy Shriver* National Institute of Child Health and Human Development (NICHD), January 31, 2017; Text beginning with the heading "I'm Pregnant. Can I Get Sexually Transmitted Diseases?" is excerpted from "Sexually Transmitted Diseases (STDs)—Fact Sheet," Centers for Disease Control and Prevention (CDC), November 10, 2016.

deficiency syndrome (AIDS) and syphilis, as a part of her prenatal care. Early treatment decreases the chances that the infant will contract the disease. While not all STDs/STIs can be cured, the mother and her healthcare provider can take steps to protect her and her infant.

To reduce the chance of certain STDs/STIs spreading to the infant during delivery, the healthcare provider might recommend a cesarean delivery. In most hospitals, infants' eyes are routinely treated with an antibiotic ointment shortly after birth. This is to prevent blindness due to exposure to gonorrhea or chlamydia bacteria during delivery if the pregnant woman had an undetected infection.

STDs/STIs during pregnancy can also cause:

- Miscarriage

- Ectopic pregnancy (when the embryo implants outside of the uterus, usually in a fallopian tube)

- Preterm labor and delivery (before 37 completed weeks of pregnancy)

- Low birth weight

- Birth defects, including blindness, deafness, bone deformities, and intellectual disability

- Stillbirth

- Illness in the newborn period (first month of life)

- Newborn death

STDs/STIs are of special concern during pregnancy and pose significant health risks to unborn infants:

- **HIV/AIDS.** HIV can be passed from mother to infant during pregnancy before birth, at the time of delivery, or after birth during breastfeeding.

- **Gonorrhea.** If a pregnant woman has a gonorrheal infection, she may give the infection to her infant as the infant passes through the birth canal during delivery. This infection in an infant can cause eye infections, pneumonia, or infections of the joints or blood. Treating gonorrhea as soon as it is detected in pregnant women will reduce the risk of transmission.

- **Chlamydia.** Similar to a gonorrheal infection, a chlamydial infection at the time of delivery can lead to eye infections or pneumonia in the infant. However, chlamydial infection during pregnancy also has been associated with an increased risk of preterm birth and its complications.

- **Genital herpes**. Pregnant women newly infected with genital herpes late in pregnancy have a 30 percent to 60 percent chance of infecting the infant they carry. The risk of infection is particularly high during delivery. Herpes infections in newborns are serious and potentially life-threatening. Infection with the herpes virus during pregnancy or at the time of delivery can lead to brain damage, blindness, and damage to other organs.

- If a pregnant woman has had genital herpes in the past, there are medications that she can take to reduce the chance that she will have an outbreak and thus reduce the risk to her infant.

- If a woman has active herpes sores when preterm labor and delivery she goes into labor, the infant can be delivered by cesarean section to reduce the chance that the infant will come in contact with the virus.

- **Hepatitis B virus**. If a woman is infected with the hepatitis B virus during pregnancy, the virus also could infect her fetus. The likelihood of this occurrence depends on when the mother was infected. If the mother acquires the infection early in her pregnancy, the chance that the virus will infect her fetus is less than 10 percent. However, if the infection occurs later in her pregnancy, the risk goes up to 90 percent. Hepatitis B can be severe in infants and can threaten their lives. It also can lead to liver scarring, failure, and cancer, which can be fatal in up to 25 percent of cases. In addition, infected newborns have a very high risk of becoming carriers of the hepatitis B virus and can spread the infection to others.

- In some cases, if a woman is exposed to hepatitis B during pregnancy, she may be treated with a special antibody to reduce the likelihood that she will get the infection. All healthy infants should be vaccinated against hepatitis B to give them lifelong protection against the virus. Infants born to women with evidence of ongoing hepatitis B infection (hepatitis B surface antigen positive) should also receive hepatitis B hyperimmune globulin as soon as possible after birth.

- **Cytomegalovirus (CMV)** is a common virus present in many body fluids that can be spread through close personal contact, such as kissing or sharing eating utensils, as well as sexual contact. The virus is common in the general population and usually does not cause health problems. However, if an expectant mother acquires the virus for the first time during pregnancy, the risk is high that she will pass it on to her infant. Unfortunately, a pregnant woman may not even know she has the infection, and she may still pass the virus on to her infant. CMV in an infant can lead to serious illness, lasting disabilities, or death. Each year in the United States, an estimated 40,000 infants are born with CMV infection, causing an estimated 400 deaths and leaving about 8,000 infants with permanent disabilities, such as hearing or vision loss, or intellectual disability. Currently, routine screening for CMV in pregnancy is not recommended. Researchers are working on treatments for CMV and also vaccines to try to prevent new infections during pregnancy and to reduce the risk of transmission to the infant.

I'm Pregnant. Can I Get Sexually Transmitted Diseases?

Yes, you can. Women who are pregnant can become infected with the same STDs as women who are not pregnant. Pregnancy does not provide women or their babies any additional protection against STDs. Many STDs are "silent," or have no symptoms, so you may not know if you are infected. If you are pregnant, you should be tested for STDs, including HIV (the virus that causes AIDS), as a part of your medical care during pregnancy. The results of an STD can be more serious, even life-threatening, for you and your baby if you become infected while pregnant. It is important that you are aware of the harmful effects of STDs and how to protect yourself and your unborn baby against infection. If you are diagnosed with an STD while pregnant, your sex partner(s) should also be tested and treated.

How Can Sexually Transmitted Diseases Affect Me and My Unborn Baby?

STDs can complicate your pregnancy and may have serious effects on both you and your developing baby. Some of these problems may be seen at birth; others may not be discovered until months or years later. In addition, it is well known that infection with an STD can make it easier for a person to get infected with HIV. Most of these problems can be prevented if you receive regular medical care during pregnancy.

This includes tests for STDs starting early in pregnancy and repeated close to delivery, as needed.

Should I Be Tested for Sexually Transmitted Diseases during My Pregnancy?

Yes. Testing and treating pregnant women for STDs is a vital way to prevent serious health complications to both mother and baby that may otherwise happen with infection. The sooner you begin receiving medical care during pregnancy, the better the health outcomes will be for you and your unborn baby. Be sure to ask your doctor about getting tested for STDs. It is also important that you have an open, honest conversation with your provider and discuss any symptoms you are experiencing and any high-risk sexual behavior that you engage in, since some doctors do not routinely perform these tests. Even if you have been tested in the past, you should be tested again when you become pregnant.

Can I Get Treated for Sexually Transmitted Diseases While I'm Pregnant?

It depends. STDs, such as chlamydia, gonorrhea, syphilis, trichomoniasis, and BV can all be treated and cured with antibiotics that are safe to take during pregnancy. STDs that are caused by viruses, like genital herpes, hepatitis B, or HIV cannot be cured. However, in some cases, these infections can be treated with antiviral medications or other preventive measures to reduce the risk of passing the infection to your baby. If you are pregnant or considering pregnancy, you should be tested so you can take steps to protect yourself and your baby.

How Can I Reduce My Risk of Getting Sexually Transmitted Diseases While Pregnant?

The only way to avoid STDs is to not have vaginal, anal, or oral sex. If you are sexually active, you can do the following things to lower your chances of getting chlamydia:

• Be in a long-term mutually monogamous relationship with a partner who has been tested and has negative STD test results;

• Use latex condoms the right way every time you have sex.

Chapter 28

Vaginitis

Vaginitis is an inflammation or infection of the vagina that can cause itching, burning, pain, discharge, or bad odor. The vagina is the tube-like passage that connects the opening of the womb to the outside of a woman's body. It is sometimes called the "birth canal." There are several types of vaginitis, each with its own causes, symptoms, and treatments.

Vaginitis is different from vulvodynia, which describes chronic pain or discomfort of the vulva, the area outside the vagina. Whereas vulvodynia affects only the vulva, vaginitis affects the vagina and can also cause itching, burning, and pain on the vulva.

What Causes Vaginitis

Vaginitis is often caused by infections. Some vaginal infections are passed through sexual contact. Some infections occur if there is a change in the balance of organisms normally found in the vagina. For a majority of affected women, vaginitis is caused by one of these types of infection:

- **Bacterial vaginosis** (BV) is the most common vaginal infection in women of childbearing age. It occurs when there are too many harmful (bad) bacteria and too few protective (good) bacteria in the vagina.

This chapter includes text excerpted from "Vaginitis: Condition Information," *Eunice Kennedy Shriver* National Institute of Child Health and Human Development (NICHD), December 1, 2016.

- **Candida or "yeast" infection** occurs when too much Candida grows in the vagina. Candida is yeast, which is a type of fungus frequently present in the vagina.

- **Trichomoniasis.** Trichomoniasis is a sexually transmitted disease caused by a single-cell parasite.

Vaginitis has other causes, too. For instance, some women are sensitive or allergic to vaginal sprays, douches, spermicides, soaps, detergents, and fabric softeners. These products can cause burning, itching, and discharge, even if there is no infection. Women also can have vaginal irritation caused by the natural lessening in estrogen levels during breastfeeding and after menopause. A woman may have more than one cause of vaginitis at the same time.

What Are the Symptoms of Vaginitis?

Symptoms depend on the type of vaginitis a woman has:

- **BV** often causes a thin, milky discharge from the vagina that may have a "fishy" odor. It may also cause itching. Most women have no symptoms and only find out they have it during a routine gynecological exam.

- **Yeast infections** produce a thick, white discharge from the vagina that can look like cottage cheese. The discharge can be watery and often has no smell. Yeast infections usually cause the vagina and vulva to become itchy and red.

- **Trichomoniasis** can cause itching, burning, and soreness of the vagina and vulva, as well as burning during urination. Some women have a "frothy" gray-green discharge, which may smell bad. Many women have no symptoms.

How Do Healthcare Providers Diagnose Vaginitis?

To find out the cause of a woman's symptoms, the healthcare provider will

- Examine the vagina, the vulva, and the cervix (opening to the womb)

- Look for vaginal discharge, noting its color, qualities, and any odor

- Study a sample of vaginal fluid under a microscope

Other lab tests are also sometimes used to diagnose vaginitis

How Is Vaginitis Treated?

The treatment needed depends on the type of vaginitis a woman has. Some women try to treat symptoms on their own rather than see a doctor, but an exam and lab tests are needed to learn the specific type of vaginitis.

BV is treated with an antibiotic that gets rid of the harmful bacteria and leaves the good bacteria. Women need a prescription for this medicine. There is no over-the-counter (OTC) treatment for BV. Treatment is recommended for women with symptoms. During treatment, women should either not have sex or use a condom during sex.

Yeast Infections are usually treated with a topical cream or with medicine that is placed inside the vagina. A healthcare provider can write a prescription for most yeast-infection treatments. Although yeast-infection treatments can be purchased over the counter, women should see a healthcare provider to confirm the cause of vaginal symptoms. Medicines used to treat yeast infection will not cure other types of vaginitis.

Trichomoniasis and other sexually transmitted infections (STIs) need to be treated right away. Trichomoniasis is usually treated with a single-dose antibiotic medicine. Both a woman and her partner(s) need to be treated to prevent spreading the infection to others and to keep from getting it again. Some other STIs that cause vaginal discomfort cannot be cured, but their symptoms can be controlled with treatment.

Allergy or Sensitivity causes vaginitis and this can be treated by not using the product that causes symptoms. A woman's healthcare provider may also give her a medicated cream to relieve symptoms until the reaction goes away.

Can Vaginitis Lead to Other Health Problems?

Without treatment, symptoms of vaginitis can worsen. Some types of vaginitis can increase a woman's risk of other health problems.

BV increases a woman's risk of getting other sexually transmitted diseases, including human immunodeficiency virus (HIV), if she is exposed to the pathogens that cause them. BV also is associated with **PID**, a serious disease that can harm a woman's reproductive organs and cause infertility. Having BV increases a woman's risk of preterm labor and preterm birth. Women who have it also are more likely to get an infection after having surgery such as abortion or hysterectomy. **Trichomoniasis** increases a woman's risk of getting or spreading other sexually transmitted diseases (STDs) such as HIV. Trichomoniasis also may cause preterm labor or preterm birth.

Does Vaginitis Affect a Pregnant Woman and Her Infant?

Some types of vaginitis can cause problems during pregnancy. Pregnant women with BV are more likely to go into labor and give birth too early (preterm). Preterm infants may face a number of health challenges, including low birth weight and breathing problems. However, treating BV in women who are pregnant has not been consistently found to reduce rates of preterm birth. For this reason, most pregnant women without symptoms are not screened for BV. Evidence does not support routine screening for BV in asymptomatic pregnant women at high risk for preterm delivery. *Eunice Kennedy Shriver* National Institute of Child Health and Human Development (NICHD) scientists are trying to clarify the link between BV and pregnancy problems to help prevent them. Sexually transmitted types of vaginitis can be very harmful to a pregnant woman and her unborn child. Trichomoniasis can cause preterm labor and preterm birth. Some sexually transmitted infections can be passed from a mother to her infant before, during, or after birth. A pregnant woman should tell her doctor about symptoms of vaginitis. She also should get routine prenatal care, including screening tests for sexually transmitted infections.

Can Vaginitis Be Prevented?

These steps can help prevent vaginitis:

- Women who often get yeast infections may want to avoid clothes that hold in heat and moisture, such as pantyhose without a cotton lining, nylon panties, or tight jeans.

- Do not douche or use vaginal sprays because they can kill "good" bacteria or cause irritation.

- Practicing safe sex can help protect against sexually transmitted forms of vaginitis. Limiting the number of sex partners and using condoms are examples of safe sex.

Part Four

Sexually Transmitted Diseases Testing and Treatment Concerns

Chapter 29

Testing for Sexually Transmitted Diseases

Chapter Contents

Section 29.1

Talk. Test. Treat

This section includes text excerpted from "How YOU Can Talk. Test. Treat," Centers for Disease Control and Prevention (CDC), May 2, 2016.

The only way to avoid getting an sexually transmitted disease (STD) is to not have vaginal, anal, or oral sex. If you are sexually active, or thinking of becoming sexually active, it is important that you Talk. Test. Treat. to protect your health. Understanding what you can do to lower your risk of getting infected is the first step. After all, STD prevention begins with you.

Talk about Your Sexual Health and Sexually Transmitted Diseases

Talk openly and honestly to your partner(s) and your healthcare provider about sexual health and STDs.

Talk with your partner BEFORE having sex. Not sure how? You can check the next section of this chapter which have tips to help you start the conversation. Make sure your discussion covers several important ways to make sex safer:

- Talk about when you were last tested and suggest getting tested together. If you have an STD (like herpes or HIV), tell your partner.

- Agree to only have sex with each other.

- Use latex condoms and dental dams the right way every time you have sex.

Talk with your healthcare provider about your sex life, and ask what STD tests you should be getting and how often.

- Not all medical checkups include STD testing, so unless you discuss if you're being tested, you shouldn't assume that you have been.

- Vaccines for hepatitis B and HPV vaccine are available. Ask your doctor whether these are right for you.

Get Tested

Get tested. It's the only way to know for sure if you have an STD.

Many STDs don't cause any symptoms. If you're having sex, getting tested is one of the most important things you can do to protect your health.

Find out which STD tests the Centers for Disease Control and Prevention (CDC) recommends that you should get. And remember, pregnancy doesn't protect against STDs. If you're having sex, you're still at risk.

If you're not comfortable talking with your regular healthcare provider about STDs, find a clinic near you that provides confidential and free or low-cost testing. You can find one at the CDC website (gettested.cdc.gov).

Get Treated

If you test positive for an STD, work with your doctor to get the correct treatment.

Some STDs can be cured with the right medicine from your doctor. It's important that you take all of the medication your doctor prescribes. To make sure your treatment works:

- Don't share your medicine with anyone.

- Avoid having sex again until you and your sex partner(s) have each completed treatment.

Other STDs aren't curable, but they are treatable. Your doctor can talk with you about which medications are right for you.

Section 29.2

Sexually Transmitted Disease Testing: Conversation Starters

This section includes text excerpted from "STD Testing: Conversation Starters," Office of Disease Prevention and Health Promotion (ODPHP), U.S. Department of Health and Human Services (HHS), October 29, 2018.

It might be hard to talk to your partner about getting tested for sexually transmitted diseases (STDs), but it's important. Chances are your partner will be glad you brought it up.

How to Talk with a Partner about Getting Tested
Talk before You Have Sex

- "Let's get tested before we have sex. That way we can protect each other."

- "Many people who have an STD don't know it. Why take a chance when we can know for sure?"

There are other things you may want to talk to your partner about, such as:

- **Sexual history.** The number of partners you've had and what kind of protection you used (for example, condoms or dental dams)

- **Risk factors.** Risk factors such as whether you've had sex without a condom or used drugs with needles

Share the Facts

- "STDs that are found and treated early are less likely to cause long-term problems."

- "Getting tested is easy. Doctors and nurses can test your urine (pee) for chlamydia and gonorrhea, two of the most common STDs."

- "Getting tested can be fast, too. For some human immunodeficiency virus (HIV) tests, you get your results within 20 minutes."

- "If you want to get tested at home, you can buy a HIV home test online or at a store."

- "If you don't feel comfortable talking about STDs with your regular doctor, you can get tested at a clinic instead."

Show That You Care

- "I really care about you. I want to make sure we are both healthy."

- "I've been tested for STDs, including HIV. Are you willing to do the same?"

- "Let's get tested together."

Agree to Stay Safe

- "If we're going to have sex, using condoms and dental dams is the best way to protect us from STDs. Let's use condoms every time we have sex."

- "We can enjoy sex more if we know it's safe."

Section 29.3

Screening Recommendations

This section includes text excerpted from "STD and HIV Screening Recommendations," Centers for Disease Control and Prevention (CDC), June 30, 2014. Reviewed February 2019.

If you are sexually active, getting tested for sexually transmitted diseases (STDs) is one of the most important things you can do to protect your health. Make sure you have an open and honest conversation about your sexual history and STD testing with your doctor and ask whether you should be tested for STDs. If you are not comfortable talking with your regular healthcare provider about STDs, there are many clinics that provide confidential and free or low-cost testing.

Below is a brief overview of STD-testing recommendations.

- All adults and adolescents from ages 13 to 64 should be tested at least once for human immunodeficiency virus (HIV).

- Annual chlamydia screening of all sexually active women younger than 25 years, as well as older women with risk factors such as new or multiple sex partners, or a sex partner who has a sexually transmitted infection (STI).

- Annual gonorrhea screening for all sexually active women younger than 25 years, as well as older women with risk factors such as new or multiple sex partners, or a sex partner who has a STI.

- Syphilis, HIV, and hepatitis B screening for all pregnant women, and chlamydia and gonorrhea screening for at-risk pregnant women starting early in pregnancy, with repeat testing as needed, to protect the health of mothers and their infants.

- Screening at least once a year for syphilis, chlamydia, and gonorrhea for all sexually active gay, bisexual, and other men who have sex with men (MSM). MSM who have multiple or anonymous partners should be screened more frequently for STDs (e.g., at three- to six-month intervals).

- Sexually active gay and bisexual men may benefit from more frequent HIV testing (e.g., every three to six months).

- Anyone who has unsafe sex or shares injection-drug equipment should get tested for HIV at least once a year.

Section 29.4

How Healthcare Providers Diagnose Sexually Transmitted Diseases or Sexually Transmitted Infections

This section includes text excerpted from "Sexually Transmitted Disease (STD)" *Eunice Kennedy Shriver* National Institute of Child Health and Human Development (NICHD), January 31, 2017.

Any person who is sexually active should discuss her or his risk factors for sexually transmitted diseases (STDs) or sexually transmitted infections (STIs) with a healthcare provider and ask about getting tested. If you are sexually active, it is important to remember that you may have an STD/STI and not know it because many STDs/STIs do not cause symptoms. You should get tested and have regular checkups with a healthcare provider who can help assess and manage your risk, answer your questions, and diagnose and treat an STD/STI if needed.

Starting treatment quickly is important to prevent transmission of infections to other people and to minimize the long-term complications of STDs/STIs. Recent sexual partners should also be treated to prevent reinfection and further transmission.

Tests for Diagnosis of Sexually Transmitted Diseases and Sexually Transmitted Infections

Physical and Microscopic Examination

Some STDs/STIs may be diagnosed during a physical exam or through microscopic examination of a sore or fluid swabbed from the vagina, penis, or anus. This fluid can also be cultured over a few days to see whether infectious bacteria or yeast can be detected.

Pap Smear Tests

The effects of human papillomavirus (HPV), which causes genital warts and cervical cancer, can be detected in a woman when her healthcare provider performs a pap smear test and takes samples of cells from the cervix to be checked microscopically for abnormal changes.

Blood Tests

Blood tests are used to detect infections such as hepatitis A, B, and C or human immunodeficiency virus (HIV) or acquired immunodeficiency syndrome (AIDS).

Importance of Getting Tested

Because STDs are passed from person to person and can have serious health consequences, the health department notifies people if they have been exposed to certain STDs/STIs. Not all STDs/STIs are reported, though. If you receive a notice, it is important to see a healthcare provider, be tested, and start treatment right away.

Screening is especially important for pregnant women, because many STDs/STIs can be passed on to the fetus during pregnancy or delivery. During an early prenatal visit, with the help of her healthcare provider, an expectant mother should be screened for these infections, including HIV and syphilis. Some of these STDs/STIs can be cured with drug treatment, but not all of them. However, even if the infection is not curable, a pregnant woman can usually take measures to protect her infant from infection.

Section 29.5

Frequently Asked Questions on Sexually Transmitted Disease Testing

This section includes text excerpted from "Frequently Asked Questions—Get Tested," Centers for Disease Control and Prevention (CDC), August 4, 2014. Reviewed February 2019.

What Are Sexually Transmitted Diseases and Should I Be Tested?

The Centers for Disease Control and Prevention (CDC) estimates that there are approximately 19 million new sexually transmitted disease (STD) infections each year—almost half of them among young people 15 to 24 years of age. Most infections have no symptoms and often go undiagnosed and untreated, which may lead to severe health consequences, especially for women.

Knowing your STD status is a critical step to stopping STD transmission. If you know you are infected, you can take steps to protect yourself and your partners. Many STDs can be easily diagnosed and treated. If either you or your partner is infected, both of you may need to receive treatment at the same time to avoid getting reinfected.

What Is Human Immunodeficiency Virus and Should I Be Tested?

HIV stands for "human immunodeficiency virus." It is the virus that can lead to acquired immunodeficiency syndrome, or AIDS. Unlike some other viruses, the human body cannot get rid of HIV. That means that once you have HIV, you have it for life.

Only certain body fluids; blood, semen (cum), preseminal fluid (precum), rectal fluids, vaginal fluids, and breast milk from a person who has HIV can transmit HIV. These fluids must come in contact with a mucous membrane or damaged tissue or be directly injected into the bloodstream (from a needle or syringe) for transmission to occur. Mucous membranes are found inside the rectum, vagina, penis, and mouth. Early HIV infection often times has no symptoms. The only way to know if you are infected with HIV is to be tested. There is no effective cure that exists for HIV. However, with proper medical care, HIV can be controlled.

The CDC recommends that everyone between the ages of 13 and 64 get tested at least once as a part of their routine healthcare. People with higher risk factors, such as more than one sex partner, other STDs, gay and bisexual men, and individuals who inject drugs should be tested at least once a year.

How Do I Know if I Am at Risk to Get Human Immunodeficiency Virus?

Knowing your risk can help you make important decisions to prevent exposure to HIV. The CDC has developed the HIV Risk Reduction Tool (wwwn.cdc.gov/hivrisk) to help you know risk and for better understanding of how different prevention methods like using condoms or taking PrEP, can reduce your risk. Overall, an American has a 1 in 99 chance of being diagnosed with HIV at some point in his or her lifetime. However, the lifetime risk is much greater among some populations. If current diagnosis rates continue the lifetime risk of getting HIV is:

- 1 in 6 for gay and bisexual men overall
- 1 in 2 for African American gay and bisexual men
- 1 in 4 for Hispanic gay and bisexual men
- 1 in 11 for white gay and bisexual men
- 1 in 20 for African American men overall
- 1 in 48 for African American women overall
- 1 in 23 for women who inject drugs
- 1 in 36 for men who inject drugs

Your health behaviors also affect your risk. You can get or transmit HIV only through specific activities. HIV is commonly transmitted through anal or vaginal sex without a condom or sharing injection and other drug injection equipment with a person infected with HIV. Substance use can increase the risk of exposure to HIV because alcohol and other drugs can affect your decision to use condoms during sex.

What Is Viral Hepatitis and Should I Be Tested?

Viral Hepatitis refers to a group of viral infections that affect the liver. The most common types are:

- Hepatitis A
- Hepatitis B
- Hepatitis C

Hepatitis A, hepatitis B, and hepatitis C are diseases caused by three different viruses. Although each can cause similar symptoms, they have different modes of transmission and can affect the liver differently. Hepatitis A appears only as an acute or newly occurring infection and does not become chronic. People with hepatitis A usually improve without treatment. Hepatitis B and hepatitis C can also begin as acute infections, but in some people, the virus remains in the body, resulting in chronic disease and long-term liver problems. There are vaccines to prevent hepatitis A and B; however, there is not one for hepatitis C. Recommendations for testing depend on many different factors and on the type of hepatitis.

What Puts Me at Risk for Human Immunodeficiency Virus, Viral Hepatitis, and Sexually Transmitted Diseases?
HIV Risk

The most common ways HIV is transmitted in the United States is through anal or vaginal sex or sharing drug injection equipment with a person infected with HIV. Although the risk factors for HIV are the same for everyone, some racial/ethnic, gender, and age groups are far more affected than others.

Risks for Hepatitis A

Hepatitis A is usually spread when a person ingests fecal matter—even in microscopic amounts—from contact with objects, food, or drinks contaminated by the feces or stool of an infected person. Due to routine vaccination of children, hepatitis A has decreased dramatically in the United States. Although anyone can get hepatitis A, certain groups of people are at higher risk, including men who have sex with men, people who use illegal drugs, people who travel to certain international countries, and people who have sexual contact with someone who has hepatitis A.

Risk for Hepatitis B

Hepatitis B is usually spread when blood, semen, or another body fluid from a person infected with the hepatitis B virus enters the body of someone who is not infected. This can happen through sexual contact with an infected person or sharing needles, syringes, or other drug-injection equipment. Hepatitis B can also be passed from an infected mother to her baby at birth.

Among adults in the United States, hepatitis B is most commonly spread through sexual contact and accounts for nearly two-thirds of acute hepatitis B cases. Hepatitis B is 50 to 100 times more infectious than HIV.

Risk for Hepatitis C

Hepatitis C is usually spread when blood from a person infected with the hepatitis C virus enters the body of someone who is not infected. Today, most people become infected with the hepatitis C virus by sharing needles or other equipment to inject drugs. Hepatitis C was also commonly spread through blood transfusions and organ transplants prior to the early 1990's. At that time, widespread screening of the blood supply began in the United States, which has helped ensure a safe blood supply.

Sexually Transmitted Diseases Risk
Risks for Genital Herpes

Genital herpes is a common STD, and most people with genital herpes infection do not know they have it. You can get genital herpes from an infected partner, even if your partner has no herpes symptoms. There is no cure for herpes, but medication is available to reduce symptoms and make it less likely that you will spread herpes to a sex partner.

Risks for Genital Human Papillomavirus

HPV is so common that most sexually active people get it at some point in their lives. Anyone who is sexually active can get HPV, even if you have had sex with only one person. In most cases, HPV goes away on its own and does not cause any health problems. But when HPV does not go away, it can cause health problems such as genital warts and cancer. HPV is passed on through genital contact (such as vaginal and anal sex). You can pass HPV to others without knowing it.

Risks for Chlamydia

Most people who have chlamydia don't know it, since the disease often has no symptoms. Chlamydia is the most commonly reported STD in the United States. Sexually active females 25 years old and younger need testing every year. Although it is easy to cure, chlamydia can make it difficult for a woman to get pregnant if left untreated.

Risks for Gonorrhea

Anyone who is sexually active can get gonorrhea, an STD that can cause infections in the genitals, rectum, and throat. It is a very common infection, especially among young people ages 15 to 24 years. But it can be easily cured. You can get gonorrhea by having anal, vaginal, or oral sex with someone who has gonorrhea. A pregnant woman with gonorrhea can give the infection to her baby during childbirth.

Risks for Syphilis

Any sexually active person can get syphilis. It is more common among men who have sex with men. Syphilis is passed through direct contact with a syphilis sore. Sores occur mainly on the external genitals, anus, or in the rectum. Sores also can occur on the lips and in the mouth. A pregnant women with syphilis can give the infection to her unborn baby.

Risks for Bacterial Vaginosis

Bacterial vaginosis (BV) is common among women of childbearing age. Any woman can get BV, but women are at a higher risk for BV if they have a new sex partner, multiple sex partners, use an intrauterine device (IUD), and/or douche.

Risks for Trichomoniasis

Trichomoniasis is a common STD that affects both women and men, although symptoms are more common in women. You can get trichomoniasis by having vaginal sex with someone who has it. Women can acquire the disease from men or women, but men usually contract it only from women.

How Do I Protect Myself and My Partner(s) from Human Immunodeficiency Virus, Viral Hepatitis, and Sexually Transmitted Diseases?

Your life matters and staying healthy is important. It's important for you, the people who care about you, and your community. Knowing your HIV status gives you powerful information to help you take steps to keep you and your partners healthy. You should get tested for HIV, and encourage your partners to get tested too. For people who are sexually active, there are more tools available today to prevent HIV than ever before. The list below provides a number of ways that you can lower your chances of getting HIV. The more of these actions you take, the safer you can be.

- **Get tested and treated for other STDs and encourage your partners to do the same.** All adults and adolescents from ages 13 to 64 should be tested at least once for HIV and high-risk groups get tested more often. STDs can have long-term health consequences. They can also increase your chance of getting HIV or transmitting it to others. It is important to have an honest and open talk with your healthcare provider and ask whether you should be tested for STDs. Your healthcare provider can offer you the best care if you discuss your sexual history openly. Find an HIV/STD testing site.

- **Choose less risky sexual behaviors.** Oral sex is much less risky than anal or vaginal sex for HIV transmission. Anal sex is the highest-risk sexual activity for HIV transmission. If you are HIV-negative, insertive anal sex (topping) is less risky for getting HIV than receptive anal sex (bottoming). Sexual activities that do not involve the potential exchange of bodily fluids carry no risk for getting HIV (e.g., touching).

- **Use condoms and dental dams consistently and correctly.**

- **Reduce the number of people you have sex with.** The number of sex partners you have affects your HIV risk. The more partners you have, the more likely you are to have a partner with HIV whose viral load is not suppressed or to have a sex partner with a STD. Both of these factors can increase the risk of HIV transmission.

- **Talk to your doctor about pre-exposure prophylaxis (PrEP).** The CDC recommends that PrEP be considered for people who are HIV-negative and at substantial risk for HIV. For sexual transmission, this includes HIV-negative persons who are in an ongoing relationship with an HIV-positive partner. It also includes anyone who:

  - Is not in a mutually monogamous* relationship with a partner who recently tested HIV-negative

  - Is a gay or bisexual man who has had anal sex without a condom or been diagnosed with an STD in the past six months; or heterosexual man or woman who does not regularly use condoms during sex with partners of unknown HIV status who are at substantial risk of HIV infection (e.g., people who inject drugs or have bisexual male partners)

For people who inject drugs, this includes those who have injected illicit drugs in the past six months and who have shared injection

---

* *Mutually monogamous means that you and your partner only have sex with each other and do not have sex outside the relationship.*

equipment or been in drug treatment for injection drug use in the past six months.

- Talk to your doctor right away (within three days) about postexposure prophylaxis (PEP) if you have a possible exposure to HIV. An example of a possible exposure is if you have anal or vaginal sex without a condom with someone who is or may be HIV-positive, and you are HIV-negative and not taking PrEP. Your chance of exposure to HIV is lower if your HIV-positive partner is taking antiretroviral therapy (ART) consistently and correctly, especially if her or his viral load is undetectable. Starting medicine immediately (known as post-exposure prophylaxis, or PEP) and taking it daily for four weeks reduces your chance of getting HIV.

- If your partner is HIV-positive, encourage your partner to get and stay on treatment. ART reduces the amount of HIV virus (viral load) in blood and body fluids. ART can keep people with HIV healthy for many years, and greatly reduce the chance of transmitting HIV to sex partners if taken consistently and correctly.

Hepatitis Prevention

The best way to prevent both hepatitis A and B is by getting vaccinated. There is no vaccine available to prevent hepatitis C. The best way to prevent hepatitis C is by avoiding behaviors that can spread the disease, such as sharing needles or other equipment to inject drugs.

STD Prevention

The only way to avoid STDs is to not have vaginal, anal, or oral sex. If you are sexually active, you can do several things to lower your chances of getting an STD, including:

- **Get tested for STDs and encourage your partner(s) to do the same.** It is important to have an honest and open talk with your healthcare provider and ask whether you should be tested for STDs. Your healthcare provider can offer you the best care if you discuss your sexual history openly. Find an STD testing site.

- **Get vaccinated.** Vaccines are safe, effective, and recommended ways to prevent hepatitis A, hepatitis B, and HPV.

- **Be in a sexually active relationship with only one person**, who has agreed to be sexually active only with you.

- **Reduce your number of sex partners.** By doing so, you decrease your risk for STDs. It is still important that you and your partner get tested, and that you share your test results with one another.

- **Use a condom every time you have vaginal, anal, or oral sex.** Correct and consistent use of the male latex condom is highly effective in reducing STD transmission.

How Do Human Immunodeficiency Virus, Viral Hepatitis, and Sexually Transmitted Diseases Relate to Each Other?

Persons who have an STD are at least two to five times more likely than uninfected persons to acquire HIV infection if they are exposed to the virus through sexual contact. In addition, if a person who is HIV positive also has an STD, that person is more likely to transmit HIV through sexual contact than other HIV-infected persons.

Hepatitis B virus and HIV are blood-borne viruses transmitted primarily through sexual contact and injection drug use. Because of these shared modes of transmission, a high proportion of adults at risk for HIV infection are also at risk for HBV infection. HIV-positive persons who become infected with HBV are at increased risk for developing chronic HBV infection and should be tested. In addition, persons who are co-infected with HIV and HBV can have serious medical complications, including an increased risk for liver-related morbidity and mortality.

Hepatitis C virus (HCV) is one of the most common causes of chronic liver disease in the United States. For persons who are HIV infected, coinfection with HCV can result in a more rapid occurrence of liver damage and may also impact the course and management of HIV infection.

Chapter 30

Talking to Your Healthcare Professional about Sexually Transmitted Diseases

Chapter Contents

Section 30.1

Questions to Ask Your Doctor

This section includes text excerpted from "Questions to Ask Your Doctor," Agency for Healthcare Research and Quality (AHRQ), U.S. Department of Health and Human Services (HHS), September 2018.

Questions Are the Answer

Your health depends on good communication.

Asking questions and providing information to your doctor and other care providers can improve your care. Talking with your doctor builds trust and leads to better results, quality, safety, and satisfaction.

Quality healthcare is a team effort. You play an important role. One of the best ways to communicate with your doctor and healthcare team is by asking questions. Because time is limited during medical appointments, you will feel less rushed if you prepare your questions before your appointment.

Your Doctor Wants Your Questions

Doctors know a lot about a lot of things, but they don't always know everything about you or what is best for you.

Your questions give your doctor and healthcare team important information about you, such as your most important healthcare concerns. That is why they need you to speak up.

Before Your Appointment

You can make sure you get the best possible care by being an active member of your healthcare team. Being involved means being prepared and asking questions.

Asking questions about your diagnoses, treatments, and medicines can improve the quality, safety, and effectiveness of your healthcare.

Taking steps before your medical appointments will help you to make the most of your time with your doctor and healthcare team.

Prepare Your Questions

Time is limited during doctor visits. Prepare for your appointment by thinking about what you want to do during your next visit. Do you want to:

- Talk about a health problem?

- Get or change a medicine?

- Get medical tests?

- Talk about surgery or treatment options?

Write down your questions to bring them to your appointment. The answers can help you make better decisions, get good care, and feel better about your healthcare.

During Your Appointment

During your appointment, make sure to ask the questions you prepared before your appointment. Start by asking the ones that are most important to you.

To get the most from your visit, tell the nurse or person at the front desk that you have questions for your doctor. If your doctor does not ask you if you have questions, ask your doctor when the best time would be to ask them.

Understand the Answers and Next Steps

Asking questions is important but so is making sure you hear—and understand—the answers you get. Take notes. Or bring someone to your appointment to help you understand and remember what you heard. If you don't understand or are confused, ask your doctor to explain the answer again.

It is very important to understand the plan or next steps that your doctor recommends. Ask questions to make sure you understand what your doctor wants you to do.

The questions you may want to ask will depend on whether your doctor gives you a diagnosis; recommends a treatment, medical test, or surgery; or gives you a prescription for medicine.

Questions could include:

- What is my diagnosis?

- What are my treatment options? What are the benefits of each option? What are the side effects?

- Will I need a test? What is the test for? What will the results tell me?

- What will the medicine you are prescribing do? How do I take it? Are there any side effects?

321

- Why do I need surgery? Are there other ways to treat my condition? How often do you perform this surgery?

- Do I need to change my daily routine?

Find out what you are to do next. Ask for written instructions, brochures, videos, or websites that may help you learn more.

After Your Appointment

After you meet with your doctor, you will need to follow her or his instructions to keep your health on track.

Your doctor may have you fill a prescription or make an another appointment for tests, lab work, or a follow-up visit. It is important for you to follow your doctor's instructions.

It also is important to call your doctor if you are unclear about any instructions or have more questions.

Prioritize Your Questions

Create a list of follow-up questions to ask if you:

- Have a health problem

- Need to get or change a medicine

- Need a medical test

- Need to have surgery

Other Times to Call Your Doctor

There are other times when you should follow up on your care and call your doctor. Call your doctor:

- If you experience any side effects or other problems with your medicines

- If your symptoms get worse after seeing the doctor

- If you receive any new prescriptions or start taking any over-the-counter (OTC) medicines

- To get results of any tests you've had. Do not assume that no news is good news.

- To ask about test results you do not understand

Your questions help your doctor and healthcare team learn more about you. Your doctor's answers to your questions can help you make better decisions, receive a higher level of care, avoid medical harm, and feel better about your healthcare. Your questions can also lead to better results for your health.

Section 30.2

General Questions to Ask Your Healthcare Professional about Sexually Transmitted Diseases

"Talking to Your Healthcare Professional about STDs,"
© 2016 Omnigraphics. Reviewed February 2019.

Talking about Sexual Health

Talking to a healthcare professional about your sexual health may be highly intimidating and outside of your comfort zone. You may feel hesitant or scared to talk about it, but it is important to understand that talking with your healthcare professional about your sexual health is as important as talking about your physical health.

Why Should I talk to My Healthcare Provider about Sexually Transmitted Diseases?

The only way to be certain about whether or not you have a sexually transmitted disease (STD) is to talk to your healthcare professional about being tested for an STD. Many STD symptoms are nonspecific, meaning the symptoms could be caused by a number of STDs or a totally unrelated disease. Whether you have symptoms that lead you to believe you have an STD or if you are just unsure, the only way to be certain is to be tested specifically for an STD.

Talking to Your Healthcare Professional

When you meet with your healthcare professional, do not shy away from telling the truth. If necessary, set boundaries with your professional and let them know what you are comfortable with when dealing with and discussing your body.

By being honest and establishing trust with your healthcare professional you will help them diagnose the problem correctly, and provide you with the best possible treatment options. The good news is STDs are curable!

Questions to Ask Your Healthcare Professional

Preparing yourself before meeting your healthcare professional is very important. It will help you get a complete picture of your sexual health. Some possible questions you can ask your healthcare professional include:

- What is an STD? What should I do to be absolutely sure of preventing it?

- How will I know if I have an STD?

- Some of my symptoms points toward STD. Do I have an STD?

- How will I know if my partner has an STD?

- Should my partner and I get tested for STDs before having sex?

- How often should I check for sexually transmitted infections (STIs)?

- Can contraception or vaccines protect me from getting STDs?

- There is a change in my sex drive. Do you think I may have an STD?

- What are the recommended screenings for STDs? Where can I get them done?

- What are the costs for STDs testing? Does my insurance cover them?

- Are STDs curable?

- Should I notify my partner on my STD status?

- Can I get any help from Partner Services to notify my partner on my STD status?

- Can I recover completely with proper treatment?

Remember that your healthcare professional is there to help you. Their experience will help you deal with your problem.

References

1. "Ten Questions to Ask," American Sexual Health Association (ASHA), 2016.

2. "Know the Facts, Keep Yourself Healthy," Within Reach, 2015.

3. "Frequently Asked Questions about STDs," Vermont Department of Health, 2016.

4. "STD Testing," Healthline, 2014.

Section 30.3

For Teens: How Do I Discuss Embarrassing Things with My Doctor?

This section includes text excerpted from "Talking with your doctor," girlshealth.gov, Office on Women's Health (OWH), October 31, 2013. Reviewed February 2019.

Talking freely with your doctor can make you feel better and gives your doctor the information she or he needs to give you the best care. You can even discuss personal things about your health with your doctor. Don't be afraid or embarrassed to discuss something that is bothering you.

Tips for Talking with Your Doctor

Stay positive. Go to your doctor's visits with a good attitude. Remember, your doctor and other caregivers are on your side. Think teamwork! Think positive!

Keep track of how you are feeling. Before your doctor visit, keep notes on how you are feeling. This will make it easier for you to answer questions about your symptoms and how medicines make you feel. It also makes it easier for you to bring up anything that you are worried about. Make sure to be honest about how you feel and how long you've felt that way. Also, let your doctor know if you are you scared, worried, or sad. Your care will be better if your doctor knows how you are feeling. Your doctor can also tell you about counselors and support groups to help you talk about your feelings.

Bring your medical history, including a list of your current medicines. If you're seeing a doctor for the first time, bring your medical history. Your medical history is a list of your illnesses, dates of operations, treatments (including medicines), names of doctors you've seen, what the doctors told you to do, and anything else you think your doctor should know. If you take medicines that you buy at the pharmacy without a prescription (an order from the doctor), make sure to also include them in your list. That includes things like vitamins, herbal medicines, and aspirin. Also, if you are allergic to any medicines, such as penicillin, be sure to mention that to your doctor.

Ask questions. Do not be afraid to ask your doctor any questions you have. This will help you understand your own health better. Maybe you've been reading a lot about your health condition and that has caused you to think of some questions. To remember all the questions you have when you are not in the doctor's office, write them down and bring the list with you to your appointment. Be sure to talk with your parents about the things you want to ask the doctor. This will make getting answers even easier!

At your appointment, your doctor may talk about a new treatment that he or she wants you to try. It may involve medicine, surgery, changes in daily habits such as what you eat, or a few of these together. You will get the most out of your treatments if you understand what's involved and why you need them. In case your doctor talks about a new treatment at your next visit, here are some questions you can print or write down to take with you:

- How long will it take?

- What will happen? (Is it a shot, pill, or operation?)

- Will it hurt?

- How many treatments do I have to have?

- Will I be able to go to school?

- Are there things I won't be able to do, such as ride a bike?

- Is this treatment to try to cure my health problem or help take away some of my symptoms?

- Will these treatments make me tired or feel pain? How long will this last?

- What happens if I miss a treatment?

- What will we do if the treatments don't work?

- Is this the best treatment out there for me?

- What will happen to me if I don't have this treatment?

If the treatment you get makes you feel bad, ask if there are others you can try. There may not be others. But you and your doctor can talk about it.

Remember, there's no such thing as a stupid question. If you don't understand the answer to a question, ask the doctor to explain it again until you do understand.

Write down what the doctor says. This will help you remember important information later on. You might even bring a tape recorder and record what the doctor says. But if you bring a tape recorder, be sure to ask the doctor first if it's okay to use it.

Use a treatment planner to keep track of anything your doctor, counselor, or therapist tells you.

Talking about Personal Things

It's okay to be nervous about talking to your doctor about things that embarrass you. Who wants to talk to a strange adult about sex, feeling sad, or what you eat? But it's easier than you think. Doctors are there to talk about everything that is going on with your body. They will not think any less of you no matter what you ask or what your problem is. In fact, they are very used to personal issues (and they likely have had to seek help for their own!). Telling them everything that is going on with you is very important for your health. By not telling them about a strange smell, rash, pain, or anything else going on with your body, you could be making a health problem worse.

Talking about personal issues with your doctor can be confidential, which means that your doctor has to keep everything you say secret. Doctors might feel they have to tell your parents what you say if they think you are in danger or aren't able to make choices on your own. Ask your doctor about the privacy policy before you begin.

Chapter 31

Confidentiality Issues Associated with Sexually Transmitted Disease Testing

Chapter Contents

Section 31.1

Will Other People Know Your Test Result?

This section includes text excerpted from "Understanding HIV Test Results," HIV.gov, U.S. Department of Health and Human Services (HHS), May 14, 2018.

If you take an anonymous test, no one but you will know the result. If you take a confidential test, your test result will be part of your medical record, but it is still protected by state and federal privacy laws. Most testing is done confidentially.

- **Anonymous testing** means that nothing ties your test results to you. When you take an anonymous human immunodeficiency virus (HIV) test, you get a unique identifier that allows you to get your test results. These tests are not available at every place that provides HIV testing.

- **Confidential testing** means that your name and other identifying information will be attached to your test results. The results will go in your medical record and may be shared with your healthcare providers and your health insurance company. Otherwise, the results are protected by state and federal privacy laws, and they can be released only with your permission.

With confidential testing, if you test positive for HIV, the test result and your name will be reported to the state or local health department to help public-health officials get better estimates of the rates of HIV in the state. The state health department will then remove all personal information about you (name, address, etc.) and share the remaining nonidentifying information with the Centers for Disease Control and Prevention (CDC). The CDC does not share this information with anyone else, including insurance companies.

As a followup to a positive HIV test, the local health department may contact you to make sure that you received the test results and understood them, and to find out whether you received referrals to HIV medical care and social services and whether you have received HIV medical care and treatment. The health department representative may talk with you about the need to tell your sexual or needle-sharing partner(s) about their possible exposure to HIV. They may also offer partner services to assist you with these conversations. If you want, the health department can try to attempt to locate any or all of your partners to let them know they may have been exposed to HIV. They will be able to help them find a place to get tested and give them information about pre-exposure prophylaxis (or PrEP), postexposure prophylaxis (PEP), and other ways that they can protect themselves and access other prevention and care services.

If you are HIV-positive, it is important to disclose your HIV status to your healthcare providers (doctors, dentists, etc.) so that they can give you the best possible care. You may also consider disclosing your status to others.

Section 31.2

At-Home/Mail-Order Sexually Transmitted Disease Tests Protect Patient Confidentiality

This section includes text excerpted from "Information Regarding the Home Access HIV-1 Test System," U.S. Food and Drug Administration (FDA), March 7, 2018.

What Is the Home-Access Human Immunodeficiency Virus-1 Test System?

The Home-Access HIV-1 Test System is a laboratory test sold over-the-counter (OTC) that uses fingerstick blood mailed to the testing laboratory. The test kit consists of multiple components, including materials for specimen self-collection, prepaid materials for mailing the specimen to a laboratory for testing, testing directions, an information booklet ("Things You Should Know About HIV and AIDS"), an anonymous registration system, and a call center to receive your test results and follow-up counseling by telephone.

This approved system uses a finger-prick process for home blood collection which results in dried blood spots on special paper. The dried blood spots are mailed to a laboratory with a confidential and anonymous unique personal identification number (PIN) and are analyzed by trained clinicians in a laboratory using the same tests that are used for samples taken in a doctor's office or clinic. Test results are obtained through a toll-free telephone number using the PIN, and posttest counseling are provided by telephone when results are obtained.

When Should I Take a Test for Human Immunodeficiency Virus?

If you actively engage in behavior that puts you at risk for HIV infection, or your partner engages in such behavior, then you should consider testing on a regular basis. It may take some time for the immune system to produce sufficient antibodies for the test to detect, and this time period can vary from person to person. This time frame is commonly referred to as the "window period," when a person is infected with HIV but antibodies to the virus cannot be detected, however, the person may be able to infect others. According to the Centers for Disease Control and Prevention (CDC), it can take up to six months to develop antibodies to HIV, although most people (97%) will develop detectable antibodies in the first three months following the time of their infection.

How Reliable Is the Home-Access Human Immunodeficiency Virus-1 Test System?

Clinical studies reported to the U.S. Food and Drug Administration (FDA) showed that the sensitivity (i.e., the percentage of results that will be positive when HIV is present) was estimated to be greater than 99.9 percent. The specificity (i.e., the percentage of results that will be negative when HIV is not present) was also estimated to be greater than 99.9 percent. Results reported as positive have undergone testing using both a screening test and another test to confirm the positive result.

What about Counseling

The Home-Access HIV-1 Test System has a built-in mechanism for pretest and posttest counseling provided by the manufacturer. This counseling is anonymous and confidential. Counseling, which uses both printed material and telephone interaction, provides the user with an interpretation of the test result. Counseling also provides information on how to keep from getting infected if you are negative, and how to prevent further transmission of disease if you are infected. Counseling provides you with information about treatment options if you are infected, and can even provide referrals to doctors who treat HIV-infected individuals in your area.

If the Test Results Are Positive, What Should I Do?

The counselors can provide you with information about treatment options and referrals to doctors who treat HIV-infected individuals in your area.

Do I Need a Confirmatory Test?

No, a positive result from the Home-Access HIV-1 Test System means that antibodies to the HIV-1 virus are present in the blood sample submitted to the testing laboratory. The Home-Access HIV-1 Test System includes confirmatory testing for HIV-1, and all confirmation testing is completed before the results are released and available to users of the test system.

How Quickly Will I Get the Results of the Home-Access Human Immunodeficiency Virus-1 Test System?

You can anonymously call for the results approximately seven business days (three business days for the Express System) after shipping your specimen to the laboratory by using the unique PIN on the tear-off label included with your test kit. This label includes both the unique PIN and the toll-free number for the counseling center.

How Are Unapproved Test Systems Different?

The manufacturers of unapproved test systems have not submitted data to the FDA to review to determine whether or not their test systems can reliably detect HIV infection. Therefore, the FDA cannot give the public any assurance that the results obtained using an unapproved test system are accurate.

Chapter 32

Is There a Cure for Sexually Transmitted Diseases or Sexually Transmitted Infections?

Viruses such as human immunodeficiency virus (HIV), genital herpes, human papillomavirus (HPV), hepatitis, and cytomegalovirus cause sexually transmitted diseases (STDs) or sexually transmitted infections (STIs) that cannot be cured. People with an STI caused by a virus will be infected for life and will always be at risk of infecting their sexual partners. However, treatments for these viruses can significantly reduce the risk of passing on the infection and can reduce or eliminate symptoms. STIs caused by bacteria, yeast, or parasites can be cured using appropriate medication.

What Are the Treatments for Sexually Transmitted Diseases and Sexually Transmitted Infections?

STDs/STIs caused by bacteria or parasites can be treated with antibiotics. These antibiotics are most often given by mouth (orally).

This chapter includes text excerpted from "Sexually Transmitted Disease (STD)," *Eunice Kennedy Shriver* National Institute of Child Health and Human Development (NICHD), January 31, 2017.

However, sometimes they are injected or applied directly to the affected area.

The treatments, complications, and outcomes for viral STIs depend on the particular virus (HIV, genital herpes, HPV, hepatitis, or cytomegalovirus). Treatments can reduce the symptoms and the progression of most of these infections. For example, medications are available to limit the frequency and severity of genital herpes outbreaks while reducing the risk that the virus will be passed on to other people.

Individuals with HIV need to take special antiretroviral drugs that control the amount of virus they carry. These drugs, called "highly active antiretroviral therapy," or "HAART," can help people live longer, healthier lives and can prevent onward transmission of HIV to others. If a woman with HIV becomes pregnant, these medicines also can reduce the chance that her fetus or infant will get the infection.

Getting tested and treated for STIs is especially important for pregnant women because some STIs may be passed on during pregnancy or delivery. Testing women for these STIs early in their pregnancy is important so that steps can be taken to help ensure delivery of a healthy infant. The necessary treatment will depend on the type of STI involved.

Whatever the infection, and regardless of how quickly the symptoms resolve after beginning treatment, infected people and their partner(s) must take all of the medicine prescribed by the healthcare provider to ensure that the STI is completely treated. Likewise, they should follow healthcare provider recommendations about how long to abstain from sex after the treatment is completed to avoid passing the infection back and forth.

What Are Some Types of and Treatments for Sexually Transmitted Diseases or Sexually Transmitted Infections?

Approximately 20 different infections are known to be transmitted through sexual contact.

Here are descriptions of the treatments for some of the common STIs.

Bacterial Vaginosis

Bacterial vaginosis (BV) occurs when problematic bacteria that are normally present in only small amounts in the body increase in number. Their levels get so high that they replace normal vaginal bacteria and upset the usual balance. It can be treated with antibiotics, typically metronidazole or clindamycin. Generally, sexual partners of women with BV do not need to be treated because treatment of partners has not been shown to reduce the risk of recurrence. Treatment is recommended for all pregnant women who show symptoms.

Chlamydia

Caused by the bacterium *Chlamydia trachomatis*, chlamydia can be treated with antibiotics. Because chlamydia and gonorrhea often occur together, people who have one infection are typically treated for both by their healthcare provider. If untreated, can cause pelvic inflammatory disease (PID), which can lead to chronic pelvic pain and permanent damage to a woman's reproductive organs. This damage may lead to ectopic pregnancy (in which the fetus develops outside of the womb, a condition that can be life-threatening) and infertility.

Gonorrhea

Gonorrhea is caused by the bacterium *Neisseria gonorrhoeae*, which can grow and multiply rapidly in the warm, moist areas of the reproductive tract. It can be treated with antibiotics. Because chlamydia and gonorrhea often occur together, people who have one infection are typically treated for both by their healthcare provider. Like chlamydia, if left untreated, gonorrhea can cause PID, which can lead to chronic pelvic pain and permanent damage to a woman's reproductive organs. This damage may lead to ectopic pregnancy (in which the fetus develops outside of the womb, a condition that can be life-threatening) and infertility.

Genital Herpes

Genital herpes is caused by the herpes simplex virus (HSV). Unfortunately it cannot be cured, but can be controlled with medication. One medication can be taken daily to make it less likely that the infection will pass on to sex partner(s) or to infants during childbirth.

Human Immunodeficiency Virus and Acquired Immunodeficiency Syndrome

Human immunodeficiency virus (HIV) is the virus that causes acquired immunodeficiency syndrome (AIDS). HIV can spread from mother to fetus during pregnancy and from mother to infant during delivery and breastfeeding. However, treatments are available that can virtually eliminate these types of transmission. People who may be at very high risk of HIV infection may be able to obtain HIV pre-exposure prophylaxis or PrEP, which consists of the HIV medication called "Truvada," from their doctor to take every day so they can prevent HIV infection. PrEP will not work if it is not taken consistently.

Human Papillomavirus

Human papillomavirus (HPV) is the most common STI. More than 40 HPV types exist, and all of them can infect both men and women. Though it cannot be cured, it can however, be prevented with vaccines and controlled with medications. Two available vaccines protect against most (but not all) HPV types that cause cervical cancer. A group advising the Centers for Disease Control and Prevention recommends this vaccine for boys and girls starting at 11 or 12 years old.

Syphilis

Syphilis is caused by the bacterium *Treponema pallidum*. It can be treated with antibiotics:

- If recognized during the early stages, usually within the first year of infection, syphilis can be treated with a single injection of antibiotic.

- If not recognized early, or not treated immediately, syphilis may need longer treatment with antibiotics.

Those being treated for syphilis must avoid sexual contact until the syphilis sores are completely healed to avoid infecting other people.

Trichomoniasis

Trichomoniasis is caused by the single-celled parasite *Trichomonas vaginalis*. It can be treated with a single dose of an antibiotic, usually either metronidazole or tinidazole, taken by mouth. Because of reinfection, it is important to make sure that the diagnosed individual and all sexual partners are treated at the same time.

Chapter 33

Understanding Antibiotic Resistance and Sexually Transmitted Disease Treatment

Chapter Contents

Section 33.1

Resistance to Antibiotics Is a Major Threat

This section contains text excerpted from the following
sources: Text under the heading "Biggest Threats and Data" is
excerpted from "Antibiotic/Antimicrobial Resistance (AR/AMR),"
Centers for Disease Control and Prevention (CDC), November
26, 2018; Text beginning with the heading "Antibiotic Resistance
Threatens Gonorrhea Treatment" is excerpted from "Antibiotic
Resistance Threatens Gonorrhea Treatment," Centers for Disease
Control and Prevention (CDC), January 25, 2017.

Biggest Threats and Data

Antibiotic resistance (AR) is one of the biggest public-health challenges of our time. In 2013, the Centers for Disease Control and Prevention (CDC) published a comprehensive analysis outlining the top
18 AR threats in the United States titled *Antibiotic Resistance Threats
in the United States*, 2013. The report sounded the alarm to the danger
of AR, stating that each year in the United States, at least 2 million
people get an AR infection, and at least 23,000 people die.

The report ranked the 18 threats (bacteria and fungi) into three
categories based on the level of concern to human health—urgent,
serious, and concerning—and identified:

- Minimum estimates of morbidity and mortality from AR
  infections

- People at especially high risk

- Gaps in knowledge about AR

- Core actions to prevent infections caused by AR bacteria, and
  slow spread of resistance

- What the CDC was doing at that time to combat the threat of AR

The data below is pulled from the *2013 Threats Report*.

Resistance to Antibiotics Threatens Gonorrhea Treatment

Resistance to azithromycin, an antibiotic used to treat gonorrhea, is
emerging, according to CDC findings published in the *Morbidity and
Mortality Weekly Report*.

The CDC recommends a combination gonorrhea treatment with two antibiotics—an oral dose of azithromycin and single shot of ceftriaxone. Findings released from the CDC's surveillance system for monitoring the threat of AR gonorrhea show that the percentage of gonorrhea isolates with decreased susceptibility to azithromycin, an indicator of emerging resistance, increased more than 300 percent between 2013 and 2014 (from 0.6 to 2.5% of gonorrhea isolates). This is a distressing sign that the future of current treatment options may be in jeopardy and underscores the importance of the federal government's Combating Antibiotic Resistant Bacteria (CARB) Action Plan.

"The confluence of emerging drug resistance and very limited alternative options for treatment creates a perfect storm for future gonorrhea treatment failure in the U.S.," said Jonathan Mermin, M.D., Director of the CDC's National Center for HIV/AIDS, Viral Hepatitis, STD, and TB Prevention. "History shows us that bacteria will find a way to outlast the antibiotics we're using to treat it. We are running just one step ahead in order to preserve the remaining treatment option for as long as possible."

The combination therapy recommended by the CDC still works. To date, no treatment failures have been reported in the United States. But signs of emerging resistance to azithromycin suggests that this drug will be next in the long line of antibiotics to which gonorrhea bacteria have become resistant—a list that includes penicillin, tetracycline, and fluoroquinolones. Because of gonorrhea ability to outsmart the antibiotics used to treat it, the CDC has been closely monitoring early warning signs of resistance not only to azithromycin but also to cephalosporins, the class of antibiotics that includes ceftriaxone.

"It is unclear how long the combination therapy of azithromycin and ceftriaxone will be effective if the increases in resistance persist," said Gail Bolan, M.D, Director of CDC's Division of STD Prevention. "We need to push forward on multiple fronts to ensure we can continue offering successful treatment to those who need it."

Section 33.2

Antibiotic Resistance Solutions Initiative

This section contains text excerpted from the following sources:
Text in this section begins with excerpts from "What You Need
to Know about Sinus Disorders," Centers for Disease Control and
Prevention (CDC), January 11, 2019; Text under the heading
"United States National Strategy for Combating Antibiotic-Resistant
Bacteria" is excerpted from "U.S. National Strategy for Combating
Antibiotic-Resistant Bacteria (National Strategy)," Centers for
Disease Control and Prevention (CDC), September 10, 2018.

The Centers for Disease Control and Prevention's (CDC) Antibiotic Resistance Solutions Initiative invests in national infrastructure
to detect, respond, contain, and prevent resistant infections across
healthcare settings, food, and communities. The CDC funding supports
all 50 state health departments, six local health departments, and
Puerto Rico. Through these investments, the CDC is transforming
how the nation and world combat and slow antibiotic resistance (AR)
at all levels.

Purpose of Antibiotic Resistance Solution Initiative

Detect, Respond, and Contain Resistant Pathogens

- **Laboratory and diagnostics.** Gold-standard lab (GSL)
  capacity offered to all United States state and regional labs
  through the CDC's AR Laboratory Network, and on-the-ground
  lab expertise and assistance in some countries abroad

- **Epidemiology capacity for response.** Increased capacity
  in state and local health departments and some countries
  for rapid detection and faster response to outbreaks and
  emerging resistance related to healthcare-associated infections,
  food-borne bacteria, and gonorrhea—to contain and control the
  spread of antibiotic-resistant pathogens

Prevent Spread of Resistant Infections

- **Surveillance and science.** More effective tracking and
  prevention of healthcare-associated infections, food-borne
  illness, tuberculosis (TB), and gonorrhea

- **Improved antibiotic use.** Improving antibiotic use to ensure antibiotics are available and work to protect people from life-threatening infections or sepsis

Encourage Innovation for New Strategies, Drugs, and Diagnostics

- **Insights for practice.** Innovations and collaborations with academic and healthcare partners to identify and implement new ways to prevent AR infections and their spread in the United States and abroad.

- **Research and development.** Sharing isolates that inform development of new drugs and diagnostics, and making public the CDC's sequencing data from AR pathogens (germs) to spur innovation in industry.

This work is done in partnership with state and local public-health departments, academia, and healthcare partners. The CDC supports most of these activities through its AR Solutions Initiative, and leverages investments from successful programs across the agency for maximum efficiency.

United States National Strategy for Combating Antibiotic-Resistant Bacteria

The National Strategy is a plan for the United States to work with domestic and international partners to reduce the national and international threat of AR.

Guiding Principles

The National Strategy takes into account both the causes of AR and opportunities to combat the threat, including:

- Using antibiotics, including misuse and overuse, in healthcare and food production accelerate the development of AR

- Detecting and responding to AR requires the adoption of One Health (OH) approach to data collection, recognizing that the health of people is connected to the health and animals and the environment

- Implementing evidence-based infection control practices can prevent the spread of resistance

- Encouraging the development of more therapies and drugs to treat infections

- Identifying opportunities to use innovations and new technologies to develop next generation tools to support human and animal health

- Recognizing that AR is a global health problem that requires international attention and collaboration

Main Goals

The National Strategy identified five main goals to guide collaborative action taken by the U.S. federal government:

- Slow the emergence of resistant bacteria and prevent the spread of resistant infections

- Strengthen national One Health surveillance efforts to combat resistance

- Advance development and use of rapid and innovative diagnostic tests for identification and characterization of resistant bacteria

- Accelerate basic and applied research and development for new antibiotics, other therapeutics, and vaccines objectives

- Improve international collaboration and capacities for antibiotic resistance prevention, surveillance, control, and antibiotic research and development

National and International Partnerships

The National Strategy requires cooperation from the public and private sector in the United States, including:

- Healthcare providers and leaders

- Veterinarians

- Agriculture industry leaders

- Manufacturers

- Universities

- Scientists and researchers

- Policymakers

- Patients

The National Strategy also calls for partnerships with international human and animal health organizations, including:

- Ministries of health, agriculture, and food safety
- World Health Organization (WHO)
- Transatlantic Taskforce on Antimicrobial Resistance (TATFAR)
- Global Health Security Agenda (GHSA)
- Food and Agriculture Organization (FAO) of the United Nations (UN)
- World Organization for Animal Health (OIE)

Chapter 34

Beware of Fake Sexually Transmitted Diseases Treatment Products

What Are Health-Fraud Scams?

"Health-fraud scams" refer to products that claim to prevent, treat, or cure diseases or other health conditions, but are not proven safe and effective for those uses. Health-fraud scams waste money and can lead to serious delays in getting the proper diagnosis and treatment, and can cause serious or even fatal injuries.

Common Types of Health-Fraud Scams

Human immunodeficiency virus (HIV) or acquired immunodeficiency syndrome (AIDS) fraud. These conditions require individualized treatments by a physician. Relying on unproven products or treatments can be dangerous, and may cause harmful delays in getting the proper diagnosis and appropriate treatments.

Sexually transmitted diseases (STDs) fraud. Drug or supplement products are not available over-the-counter (OTC) to prevent,

This chapter includes text excerpted from "Health Fraud Scams... Are Everywhere," U.S. Food and Drug Administration (FDA), November 2011. Reviewed February 2019.

treat, or cure STDs. They are available only by prescription. Use of bogus STD products may result in inaccurate diagnosis and delayed treatment, increasing the possibility of infecting a sexual partner.

Don't Be a Victim of Health-Fraud Scams

Health-fraud scams are everywhere. You can find them on TV "info-mercials," radio, and in magazines or newspapers. Promotions for fraudulent health products are frequently found on the Internet, and you might even receive them in unsolicited emails. Fraudulent health products are also sold in stores and through mail-order catalogs. Some companies even recruit your friends, family, or coworkers to spread the word about their products through word-of-mouth marketing. Be wary of personal testimonials by "real people," or "doctors," played by actors claiming amazing results. Testimonials are not a substitute for scientific proof and can be a tip-off that it's a scam. The bottom line is this: if it's an unproven or little-known treatment, talk to your doctor or healthcare professional before using it. This is especially important if you are already taking prescription drugs.

When it comes to health-fraud scams,

- **BE SMART.** Scams often target those with chronic or incurable diseases. If it sounds too good to be true, it's probably a scam.

- **BE AWARE.** Learn the most common types of health-fraud scams and the red flag claims.

- **BE CAREFUL.** If a product claims to cure a wide range of unrelated diseases, it's probably a scam. No one product can treat or cure many different illnesses.

Tip-Offs to Rip-Offs

By learning to recognize health-fraud scams, you can help to avoid them. Be suspicious of these red flag claims:

- "Quick fix"

- "All natural, miracle cure"

- "One product does it all"

- "New discovery" or "Scientific breakthrough"

- "Secret ingredient"

- "No more herpes"

- "Shrinks tumors"
- "Lowers blood sugar"
- "Lose weight without diet or exercise"

Protect Your Information

Never give out personal information including your Medicare ID in exchange for a free offer.

Part Five

Sexually Transmitted Diseases Risks and Prevention

Chapter 35

Sexual Behaviors That Increase the Likelihood of Sexually Transmitted Disease Transmission

Chapter Contents

Section 35.1

Overview of Risky Sexual Behaviors

This section includes text excerpted from "Sexual Risk Behaviors: HIV, STD, and Teen Pregnancy Prevention," Centers for Disease Control and Prevention (CDC), June 14, 2018.

Many young people engage in sexual-risk behaviors and experiences that can result in unintended health outcomes. For example, among U.S. high-school students surveyed in 2017:

- 40 percent had sexual intercourse at least once

- 10 percent had 4 or more sexual partners

- 7 percent had been physically forced to have sexual intercourse when they did not want to

- 30 percent had had sexual intercourse during the previous 3 months, and, of these:

  - 46 percent did not use a condom the last time they had sex

  - 14 percent did not use any method to prevent pregnancy

  - 19 percent had drunk alcohol or used drugs before last sexual intercourse

  - Nearly 10 percent of all students have been tested for human immunodeficiency virus (HIV)*

The Centers for Disease Control and Prevention (CDC) data show that lesbian, gay, and bisexual high-school students are at substantial risk for serious health outcomes as compared to their peers.

Sexual-risk behaviors place youth at risk for HIV infection, other sexually transmitted diseases (STDs), and unintended pregnancy:

- Young people (aged 13 to 24) accounted for an estimated 21 percent of all new human immunodeficiency virus (HIV) diagnoses in the United States in 2016.

- Among young people (aged 13 to 24) diagnosed with HIV in 2016, 81 percent were gay and bisexual males.

- Half of the 20 million new STDs reported each year were among young people, between the ages of 15 to 24.

* The CDC recommends all adolescents and adults 13 to 64 get tested for HIV at least once as part of routine medical care.

- Nearly 210,000 babies were born to teen girls aged 15 to 19 years in 2016.

To reduce sexual-risk behaviors and related health problems among youth, schools and other youth-serving organizations can help young people adopt lifelong attitudes and behaviors that support their health and well-being—including behaviors that reduce their risk for HIV, other STDs, and unintended pregnancy. The National HIV/acquired immunodeficiency syndrome (AIDS) Strategy calls for all Americans to be educated about HIV. This includes knowing how HIV is transmitted and prevented, and knowing which behaviors place individuals at greatest risk for infection. HIV awareness and education should be universally integrated into all educational environments.

Remember, abstinence from vaginal, anal, and oral intercourse is the only 100 percent effective way to prevent HIV, other STDs, and pregnancy. The correct and consistent use of male latex condoms can reduce the risk of STD transmission, including HIV infection. However, no protective method is 100 percent effective, and condom use cannot guarantee absolute protection against any STD or pregnancy.

Section 35.2

Having Multiple Sexual Partners

This section includes text excerpted from "My Sexual Partners," Centers for Disease Control and Prevention (CDC), December 7, 2015. Reviewed February 2019.

There may be things about your sexual partners that can put you at increased risk for getting or transmitting human immunodeficiency virus (HIV). If you have sexual partners with a different HIV status than you, then every time you have anal or vaginal sex you could be at risk for getting or transmitting HIV. However, every exposure to HIV does not carry the same risk. Having a high viral load greatly increases the chance of transmitting HIV, and having a sexually transmitted disease (STD) can increase the chances of getting or transmitting HIV. Having more than one partner can increase the chance that you come into contact with a partner who has a different HIV status than you. Power differences in relationships can also that make it harder to engage in safer sex.

Do You Have Multiple Sexual Partners?

Having multiple sexual partners can be risky. STDs spread rapidly in populations where people have multiple partners who overlap in time. This happens because a newly infected person can transmit an STD to more than one uninfected partner, while the newly infected person is the most infectious.

If you or your partner have sex partners who overlap in time, your risk for getting or transmitting HIV or other STDs increases. This is because the more sexual partners you have in your lifetime, the more likely you are to have a sex partner who has HIV and whose viral load isn't suppressed or who has another STD.

What You Can Do?

Not having sex is the best way to prevent getting or transmitting HIV. If you are sexually active, you can choose to have fewer partners in the future. You can also choose sexual activities that are lower risk for HIV than anal or vaginal sex.

A monogamous relationship, which means that both you and your partner are having sex only with each other, can also reduce your risk of infection. Monogamy only reduces your risk of getting HIV if both partners are certain that they're HIV-negative and stay monogamous. You may not always know if your partner is having sex with other people or engaging in other behaviors that increase the risk for getting HIV or other STDs. Having open and honest communication with your partner is important. Talk to your partner about your decision to be monogamous and what you would do if one of you had sex with another person. Be sure you and your partner understand any agreements you have about sex, and communicate about any changes in your HIV status or sexual activity. And, if you're just beginning a monogamous relationship, it's a good idea for both of you to get tested for HIV before you have sex.

You can do other things to reduce your HIV risk, including using a condom and dental dams the right way every time you have sex and taking medicines to prevent or treat HIV. Even though it may be difficult, you can learn how to talk with your partner about protection and safer sex.

Talking openly and frequently with your partner about sex can help you make decisions that may decrease your risk of getting or transmitting HIV.

Section 35.3

Oral Sex and Human Immunodeficiency Virus Risk

This section includes text excerpted from "Oral Sex and HIV Risk," Centers for Disease Control and Prevention (CDC), July 8, 2016.

Oral sex involves using the mouth to stimulate the penis (fellatio), vagina (cunnilingus), or anus (anilingus).

Risk of Human Immunodeficiency Virus

The chance a human immunodeficiency virus (HIV)-negative person will get HIV from oral sex with an HIV-positive partner is extremely low. However, it is hard to know the exact risk because a lot of people who have oral sex also have anal or vaginal sex. The type of oral sex that may be the riskiest is mouth-to-penis oral sex. But the risk is still very low, and much lower than with anal or vaginal sex.

Though the risk of HIV transmission through oral sex is low, several factors may increase that risk, including sores in the mouth or vagina or on the penis, bleeding gums, oral contact with menstrual blood, and the presence of other sexually transmitted diseases (STDs).

Risk of Other Infections

Other STDs, such as syphilis, herpes, gonorrhea, and chlamydia, can be transmitted during oral sex. Anilingus can also transmit hepatitis A and B, intestinal parasites like *Giardia*, and bacteria like *E. coli*.

Fast Facts

- There is little to no risk of getting or transmitting HIV from oral sex.

- Other STDs and hepatitis can be transmitted during oral sex.

Latex barriers and medicines to prevent and treat HIV can further reduce the very low risk of getting HIV from oral sex.

Reducing the Risk

Individuals can further reduce the already-low risk of HIV transmission from oral sex by keeping their male partners from ejaculating in their mouth. This could be done by removing the mouth from the penis before ejaculation, or by using a condom.

Using a barrier like a condom or dental dam during oral sex can further reduce the risk of transmitting HIV, other STDs, and hepatitis. A dental dam is a thin, square piece of latex or silicone that is placed over the vagina or anus during oral sex. A latex condom can also be cut lengthwise and used like a dental dam.

The risk of HIV transmission through oral sex is even lower if the HIV-negative partner is taking medicine to prevent HIV (pre-exposure prophylaxis or PrEP) or the HIV-positive partner is taking medicine to treat HIV (antiretroviral therapy or ART) and is virally suppressed.

Chapter 36

Factors That Can Increase Human Immunodeficiency Virus Risk Other than Sex

Chapter Contents

Section 36.1

Substance Use and Sexually Transmitted Diseases

This section contains text excerpted from "Substance Use and Sexual Risk Behaviors among Youth," Centers for Disease Control and Prevention (CDC), July 11, 2018.

According to the Surgeon General's Report *Facing Addiction in America*, the misuse of substances such as alcohol and drugs is a growing problem in the United States. Although substance misuse can occur at any age, the teenage and young adult years are particularly critical at-risk periods. Research shows that the majority of adults who meet the criteria for having a substance-use disorder (SUD) started using substances during their teen and young adult years. Teen substance use is also associated with sexual-risk behaviors that put young people at risk for human immunodeficiency virus (HIV), sexually transmitted diseases (STDs), and pregnancy. To address these issues, more needs to be done to lessen risks and increase protective factors for teens.

Studies conducted among adolescents have identified an association between substance use and sexual-risk behaviors such as ever having sex, having multiple sex partners, not using a condom, and pregnancy before the age of 15 years of age.

Researchers have found that as the frequency of substance use increases, the likelihood of sex and the number of sex partners also increases. In addition, studies show that sexual-risk behaviors increase in adolescents who use alcohol, and are highest among students who use marijuana, cocaine, prescription drugs (such as sedatives, opioids, and stimulants), and other illicit drugs. Adolescents who reported no substance use are the least likely to engage in sexual risk-taking.

According to the 2017 National Youth Risk Behavior Survey (YRBS), 40 percent of high-school students have had intercourse and 29 percent of high-school students are currently sexually active. Of the students who are currently sexually active, 19 percent drank alcohol or used drugs before last sexual intercourse.

Risk Factors and Prevention Activities

Substance use and sexual-risk behaviors share some common underlying factors that may predispose youth to these behaviors. Because substance use clusters with other risk behaviors, it is important to learn whether precursors can be determined early to help identify youth who are most at risk.

Primary prevention approaches that are most effective are those that address common risk factors. Prevention programs for substance use and sexual-risk behaviors should include a focus on individuals, peers, families, schools, and communities. When students' school environments are supportive and their parents are engaged in their lives, they are less likely to use alcohol and drugs and engage in sexual behaviors that put them at risk for HIV, STDs, or pregnancy.

Substance Use Is Associated with Behaviors That Put Youth at Risk for Human Immunodeficiency Virus, Sexually Transmitted Diseases, and Pregnancy

Common risk factors for substance use and sexual-risk behaviors include:

- Extreme economic deprivation (poverty, overcrowding)
- Family history of the problem behavior, family conflict, and family-management problems
- Favorable parental attitudes towards the problem behavior and/ or parental involvement in the problem behavior
- Lack of positive parent engagement
- Association with substance-using peers
- Alienation and rebelliousness
- Lack of school connectedness

For primary prevention activities targeting substance use and sexual-risk behaviors to be effective, they should include:

- School-based programs that promote social and emotional competence
- Peer-led drug and alcohol-resistance programs
- Parenting skills training
- Parent engagement
- Family support programs

Section 36.2

Substance Use and Human Immunodeficiency Virus Risk

This section includes text excerpted from "HIV and Substance Use in the United States," Centers for Disease Control and Prevention (CDC), September 21, 2018.

Substance-use disorders (SUD), which are problematic patterns of using alcohol or another substance, such as crack cocaine, methamphetamine ("meth"), amyl nitrite ("poppers"), prescription opioids, and heroin, are closely associated with human immunodeficiency virus (HIV) and other sexually transmitted diseases (STD).

Injection-drug use (IDU) can be a direct route of HIV transmission if people share needles, syringes, or other injection materials that are contaminated with HIV. However, drinking alcohol and ingesting, smoking, or inhaling drugs are also associated with increased risk for HIV. These substances alter judgment, which can lead to risky sexual behaviors (e.g., having sex without a condom, having multiple partners) that can make people more likely to get and transmit HIV.

In people living with HIV, substance use can hasten disease progression, affect adherence to antiretroviral therapy (ART) (HIV medicine), and worsen the overall consequences of HIV.

Commonly Used Substances and Human Immunodeficiency Viruses Risk

Some of the commonly used substances that can increase the risk of HIV include:

- **Alcohol.** Excessive alcohol consumption, notably binge drinking, can be a major risk factor for HIV because it is linked to risky sexual behaviors and, among people living with HIV, can hurt treatment outcomes.

- **Opioids.** Opioids, a class of drugs that reduce pain, include both prescription drugs and heroin. They are associated with HIV-risk behaviors such as needle sharing when infected and risky sex and have been linked to a recent HIV outbreak.

- **Methamphetamine.** "Meth" is linked to risky sexual behavior that places people at greater HIV risk. It can be injected, which also increases HIV risk if people share needles and other injection equipment.

- **Crack cocaine.** Crack cocaine is a stimulant that can create a cycle in which people quickly exhaust their resources and turn to other ways to get the drug, including trading sex for drugs or money, which increases HIV risk.

- **Inhalants.** Use of amyl nitrite ("poppers") has long been linked to risky sexual behaviors, illegal drug use, and sexually transmitted diseases among gay and bisexual men.

Prevention Challenges

A number of behavioral, structural, and environmental factors make it difficult to control the spread of HIV among people who use or misuse substances:

- **Complex health and social needs.** People who are alcohol dependent or use drugs often have other complex health and social needs. Research shows that people who use substances are more likely to be homeless, face unemployment, live in poverty, and experience multiple forms of violence, creating challenges for HIV-prevention efforts.

- **Stigma and discrimination associated with substance use.** Often, illicit-drug use is viewed as a criminal activity rather than a medical issue that requires counseling and rehabilitation. Fear of arrest, stigma, feelings of guilt, and low self-esteem may prevent people who use illicit drugs from seeking treatment services, which places them at greater risk for HIV.

- **Lack of access to the healthcare system.** Since HIV testing often involves questioning about substance-use histories, those who use substances may feel uncomfortable getting tested. As a result, it may be harder to reach people who use substances with HIV-prevention services.

- **Poor adherence to HIV treatment.** People living with HIV who use substances are less likely to take antiretroviral therapy as prescribed due to side effects from a drug interaction. Not taking ART as prescribed can worsen the effects of HIV and increase the likelihood of spreading HIV to sex and drug-sharing partners.

Section 36.3

Alcohol and Human Immunodeficiency Virus Risk

This section includes text excerpted from "Alcohol and HIV Risk," HIV.gov, U.S. Department of Health and Human Services (HHS), August 27, 2018.

How Can Alcohol Put You at Risk for Getting or Transmitting Human Immunodeficiency Viruses?

Drinking alcohol, particularly binge drinking, affects your brain, making it hard to think clearly. When you're drunk, you may be more likely to make poor decisions that put you at risk for getting or transmitting human immunodeficiency virus (HIV), such as having sex without a condom or dental dam.

You also may be more likely to have a harder time using a condom or dental dam the right way every time you have sex, have more sexual partners or use other drugs. Those behaviors can increase your risk of exposure to HIV and other sexually transmitted diseases (STDs). Or, if you have HIV, they can also increase your risk of transmitting HIV to others.

What Can You Do?

If you drink alcohol:

- **Drink in moderation.** Moderate drinking is up to 1 drink per day for women and up to 2 drinks per day for men. One drink is a 12-ounce bottle of beer, a 5-ounce glass of wine, or a shot of liquor.

- **Visit Rethinking Drinking**, a website from the National Institutes of Health (NIH) National Institute on Alcohol Abuse and Alcoholism (NIAAA). This website can help you evaluate your drinking habits and consider how alcohol may be affecting your health.

- **Don't have sex** if you're drunk or high from other drugs.

- **Use a condom every time you have sex**. You can also consider sexual activities that are at lower risk for HIV than anal or vaginal sex (such as oral sex).

- If you are HIV-negative, talk to your healthcare provider about pre-exposure prophylaxis (PrEP). PrEP is when people at very high risk for HIV take HIV medicine (called antiretroviral therapy or ART) daily to lower their chances of getting HIV. PrEP must be taken every day as prescribed and alcohol use can make it hard to stick to a daily HIV regimen. Be open and honest about your alcohol use so you and your doctor can develop a plan for you to stick to your HIV medicine.

- If you are living with HIV, taking ART every day, exactly as prescribed is also important to stay healthy and prevent transmission. People living with HIV who take HIV medication daily as prescribed and get and keep an undetectable viral load have effectively no risk of sexually transmitting HIV to their HIV-negative partners. Like PrEP, ART must be taken every day, exactly as prescribed.

Section 36.4

Viral Load

This section includes text excerpted from "Viral Load," Centers for Disease Control and Prevention (CDC), December 7, 2015. Reviewed February 2019.

Not Having a Low Viral Load (Not Being Virally Suppressed)?

When your viral load is high, you have more human immunodeficiency virus (HIV) in your body. Someone who maintains a high viral load will have health problems and is also much more likely to transmit HIV to sexual and drug-using partners. Without HIV treatment, someone who is not virally suppressed will eventually develop acquired immunodeficiency syndrome (AIDS). With HIV treatment and viral suppression, people with HIV can live long, healthy lives and are much less likely to transmit HIV to their partners.

What You Can Do

If you're HIV-positive, enrolling in a medical treatment program and taking medicine to treat HIV the right way, every day will give you the greatest chance to be and stay virally suppressed, live a longer, healthier life, and reduce the chance of transmitting HIV to your partners.

If you're HIV-negative and have an HIV-positive partner, encourage your partner to enroll in a medical treatment program and take HIV treatment medicines.

Taking other actions, like using a condom the right way every time you have sex or taking daily medicine to prevent HIV (called pre-exposure prophylaxis or PrEP) if you're HIV-negative, can lower your chances of transmitting or getting HIV even more.

Acute Human Immunodeficiency Viruses Infection

Acute HIV infection is the phase of infection right after people are infected, but before they develop antibodies to HIV. Some people with acute infection get flu-like symptoms, but not everyone with acute infection feels sick.

When people have an acute infection, they're much more likely to transmit HIV to others because the amount of virus in their blood is very high. This means that a person is much more likely to get HIV from someone who has an acute infection than from someone who has been infected with HIV longer, even if the person who has been infected longer is not taking HIV medicines. The difference in transmission risk between a person living with acute HIV and someone on treatment and virally suppressed is even greater.

During acute infection, you may seem to be HIV-negative (uninfected) because you have not yet developed antibodies to HIV—but you're infected. Most current HIV tests work by detecting the HIV antibodies a person develops after becoming infected. But there is a window period during which a person is infected but doesn't yet have detectable antibodies. A fourth-generation or nucleic acid test (NAT) can be used to find out whether someone may have an acute infection.

What You Can Do

If you feel like you have the flu and you had a potential HIV exposure in the past month, talk to your healthcare provider about what type of HIV test you should take and what its window period is. Some healthcare providers may not know about the NAT, but it can detect the virus earlier than any other test, about ten days after infection. You should avoid potentially exposing other people to HIV through sex and drug use until you get tested and know your results.

If you find out you are HIV-positive, enrolling in a medical treatment program and taking medicine to treat HIV the right way, every day will give you the greatest chance to get and stay virally suppressed, live a longer, healthier life, and reduce the chance of transmitting HIV to your partners.

If you're HIV-negative and have an HIV-positive partner, encourage your partner to get in care and take HIV treatment medicines.

Taking other actions, such as using a condom and dental dam the right way every time you have sex or having your partner take daily medicine to prevent HIV (called PrEP) if you're HIV-negative, can lower your chances of transmitting or getting HIV even more.

Chapter 37

Other Behaviors That Increase Sexually Transmitted Disease Risk

Chapter Contents

Section 37.1

Douching May Increase Risk of Sexually Transmitted Diseases

This section includes text excerpted from "Douching," Office on Women's Health (OWH), U.S. Department of Health and Human Services (HHS), May 22, 2018.

What Is Douching?

The word "douche" means to wash or soak. Douching is washing or cleaning out the inside of the vagina with water or other mixtures of fluids. Most douches are sold in stores as prepackaged mixes of water and vinegar, baking soda, or iodine. The mixtures usually come in a bottle or bag. You squirt the douche upward through a tube or nozzle into your vagina. The water mixture then comes back out through your vagina.

Douching is different from washing the outside of your vagina during a bath or shower. Rinsing the outside of your vagina with warm water will not harm your vagina. But, douching can lead to many different health problems.

Most doctors recommend that women do not douche.

How Common Is Douching?

In the United States, almost one in five women 15 to 44 years old douche.

More African American and Hispanic women douche than White women. Douching is also common in teens of all races and ethnicities.

Studies have not found any health benefit to douching. But, studies have found that douching is linked to many health problems.

Why Should Women Not Douche?

Most doctors recommend that women do not douche. Douching can change the necessary balance of vaginal flora (bacteria that live in the vagina) and natural acidity in a healthy vagina.

A healthy vagina has good and harmful bacteria. The balance of bacteria helps maintain an acidic environment. The acidic environment protects the vagina from infections or irritation.

Douching can cause an overgrowth of harmful bacteria. This can lead to a yeast infection or bacterial vaginosis (BV). If you already have a vaginal infection, douching can push the bacteria causing the infection up into the uterus, fallopian tubes, and ovaries. This can lead to pelvic inflammatory disease (PID), a serious health problem. Douching is also linked to other health problems.

What Health Problems Are Linked to Douching?

Health problems linked to douching include:

- BV, which is an infection in the vagina. Women who douche often (once a week) are five times more likely to develop BV than women who do not douche.
- PID, an infection in the reproductive organs that is often caused by a sexually transmitted infection (STI)
- Problems during pregnancy, including preterm birth and ectopic pregnancy
- STIs, including human immunodeficiency virus (HIV)
- Vaginal irritation or dryness

Researchers are studying whether douching causes these problems or whether women at higher risk for these health problems are more likely to douche.

Should I Douche to Get Rid of Vaginal Odor or Other Problems?

No. You should not douche to try to get rid of vaginal odor or other vaginal problems such as discharge, pain, itching, or burning.

Douching will only cover up odor for a short time and will make other problems worse. Call your doctor or nurse if you have:

- Vaginal discharge that smells bad
- Vaginal itching and thick, white, or yellowish-green discharge with or without an odor
- Burning, redness, and swelling in or around the vagina
- Pain when urinating
- Pain or discomfort during sex

These may be signs of a vaginal infection or an STI. Do not douche before seeing your doctor or nurse. This can make it hard for the doctor or nurse to find out what may be wrong.

Should I Douche to Clean inside My Vagina?

No. Doctors recommend that women do not douche. You do not need to douche to clean your vagina. Your body naturally flushes out and cleans your vagina. Any strong odor or irritation usually means something is wrong.

Douching also can raise your chances of a vaginal infection or an STI. If you have questions or concerns, talk to your doctor.

What Is the Best Way to Clean My Vagina?

It is best to let your vagina clean itself. The vagina cleans itself naturally by making mucous. The mucous washes away blood, semen, and vaginal discharge.

If you are worried about vaginal odor, talk to your doctor or nurse. But you should know that even healthy, clean vaginas have a mild odor that changes throughout the day. Physical activity also can give your vagina a stronger, muskier scent, but this is still normal.

Keep your vagina clean and healthy by:

• Washing the outside of your vagina with warm water when you bathe. Some women also use mild soaps. But, if you have sensitive skin or any current vaginal infections, even mild soaps can cause dryness and irritation.

• Avoiding scented tampons, pads, powders, and sprays. These products may increase your chances of getting a vaginal infection.

Can Douching before or after Sex Prevent Sexually Transmitted Infections?

No. Douching before or after sex does not prevent STIs. In fact, douching removes some of the normal bacteria in the vagina that protect you from infection. This can actually increase your risk of getting STIs, including HIV, the virus that causes acquired immunodeficiency syndrome (AIDS).

Should I Douche If I Had Sex without Using Protection or If the Condom Broke?

No. Douching removes some of the normal bacteria in the vagina that protect you from infection. This can increase your risk of getting STIs, including HIV. Douching also does not protect against pregnancy.

If you had sex without using protection or if the condom broke during sex, see a doctor right away. You can get medicine to help prevent HIV and unwanted pregnancy.

Should I Douche If I Was Sexually Assaulted?

No, you should not douche, bathe, or shower. As hard as it may be to not wash up, you may wash away important evidence if you do. Douching may also increase your risk of getting STIs, including HIV. Go to the nearest hospital emergency room as soon as possible. The National Sexual Assault Hotline at 800-656-HOPE (800-656-4673) can help you find a hospital able to collect evidence of sexual assault. Your doctor or nurse can help you get medicine to help prevent HIV and unwanted pregnancy.

Can Douching after Sex Prevent Pregnancy?

No. Douching does not prevent pregnancy. It should never be used for birth control. If you had sex without using birth control or if your birth control method did not work correctly (failed), you can use emergency contraception to keep from getting pregnant.

If you need birth control, talk to your doctor or nurse about which type of birth control method is best for you.

How Does Douching Affect Pregnancy?

Douching can make it harder to get pregnant and can cause problems during pregnancy:

- **Trouble getting pregnant.** Women who douched at least once a month had a harder time getting pregnant than women who did not douche.

- **Higher risk of ectopic pregnancy.** Douching may increase a woman's chance of damaged fallopian tubes and ectopic pregnancy. Ectopic pregnancy is when the fertilized egg attaches to the inside of the fallopian tube instead of the uterus. If left untreated, ectopic pregnancy can be life-threatening. It can also make it hard for a woman to get pregnant in the future.

- **Higher risk of early childbirth.** Douching raises your risk for premature birth. One study found that women who douched during pregnancy were more likely to deliver their babies early. This raises the risk for health problems for you and your baby.

Section 37.2

Body Art Allows Exposure to Bloodborne Pathogens Such as Human Immunodeficiency Virus

This section includes text excerpted from "Body Art," Centers for Disease Control and Prevention (CDC), November 23, 2016.

Body art.... This may seem like an odd topic, but not when you consider the artists' risk of exposure to blood-borne pathogens. Body art is popular and growing, with an estimated 16,000 body artists working in the United States. Body art, which typically consists of tattoos and body piercings, is an art form where the artists' canvas is the human body.

When working on this unique medium, artists may come in contact with a client's blood if they are stuck with the needle that they are using on a client (or stuck with a used needle during disposal), or if the client's blood splashes into the eyes, nose, or mouth. Contact with another person's blood may expose workers to blood-borne pathogens such as hepatitis B virus (HBV), hepatitis C virus (HCV), or human immunodeficiency virus (HIV). These blood-borne pathogens can be dangerous and may cause permanent illness. If an artist gets one of these viruses, he or she may become ill and be unable to support his or her family. Also, since blood-borne pathogens can be spread through contact with blood and other bodily fluids such as semen and vaginal secretions, sexual partners could also be at risk of getting a blood-borne disease.

In the early 1990s as the body-art industry grew, professional associations were formed to promote better business practices in the industry and address safety and health issues. Because of concerns voiced by artists in the industry, the National Institute for Occupational Safety and Health (NIOSH) researchers visited several tattooing and piercing studios and found certain practices used in body piercing and tattooing could increase the chance of an artist coming in contact with blood. NIOSH met with many of the tattooing and piercing professional organizations, other government agencies, scientists and the artists themselves to learn more about body-artwork practices and what could be done to lower artists' chance of exposure to blood-borne diseases.

To lower exposure to blood, NIOSH recommends using safe work practices and staying informed about problems affecting body artists.

Recommendations for protecting tattoo artists and body piercers from blood-borne pathogens include:

- **Seek emergency medical assistance if an artist is exposed to another person's blood.** If a tattooist or piercer is exposed to another person's blood, the artist should notify the shop owner and immediately seek medical attention. If treatment is needed, it is more likely to be effective if it begins soon after the exposure happens.

- **Use single-use, disposable needles and razors.** Disposable piercing needles, tattoo needles, and razors are used on one person and then thrown away. Reusing needles or razors is not safe.

- **Safely dispose of needles and razors.** Used needles and razors should be thrown away in a sharps disposal container to protect both the client and the person changing or handling the trash bag from getting cut. Sharps disposal containers must be closeable, puncture resistant, leak-proof, and labeled.

- **Wash hands before and after putting on disposable gloves.** Gloves are always worn while working with equipment and clients, changed when necessary, and are not reused.

- **Clean and sterilize reusable tools and equipment.** Some tools and equipment can be reused when tattooing or piercing. Reusable tools and equipment should be cleaned and then sterilized to remove viruses and bacteria.

- **Frequently clean surfaces and work areas.** Chairs, tables, workspaces, and counters should be disinfected between procedures to protect both the health of the client and the artist. Cross-contamination (spreading bacteria and viruses from one surface to another) can occur if surfaces are not disinfected frequently and between clients. Any disinfectant that claims to be able to eliminate the tuberculosis germ can also kill HIV, hepatitis B, and hepatitis C viruses. Use a commercial disinfectant, following the manufacturer's instructions, or a mixture of bleach and water (1 part bleach to 9 parts water).

Body artists face unique risks for exposure to blood-borne pathogens, but when proper safety and health practices are followed, these risks can be greatly reduced.

Section 37.3

Injection-Drug Use

This section includes text excerpted from "Injection Drug
Use and HIV Risk," Centers for Disease Control
and Prevention (CDC), November 9, 2018.

Sharing needles, syringes, or other injection equipment (works)
to inject drugs puts people at risk for getting or transmitting human
immunodeficiency virus (HIV) and other infections. About one in ten
new HIV diagnoses in the United States are attributed to injection
drug use or male-to-male sexual contact and injection drug use.

Risk of Human Immunodeficiency Virus

The risk for getting or transmitting HIV is very high if an HIV-negative person uses injection equipment that someone living with HIV
has used. This is because the needles or works may have blood in them,
and blood can carry HIV. HIV can survive in a used needle for up to
42 days, depending on temperature and other factors.

Substance misuse can also increase the risk of getting HIV through
sex. When people are high, they are more likely to have risky anal or
vaginal sex, such as having sex without a condom or without medicines
to prevent or treat HIV, having sex with multiple partners, or trading
sex for money or drugs.

Risk of Other Infections and Overdose

Sharing needles or works also puts people at risk for getting viral hepatitis. People who inject drugs should talk to a doctor about getting vaccinated for hepatitis A and B and getting a blood test for hepatitis B and C.

In addition to being at risk for HIV and viral hepatitis, people who
inject drugs can get other serious health problems, such as skin infections or abscesses. People can also overdose and get very sick or even
die from having too many drugs in their body or from products that
may be mixed with the drugs without their knowledge (for example,
illegally made fentanyl).

Reducing the Risk

The best way to reduce the risk of getting or transmitting HIV
through injection drug use is to stop injecting drugs. Talk with a

counselor, doctor, or other healthcare providers about substance-use disorder (SUD) treatment, including medication-assisted treatment. To find a treatment center near you, check out the locator tools on Substance Abuse and Mental Health Services Administration (SAMHSA) or www.hiv.gov, or call 800-662-4357.

If you continue injecting drugs, never share needles or works. Many communities have syringe services programs (SSPs) where you can get free sterile needles and syringes and safely dispose of used ones. They can also refer you to SUD treatment and help you get tested for HIV and hepatitis. Contact your local health department or North American Syringe Exchange Network (NASEN) to find an SSP. Also, some pharmacies may sell needles without a prescription.

Other things you can do to lower your risk of getting or transmitting HIV if you continue to inject drugs, include:

- Cleaning used needles with bleach. This may reduce the risk of HIV but doesn't eliminate it.

- Using sterile water to fix drugs.

- Cleaning your skin with a new alcohol swab before you inject.

- Being careful not to get someone else's blood on your hands or your needle or works.

- Disposing of needles safely after one use. Use a sharps container, or keep used needles away from other people.

- Getting tested for HIV at least once a year.

- Asking your doctor about taking daily medicine to prevent HIV (called pre-exposure prophylaxis or PrEP).

- Using a condom the right way every time you have anal or vaginal sex. Learn the right way to use a condom.

Chapter 38

How Can We Reduce Sexually Transmitted Disease Risks?

Chapter Contents

Section 38.1

What Are the Best Ways to Decrease My Chances of Getting or Transmitting Human Immunodeficiency Virus?

This section includes text excerpted from "What Are the Best Ways to Decrease My Chances of Getting or Transmitting HIV?—HIV Risk Reduction Tool," Centers for Disease Control and Prevention (CDC), December 7, 2015. Reviewed February 2019.

Your life matters and staying healthy is important. Staying healthy starts with getting tested for human immunodeficiency virus (HIV) and knowing your HIV status. The Centers for Disease Control and Prevention (CDC) recommends that everyone between the ages of 13 and 64 gets tested for HIV at least once as part of routine healthcare and that people with certain risk factors get tested more often. Some people are more likely to be at higher risk and should get tested at least once a year, including people with more than one sex partner, sexually active gay and bisexual men, people with other sexually transmitted diseases (STD), and people who inject drugs.

Some gay and bisexual men may benefit from even more frequent testing, depending on their risk. If you haven't been tested for HIV in the past year, get tested for HIV, and encourage your partners to get tested too.

If you test positive, the most important thing you can do is take antiretroviral therapy (ART) the right way, every day. ART is recommended for all people with HIV, regardless of how long they've had the virus or how healthy they are.

If you are HIV-positive, talk about your HIV status with all of your sexual partners and take steps to protect your health and your partners' health.

The only way to be completely certain that HIV transmission will not occur through sex is to not have sex. However, there are more tools available nowadays to prevent HIV transmission than ever before. The more of these actions you take, the safer you can be. Here's what you can do:

- Use condoms the right way every time you have sex.

- Choose less risky sexual behaviors.

- Reduce the number of people with whom you have risky sex.

- If you're HIV-negative, consider pre-exposure prophylaxis (PrEP) and taking HIV medicines daily to prevent HIV infection.

- If you're HIV-negative, talk to your doctor right away (within three days) about postexposure prophylaxis (PEP) if you have had a recent possible exposure to HIV.

- Get tested and treated for other STDs and encourage your partners to do the same. Find an STD testing site.

- If you're HIV-positive, take ART.

- If you're taking ART, follow your healthcare provider's advice.

- If your partner is HIV-positive, encourage your partner to enroll and remain in treatment.

You can also reduce your risk of getting or transmitting HIV by not sharing needles or works. You're at very high risk of getting or transmitting HIV if someone else uses your needle or works after you've used it. People use needles for many reasons—to inject drugs for medical purposes (such as insulin to treat diabetes), get high, change their appearance, or for tattoos and piercings. No matter the reason, never share your needles or works with anyone to lower your chances of getting or transmitting HIV.

Section 38.2

Sex and Risk Reduction

This section contains text excerpted from the following sources:
Text beginning with the heading "What We Know about Choosing
Less Risky Sexual Activities" is excerpted from "Choosing Less
Risky Sexual Activities—HIV Risk Reduction Tool," Centers for
Disease Control and Prevention (CDC), December 7, 2015. Reviewed
February 2019; Text beginning with the heading "Vaginal Sex
and Human Immunodeficiency Virus Risk-Reducing the Risk" is
excerpted from is excerpted from "HIV Risk and Prevention," Centers
for Disease Control and Prevention (CDC), November 13, 2018.

What We Know about Choosing Less Risky Sexual Activities

Human immunodeficiency virus (HIV) is mainly spread by having
sex without using a condom or without taking medicines to prevent
or treat. Anal sex is the riskiest type of sex for transmitting HIV. It's
possible for either partner—the partner inserting the penis in the anus
or the partner receiving the penis in the anus—to get HIV, but it is
much riskier for an HIV-negative partner to be the receptive partner.

Vaginal sex is less risky than anal sex, and oral sex and touching are
much less risky than anal or vaginal sex for getting or transmitting HIV.

What You Can Do

Choosing activities with little to no risk, such as oral sex instead
of higher-risk activities such as anal or vaginal sex can lower your
chances of getting or transmitting HIV. You can do other things to
reduce your risk, including taking medicines to prevent or treat HIV
and using condoms the right way every time you have sex. Even if you
take medicines and use condoms, it's safer if the HIV-positive partner
is always on the bottom during anal sex.

Vaginal Sex and Human Immunodeficiency Virus Risk-Reducing the Risk
Condoms and Lubrication

Latex or polyurethane male condoms are highly effective in preventing HIV and certain other STDs when used correctly from start
to finish for each act of vaginal sex. People who report using condoms

consistently reduced their risk of getting HIV through vaginal sex, on average, by 80 percent. Condoms are much less effective when not used consistently. It is also important that sufficient water- or silicone-based lubricant be used during vaginal sex to prevent condom breakage and tearing of tissue. Female nitrile condoms can also prevent HIV and some other sexually transmitted diseases (STDs). Since condoms are not 100 percent effective, consider using other prevention methods to further reduce your risk.

Pre-Exposure Prophylaxis

People who are HIV-negative and at very high risk for HIV can take daily medicine to prevent HIV. Pre-exposure prophylaxis (PrEP), if taken consistently, can reduce the risk of getting HIV from sex by more than 90 percent. PrEP is much less effective when it is not taken consistently. Since PrEP is not 100 percent effective at preventing HIV, consider using other prevention methods to further reduce your risk. Only condoms can help protect against other STDs.

Postexposure Prophylaxis

Postexposure prophylaxis (PEP) means taking antiretroviral medicines—medicines used to treat HIV—after being potentially exposed to HIV during sex to prevent becoming infected. PEP should be used only in emergency situations and must be started within 72 hours after possible exposure to HIV, but the sooner the better. PEP must be taken once or twice daily for 28 days. When administered correctly, PEP is effective in preventing HIV, but not 100 percent. To obtain PEP, contact your healthcare provider, your local or state health department, or go to an emergency room (ER).

Antiretroviral Therapy

For people with HIV, antiretroviral therapy (ART) can reduce the amount of virus in the blood and body fluids to very low levels, if taken as prescribed. This is called "viral suppression"—usually defined as having less than 200 copies of HIV per milliliter of blood. HIV medicine can even make the viral load so low that a test can't detect it. This is called an "undetectable viral load." People who take HIV medicine as prescribed and get and stay virally suppressed or undetectable can stay healthy for many years, and they have effectively no risk of transmitting HIV to an HIV-negative partner through sex. Only condoms can help protect against some other STDs.

Other Ways to Reduce Your Risk

People who engage in vaginal sex can make other behavioral choices to lower their risk of getting or transmitting HIV. These individuals can:

- Choose less risky behaviors such as oral sex, which has little to no risk of transmission

- Get tested and treated for other STDs

Anal Sex and Human Immunodeficiency Virus Risk-Reducing the Risk
Condoms and Lubrication

Latex or polyurethane male condoms are highly effective in preventing HIV and certain other STDs when used correctly from start to finish for each act of anal sex. People who report using condoms consistently reduced their risk of getting HIV through insertive anal sex with an HIV-positive partner, on average, by 63 percent, and receptive anal sex with an HIV-positive partner, on average, by 72 percent. Condoms are much less effective when not used consistently. It is also important that sufficient water- or silicone-based lubricant be used during anal sex to prevent condom breakage and tearing of tissue. Female nitrile condoms can also prevent HIV and some other STDs. Since condoms are not 100 percent effective, consider using other prevention methods to further reduce your risk.

Pre-Exposure Prophylaxis

People who are HIV-negative and at very high risk for HIV can take daily medicine to prevent HIV. Pre-exposure prophylaxis (PrEP), if taken consistently, can reduce the risk of getting HIV from sex by more than 90 percent. PrEP is much less effective when it is not taken consistently. Since PrEP is not 100 percent effective at preventing HIV, consider using other prevention methods to further reduce your risk. Only condoms can help protect against other STDs.

Post-Exposure Prophylaxis

Postexposure prophylaxis (PEP) means taking antiretroviral medicines—medicines used to treat HIV—after being potentially exposed to HIV during sex to prevent becoming infected. PEP should be used only in emergency situations and must be started within 72 hours after possible exposure to HIV, but the sooner the better. PEP must be taken once or twice daily for 28 days. When administered correctly, PEP is effective in preventing HIV, but not 100 percent. To obtain PEP, contact your healthcare provider, your local or state health department, or go to an emergency room.

Antiretroviral Therapy

For people with HIV antiretroviral therapy can reduce the amount of virus in the blood and body fluids to very low levels, if taken as prescribed. This is called "viral suppression"—usually defined as having less than 200 copies of HIV per milliliter of blood. HIV medicine can even make the viral load so low that a test can't detect it. This is called an "undetectable viral load." People who take HIV medicine as prescribed and get and stay virally suppressed or undetectable can stay healthy for many years, and they have effectively no risk of transmitting HIV to an HIV-negative partner through sex. Only condoms can help protect against some other STDs.

Other Ways to Reduce Your Risk

People who engage in anal sex can make other behavioral choices to lower their risk of getting or transmitting HIV. These individuals can:

- Choose less risky behaviors like oral sex, which has little to no risk of transmission.
- Get tested and treated for other STDs.

Section 38.3

Using Condoms and Dental Dams

This section contains text excerpted from the following sources: Text beginning with the heading "Male Condoms" is excerpted from "Male Condoms—HIV Risk Reduction Tool," Centers for Disease Control and Prevention (CDC), December 7, 2015. Reviewed February 2019; Text under the heading "Tips for Using Condoms and Dental Dams" is excerpted from "Tips for Using Condoms and Dental Dams—HIV/AIDS," HIV.gov, U.S. Department of Health and Human Services (HHS), May 2018.

Male Condoms
What We Know about Male Condoms

Condoms are very effective at reducing the risk of getting or transmitting human immunodeficiency virus (HIV) if you use them the right way every time you have sex. Latex condoms provide the best protection against HIV. Polyurethane (plastic) or polyisoprene (synthetic rubber) condoms are good options for people with latex allergies, but plastic ones break more often than latex ones. Natural membrane (such as lambskin) condoms have small holes in them, so they don't block HIV and sexually transmitted diseases (STDs).

Condoms can also help prevent other STDs you can get through body fluids, such as gonorrhea and chlamydia. However, they provide less protection against STDs spread through skin-to-skin contacts, such as human papillomavirus or HPV (genital warts), genital herpes, and syphilis.

What You Can Do

Use a condom the right way every time you have sex:

- Use a new condom every time you have sex (vaginal, anal, and oral), and keep it on the entire time you're having sex.

- Before any genital contact, put the condom on the tip of the hard penis with the rolled side out.

- Pinch the tip of the condom enough to leave a half-inch space for semen (cum) to collect. While holding the tip, unroll the condom all the way to the base of the hard penis.

- After ejaculation and before the penis gets soft, hold the bottom of the condom so it stays on and carefully pull out the penis.

Then gently pull the condom off the penis, making sure that semen doesn't spill out.

- Wrap the condom in a tissue and throw it in the trash where others won't handle it.

- If you feel the condom break at any time during sex, stop immediately, pull out the penis, take off the broken condom, and put on a new condom.

- Use enough lubricant (lube) during vaginal and anal sex to help keep the condom from tearing. Don't use oil-based lubricants (for example, vaseline, shortening, mineral oil, massage oils, body lotions, and cooking oil) because they can weaken the condom and cause it to break.

Natural membrane condoms aren't recommended for HIV or STD prevention. If you or your partner has a latex allergy, you can use male condoms made out of polyurethane or polyisoprene. Use water- or silicon-based lubricants to lower the chances that the condom will break or slip during sex.

Be aware that even if you use condoms the right way every time you have sex, there's still a chance of getting HIV, so adding other prevention methods, such as taking medicines to prevent or treat HIV, can further reduce your risk.

Female Condoms
What We Know about Female Condoms

When worn in the vagina, female condoms are comparable to male condoms at preventing HIV, other STDs, and pregnancy.

We don't currently have scientific evidence on how effective female condoms are at preventing HIV and other STDs when used by men or women for anal sex. But we do know that HIV can't travel through the nitrile barrier. It's safe to use any kind of lubricant with female condoms.

What You Can Do

You and your sexual partners might consider using a female condom instead of a male condom. Female condoms allow individuals to initiate condom use when talking about or using male condoms is difficult or impossible because of an imbalance in power between partners. Female condoms also allow couples to alternate who wears the condom, giving them more options when they have sex. If you or your partner has an allergy to latex, you can use female condoms since they are made from nitrile.

Even though it may be difficult, you can learn how to talk with your partner about condoms and safer sex. And there are many tips for learning to use a condom or a dental dam the right way. Even if you use condoms the right way every time you have sex, there's still a chance of getting HIV, so adding other prevention methods, such as taking medicines to prevent or treat HIV, can further reduce your risk.

Tips for Using Condoms and Dental Dams

Some people think that using a condom makes sex less fun. Other people have become creative and find condoms sexy. Not having to worry about infecting someone will definitely make sex much more enjoyable!

If you are not used to using condoms: practice, practice, practice. Condom dos and don'ts:

- **Shop around: Use lubricated latex condoms.** Always use latex, because lambskin condoms don't block HIV and STDs, and polyurethane condoms break more often than latex. If you are allergic to latex, polyurethane condoms are an option. Shop around and find your favorite brand. Try different sizes and shapes (yes, they come in different sizes and shapes!) There are a lot of choices—one will work for you.

- **Keep it fresh.** Store condoms loosely in a cool, dry place (not your wallet). Make sure your condoms are fresh—check the expiration date. Throw away condoms that have expired, been very hot, or been washed in the washer. If you think the condom might not be good, get a new one. You and your partner are worth it.

- **Take it easy.** Open the package carefully, so that you don't rip the condom. Be careful if you use your teeth. Make sure that the condom package has not been punctured (there should be a pocket of air). Check the condom for damaged packaging and signs of aging such as brittleness, stickiness, and discoloration.

- **Keep it hard.** Put on the condom after the penis is erect and before it touches any part of a partner's body. If the penis is uncircumcised (uncut), the foreskin must be pulled back before putting on the condom.

- **Heads up! Make sure the condom is right-side out.** It's like a sock—there's a right side and a wrong side. Before you put it on the penis, unroll the condom about half an inch to see which direction it is unrolling. Then put it on the head of the penis and hold the tip of the condom between your fingers as you roll it all the way down the shaft of the penis from head to base. This keeps out air bubbles that can cause the condom to break. It also leaves space for semen to collect after ejaculation.

- **Slippery when wet.** If you use a lubricant (lube), it should be a water-soluble lubricant (for example, ID Glide, K-Y Jelly, Slippery Stuff, Foreplay, Wet, Astroglide) in order to prevent breakdown of the condom. Products such as petroleum jelly, massage oils, butter, Crisco, Vaseline, and hand creams are not considered water-soluble lubricants and should not be used.

- **Use lubrication.** Put lubricant on after you put on the condom, not before—it could slip off. Add more lube often. Dry condoms break more easily.

- **Come and go.** Withdraw the penis immediately after ejaculation, while the penis is still erect; grasp the rim of the condom between your fingers and slowly withdraw the penis (with the condom still on) so that no semen is spilled.

- **Clean up.** Throw out the used condom right away. Tie it off to prevent spillage or wrap it in bathroom tissue and put it in the garbage. Condoms can clog toilets. Use a condom only once. Never use the same condom for vaginal and anal intercourse. Never use a condom that has been used by someone else.

Do You Have to Use a Condom for Oral Sex?

It is possible for oral sex to transmit HIV, whether the infected partner is performing or receiving oral sex. But the risk is very low compared with unprotected vaginal or anal sex.

If you choose to perform oral sex, you may:

- Use a latex condom on the penis, or

- Use a latex barrier (such as a natural rubber latex sheet, a dental dam, or a cut-open condom that makes a square) between the mouth and the vagina. A latex barrier such as a dental dam reduces the risk of blood or vaginal fluids entering the mouth. Plastic food wrap also can be used as a barrier.

- If either you or your partner is allergic to latex, plastic (polyurethane) condoms can be used.

If you choose to perform oral sex and this sex includes oral contact with your partner's anus (anilingus or rimming):

- Use a latex barrier (such as a natural rubber latex sheet, a dental dam, or a cut-open condom that makes a square) between your mouth and the anus. Plastic food wrap also can be used as a barrier. This barrier is to prevent getting another sexually transmitted disease or parasites, not HIV.

If you choose to share sex toys, such as dildos or vibrators, with your partner:

- Each partner should use a new condom on the sex toy, and be sure to clean sex toys between each use.

Internal Condom (Also Called Female Condom)

This type of condom was originally designed to be inserted into the vagina before sex. It also can be used in the anus, by either men or women, though its effectiveness in preventing HIV transmission via anal sex has not been studied.

The internal condom is a large condom fitted with larger and smaller rings at each end. The rings help keep it inside the vagina during sex; for anal sex, the inner ring usually is removed before it is inserted. It is made of nitrile, so any lubricant can be used without damaging it. It may seem a little awkward at first, but can be a useful alternative to the traditional male condom. Female condoms generally cost more than male condoms.

- Store the condom in a cool dry place, not in direct heat or sunlight.

- Throw away any condoms that have expired—the date is printed on individual condom wrappers.

- Check the package for damage and check the condom for signs of aging, such as brittleness, stickiness, and discoloration. The internal condom is lubricated, so it will be somewhat wet.

- Before inserting the condom, you can squeeze lubricant into the condom pouch and rub the sides together to spread it around.

- Put the condom in before sex play because preejaculatory fluid, which comes from the penis, may contain HIV. The condom can be inserted up to eight hours before sex.

- The internal condom has a firm ring at each end of it. To insert the condom in the vagina, squeeze the ring at the closed end between the fingers (like a diaphragm), and push it up into the back of the vagina. The open ring must stay outside the vagina at all times, and it will partly cover the lip area. For use in the anus, most people remove the internal ring before insertion.

- Do not use a male condom with the internal condom.

- Do not use an internal condom with a diaphragm.

- If the penis is inserted outside the condom pouch or if the outer ring (open ring) slips into the vagina, stop and take the condom out. Use a new condom before you start sex again.

- Don't tear the condom with fingernails or jewelry.

- Use a condom only once and properly dispose of it in the trash (not the toilet).

Dental Dams and Plastic Wrap

Even though oral sex is a low-risk sexual practice, you may want to use protection when performing oral sex on someone who has HIV.

Dental dams are small squares of latex that were made originally for use in dental procedures. They are now commonly used as barriers when performing oral sex on women, to keep in vaginal fluids or menstrual blood that could transmit HIV or other STDs.

Some people use plastic wrap instead of a dental dam. It's thinner. Here are some things to remember:

- Before using a dental dam, first, check it visually for any holes.

- If the dental dam has cornstarch on it, rinse that off with water (starch in the vagina can lead to an infection).

- Cover the woman's genital area with the dental dam.

- For oral–anal sex, cover the opening of the anus with a new dental dam.

- A new dental dam should be used for each act of oral sex; it should never be reused.

Section 38.4

Reducing Number of Partners and Male Circumcision

This section includes text excerpted from "Reducing the Number of Partners—HIV Risk Reduction Tool," Centers for Disease Control and Prevention (CDC), December 7, 2015. Reviewed February 2019.

What We Know about Reducing the Number of Partners

The more sexual partners you have in your lifetime, the more likely you are to have a sex partner who has human immunodeficiency virus (HIV) and whose viral load isn't suppressed or who has another sexually transmitted disease (STD).

What You Can Do

Not having sex is the best way to prevent getting or transmitting HIV. If you are sexually active, you can choose to have fewer partners in the future. You can also choose sexual activities that are at lower risk for HIV than anal or vaginal sex.

Limiting the number of partners you have can lower your risk of getting or transmitting HIV. You can decrease your risk even more by taking other actions, including using a condom the right way every time you have sex and taking medicines to prevent or treat HIV.

Talking openly and frequently with your partner about sex can help you make decisions that may decrease your risk of getting or transmitting HIV.

Male Circumcision
What We Know about Male Circumcision

When men are circumcised, they're less likely than uncircumcised men to get HIV from their HIV-positive female partners. There are biological reasons why, for some men, male circumcision may decrease the risk of getting HIV during vaginal sex with an HIV-positive female partner. Male circumcision also reduces the risk of a man getting herpes and human papillomavirus (HPV) from a woman who has those infections. However, there is no evidence that circumcision decreases the risk of HIV-negative receptive partners getting HIV from a circumcised HIV-positive partner.

Evidence about the benefits of circumcision among gay and bisexual men is inconclusive. More studies are underway.

What You Can Do

Male circumcision is known to decrease the risk of getting HIV only for HIV-negative circumcised men who have sex with HIV-positive women. Also, circumcised men and their partners can still get other sexually transmitted diseases. Take other actions, such as using condoms the right way every time you have sex or taking medicine to prevent or treat HIV to further reduce your chances of getting HIV.

If you're a parent, talk to your healthcare provider about the potential risks and benefits of male circumcision to your newborn.

Chapter 39

Talking to Your Child or Teen about Sexually Transmitted Diseases

Talk with your teen about how to prevent sexually transmitted diseases (STDs), even if you don't think your teen is sexually active.

If talking about sex and STDs with your teen makes you nervous, you aren't alone. It can be hard to know where to start. But it's important to make sure your teen knows how to stay safe.

How Do I Talk with My Teen about Sexually Transmitted Diseases?

These tips can help you talk to your teen about preventing STDs:

• Think about what you want to say ahead of time

• Be honest about how you feel

• Try not to give your teen too much information at once

• Use examples to start a conversation

This chapter includes text excerpted from "Talk with Your Teen about Preventing STDs," Office of Disease Prevention and Health Promotion (ODPHP), U.S. Department of Health and Human Services (HHS), January 31, 2019.

- Talk while you are doing something together

- Get ideas from other parents

You can also ask your teen's doctor to talk with your teen about preventing STDs. This is called "STD prevention counseling."

Why Do I Need to Talk with My Teen?

All teens need accurate information about how to prevent STDs. Teens whose parents talk with them about sex and how to prevent STDs are not more likely to have sex. But they will be more likely to make healthy choices about sex when they're older.

In fact, teens say that their parents have a bigger influence on their decisions about sex than the media, their siblings, or their friends.

Young People Are More Likely to Get Sexually Transmitted Diseases

About half of all STD cases in the United States happen in young people ages 15 to 24.

Teens are at a higher risk than adults of getting STDs for a number of reasons. For example, they may:

- Not know they need tests to check for STDs

- Not use condoms correctly every time they have sex

- Have sexual contact with multiple partners during the same period of time

What Do I Need to Know about Sexually Transmitted Diseases?

STDs are diseases that can spread from person to person during vaginal, anal, or oral sex. Some STDs can also spread during any kind of activity that involves skin-to-skin sexual contact.

STDs are sometimes called STIs, or sexually transmitted infections. Examples of STDs include genital herpes, chlamydia, gonorrhea, and human immunodeficiency virus (HIV).

These diseases are very common. Although many STDs can be cured, they can cause serious health problems if they aren't treated. Many STDs don't have any symptoms, so the only way to know for sure if you have an STD is to get tested.

What Do I Tell My Teen about Preventing Sexually Transmitted Diseases?

Talk to your teen about what STDs are and how to prevent them. Use the facts and resources below to talk with your teen.

It's important to learn about STDs and how they spread. Knowing the facts helps teens protect themselves.

Complete abstinence is the best way to prevent STDs. Complete abstinence means not having any kind of sexual contact. This includes vaginal, anal, or oral sex and skin-to-skin sexual contact. Complete abstinence is the only sure way to prevent STDs.

Condoms can help prevent STDs. Make sure your teen knows how to use condoms, even if you don't think he is sexually active. Offer to help get condoms if your teen doesn't know where to go.

It's important for teens to talk with their partners about STDs before having sex. Encourage your teen to talk with her partner about STD prevention before having sex. Say that you understand it may not be easy, but it's important for your teen to speak up.

Your teen may need to get tested for STDs. Ask your teen to talk honestly with the doctor or nurse about any sexual activity. That way, the doctor can decide which tests your teen may need. Sexually active teens may need to be tested for:

- Chlamydia and gonorrhea
- Syphilis
- HIV

It's important to help your teen develop a trusting relationship with the doctor or nurse. Step out of the room to give your teen a chance to ask about STD testing and prevention in private.

This is an important step in teaching teens to play an active role in their healthcare.

Keep in mind that your teen can get tested for STDs at the doctor, or go to a clinic. To find an STD clinic near you, enter your Zip code to find a local testing site at gettested.cdc.gov or call: 800-232-463.

How Can I Help My Teen Build Healthy Relationships?

Families have different rules about when it's okay for teens to start dating. Whatever your rules are, the best time to start talking about healthy relationships is before your teen starts dating.

Help your teen develop healthy expectations for relationships.

Does My LGBT Teen Need Information about Preventing Sexually Transmitted Diseases?

Yes. All teens—including lesbian, gay, bisexual, transgender (LGBT) teens—need accurate information about STDs. Remember, STDs can spread through vaginal, anal, or oral sex and skin-to-skin sexual contact.

LGBT teens may also be at higher risk for STDs than straight teens, so it's important to talk to your teen about STD prevention.

Help Your Teen

Help protect your teen from STDs by sharing the facts she or he needs to make healthy decisions.

Think about what you want to say ahead of time. It's very common to be nervous when talking to your teen about something like STDs. Learn about STDs so you'll be ready for the conversation. You may also want to practice what you'll say to your teen with another adult, like your partner or another parent.

Be honest about how you feel. Talking with your teen about how to prevent STDs may not be easy for you. It's normal for both of you to feel uncomfortable—and it's okay, to be honest with your teen about how you feel.

Remember, when you are honest with your teen, he's more likely, to be honest with you. And keep in mind that your teen may ask a question you can't answer. Tell him you aren't sure—then look up the answer together!

Try not to give your teen too much information at once. Remember, you have plenty of time to talk about preventing STDs. You don't need to fit everything into one conversation—it's actually better if you don't. Give your teen time to think—she may come back later and ask questions.

Make this the first conversation of many about preventing STDs.

Listen and ask questions. Show your teen that you are paying attention and trying to understand his thoughts and feelings. Try these tips:

- Repeat back what your teen says in your own words. For example, "So you don't think you are at risk of getting an STD?"

- Ask questions to help guide the conversation. For example, "Have you talked in school about how to prevent STDs?"

- Ask questions that check for your teen's understanding. For example, "What did you learn about how STDs are spread?"

- Talk about something that happened in a movie or TV show. For example, "It looks like they had sex without using a condom. What do you think about that?"

Talk while you are doing something together. Sometimes it's easier to have a conversation while you are doing something else at the same time. For example, try talking with your teen about sex and STDs when you are driving in the car or cooking dinner.

You can still show your teen that you are listening to him by nodding your head or repeating what he says.

Get ideas from other parents. Remember that you aren't the only person thinking about how to talk to a teen about preventing STDs. Ask other parents what they have done. You may be able to get helpful tips and ideas.

Ask your teen's doctor about STD prevention counseling. Counseling to prevent STDs is recommended for all teens who are sexually active. That means it's part of a doctor's job to help teens learn how to prevent STDs. The doctor may:

- Give your teen information about preventing STDs

- Refer your teen to a health educator or counselor for STD prevention counseling

- STD prevention counseling includes:

  - Giving your teen basic information about STDs and how they spread

  - Figuring out your teen's risk of getting or spreading an STD

Teaching your teen important skills—like how to use condoms, how to talk with a partner about STDs, and how to get tested for STDs

What about Cost

Under the Affordable Care Act (ACA), the healthcare reform law passed in 2010, health insurance plans must cover prevention counseling and screening for teens at higher risk of getting an STD.

Depending on your insurance plan, your teen may be able to get STD counseling and screening at no cost to you.

Chapter 40

Prevention of Sexually Transmitted Diseases

Chapter Contents

Section 40.1

Lowdown on How to Prevent Sexually Transmitted Diseases

This section includes text excerpted from "The Lowdown Infographic Text Only Version," Centers for Disease Control and Prevention (CDC), February 9, 2016.

Every year, there are an estimated 20 million new sexually transmitted diseases (STDs) infections in the United States.

Anyone who is sexually active can get an STD. Some groups are disproportionately affected by STDs:

- Adolescents and young adults

- Gay, bisexual, and other men who have sex with men

- Some racial and ethnic minorities

The good news is that STDs are preventable. There are steps you can take to keep yourself and your partner(s) healthy.

This section gives tips on how you can avoid giving or getting an STD.

Steps You Can Take to Prevent Sexually Transmitted Diseases

Practice Abstinence

The surest way to avoid STDs is to not have sex. This means not having vaginal, oral, or anal sex.

Use Condoms

Using a condom correctly every time you have sex can help you avoid STDs. Condoms lessen the risk of infection for all STDs. You still can get certain STDs, such as herpes or human papillomavirus infection (HPV), from contact with your partner's skin even when using a condom.

Most people say they used a condom the first time they ever had sex, but when asked about the last four weeks, less than a quarter said they used a condom every time.

Have Fewer Partners

Agree to only have sex with one person who agrees to only have sex with you. Make sure you both get tested to know for sure that neither of you has an STD. This is one of the most reliable ways to avoid STDs.

Get Vaccinated

The most common STD can be prevented by a vaccine. The HPV vaccine is safe, effective, and can help you avoid HPV-related health problems like genital warts and some cancers.

Get the HPV infection vaccine:

- Routine vaccination for boys and girls ages 11 to 12

- Catch-up vaccination for:

  - Young women ages 13 to 26 and young men ages 13 to 21

  - Gay, bisexual, and other men who have sex with men up to age 26

  - Men with compromised immune systems up to age 26

Talk with Your Partner

Talk with your sex partner(s) about STDs and staying safe before having sex. It might be uncomfortable to start the conversation, but protecting your health is your responsibility.

If Tested Positive?

Getting an STD is not the end. Many STDs are curable and all are treatable. If either you or your partner is infected with an STD that can be cured, both of you need to start treatment immediately to avoid getting reinfected.

Section 40.2

Birth-Control Methods for Sexually Transmitted Disease Prevention

This section contains text excerpted from the following sources: Text in this section begins with excerpts from "Birth Control and HIV—HIV/AIDS," Centers for Disease Control and Prevention (CDC), February 8, 2018; Text beginning with the heading "What Is Spermicide?" is excerpted from "Spermicide," U.S. Department of Health and Human Services (HHS), October 13, 2017.

The only forms of birth control that will protect against human immunodeficiency virus (HIV) are abstinence and using condoms while having sex. Other methods of birth control offer protection against unplanned pregnancy but do not protect against HIV or other sexually transmitted diseases (STDs).

Birth-control options that DO protect against HIV:

- Abstinence (not having sex)

- Male condom

- Internal or female condom

Birth-control options that DO NOT protect against HIV:

- Oral contraceptive (OC) ("the pill")

- Injectable contraceptive (shot)

- Contraceptive implant

- Intrauterine device (IUD)

- Emergency contraception (EC) ("morning-after pill")

- Diaphragm, cap, and shield

- Vasectomy (getting your tubes tied if you are a man)

- Tubal ligation (getting your tubes tied if you are a woman)

- Withdrawal

Considerations for Women with Human Immunodeficiency Virus

If you are in a monogamous relationship and your partner also is HIV positive, you may decide to use a birth control method other

404

than condoms. (These methods won't protect against other STDs or reinfection.)

Safe methods of birth control for an HIV-positive woman with an HIV-positive partner include:

- Using a diaphragm
- Tubal ligation (getting your tubes tied)
- Intrauterine device (IUD)

Use only after checking with your provider (these may interact with your anti-HIV medications):

- Birth-control pills (BCP)
- Contraceptive injection (e.g., Depo-Provera)
- Contraceptive implant (e.g., Norplant)

What Is Spermicide?

Spermicides are chemicals that prevent pregnancy by killing sperm. The only chemical available in spermicides in the United States is non-oxynol-9 (N-9). Spermicides containing N-9 are available as a cream, foam, jelly, tablet, suppository, or film.

How Do I Use It?

The spermicide is put deep inside the vagina and works to prevent pregnancy by stopping and killing sperm before they can reach an egg and fertilize it. Instructions can be different for each type of spermicide, so read the label carefully before use.

Spermicide can be inserted/used up to one hour before having sex. The spermicide should remain in the vagina at least six hours after sex. Do not rinse or douche the vagina during this time.

How Effective Is It?

Of 100 women each year who use spermicides alone for birth control, about 28 may become pregnant. Effectiveness varies. For better pregnancy protection, a spermicide should be used with a condom, diaphragm, or cervical cap.

How Do I Get It?

You do not need a prescription or personal identification to buy spermicide. Spermicide is available at pharmacies, clinics, and some grocery stores.

What Is Abstinence?

Sexual abstinence is defined as refraining from all forms of sexual activity and genital contact such as vaginal, oral, or anal sex.

How Do I Use It?

Abstinence is the only 100 percent effective way to protect against pregnancy, ensuring that there is no exchange of bodily fluids (such as vaginal secretions and semen). Abstinence prevents pregnancy by keeping semen away from the vagina so the sperm cells in semen cannot meet with an egg and fertilize it. If you are abstinent 100 percent of the time, pregnancy cannot happen. People sometimes also use abstinence to prevent pregnancy on days they are fertile (most likely to get pregnant), but they may have vaginal sex at other times.

It will be important to discuss with your partner what abstinence means to you, especially if you are developing a new relationship. Someone that cares about you will honor your choices and not push for sexual behavior that makes you uncomfortable.

How Effective Is It?

When practiced consistently, abstinence provides the most effective protection against unplanned pregnancy and sexually transmitted diseases (STDs) including HIV infection. It is only effective when both partners are completely committed and practices abstinence (no genital contact or sharing semen or vaginal fluid) 100 percent of the time. Abstinence is most effective when both partners talk and agree about their reasons to remain abstinent.

How Do I Get It?

Abstinence is a personal decision that should be discussed with your partner.

Section 40.3

Preventing Mother-to-Child Transmission

This section includes text excerpted from "Preventing Mother-to-Child Transmission of HIV," AIDS*info*, U.S. Department of Health and Human Services (HHS), December 17, 2018.

Mother-to-child transmission of human immunodeficiency virus (HIV) is the spread of HIV from a woman living with HIV to her child during pregnancy, childbirth, or breastfeeding (through breast milk). Mother-to-child transmission of HIV is also called "perinatal transmission" of HIV.

Can Mother-to-Child Transmission of Human Immunodeficiency Virus Be Prevented?

Yes. The use of HIV medicines and other strategies have helped to lower the risk of mother-to-child transmission of HIV to one percent or less in the United States and Europe. The risk of transmission is low when:

- HIV is detected as early as possible during pregnancy (or before a woman gets pregnant)

- Women with HIV receive HIV medicines during pregnancy and childbirth and, in certain situations, have a scheduled cesarean delivery (sometimes called a "C-section")

- Babies born to women with HIV receive HIV medicines for four to six weeks after birth and are not breastfeed

Is Human Immunodeficiency Virus Testing Recommended for Pregnant Women?

The Centers for Disease Control and Prevention (CDC) recommends that all women get tested for HIV before they become pregnant or as early as possible in their pregnancy. Women should be tested for HIV again during every pregnancy.

Pregnant women with HIV receive HIV medicines to reduce the risk of mother-to-child transmission of HIV and to protect their own health. HIV medicines are recommended for everyone who has HIV. HIV medicines help people with HIV live longer, healthier lives and reduce the risk of HIV transmission.

How Do Human Immunodeficiency Virus Medicines Prevent Mother-to-Child Transmission of Human Immunodeficiency Virus?

HIV medicines work by preventing HIV from multiplying, which reduces the amount of HIV in the body (also called the "viral load"). Having less HIV in the body protects a woman's health and reduces her risk of passing HIV to her child during pregnancy and childbirth.

Some HIV medicines pass from the pregnant woman to her unborn baby across the placenta (also called the "afterbirth"). This transfer of HIV medicines protects the baby from HIV infection, especially during a vaginal delivery when the baby passes through the birth canal and is exposed to any HIV in the mother's blood or other fluids. In some situations, a woman with HIV may have a cesarean delivery to reduce the risk of mother-to-child transmission of HIV during delivery.

Babies born to women with HIV receive HIV medicines for four to six weeks after birth. The HIV medicines reduce the risk of infection from any HIV that may have entered a baby's body during childbirth.

Are Human Immunodeficiency Virus Medicines Safe to Use during Pregnancy?

Most HIV medicines are safe to use during pregnancy. In general, HIV medicines don't increase the risk of birth defects. Healthcare providers can explain the benefits and risks of specific HIV medicines to help women with HIV decide which HIV medicines to use during pregnancy or while they are trying to conceive.

Are There Other Ways to Prevent Mother-to-Child Transmission of Human Immunodeficiency Virus?

Because HIV can be transmitted in breast milk, women with HIV in the United States should not breastfeed their babies. In the United States, baby formula is a safe and healthy alternative to breast milk.

There are reports of children becoming infected with HIV by eating food that was previously chewed by a person with HIV. To be safe, babies should not be fed pre-chewed food.

Section 40.4

Human Immunodeficiency Virus Vaccines

This section includes text excerpted from "HIV Vaccines,"
HIV.gov, U.S. Department of Health and Human
Services (HHS), May 15, 2017.

What Are Vaccines and What Do They Do?

A vaccine—also called a "shot" or "immunization"—is a substance that teaches your body's immune system to recognize and defend against harmful viruses or bacteria.

Vaccines given before you get infected are called "preventive vaccines" or "prophylactic vaccines," and you get them while you are healthy. This allows your body to set up defenses against those dangers ahead of time. That way, you won't get sick if you're exposed to diseases later. Preventive vaccines are widely used to prevent diseases such as polio, chicken pox, measles, mumps, rubella, influenza (flu), hepatitis A and B, and human papillomavirus (HPV).

Is There a Vaccine for Human Immunodeficiency Virus?

No. There is currently no vaccine available that will prevent human immunodeficiency virus (HIV) infection or treat those who have it.

However, scientists are working to develop one. Building on the findings of an earlier study that found for the first time, albeit modestly, that a vaccine could prevent HIV infection in 2016, a National Institute of Health (NIH)-supported clinical trial was launched to test a modified HIV vaccine. This current vaccine trial, called "HVTN 702," is testing whether an experimental vaccine regimen safely prevents HIV infection among South African adults.

Why Do We Need a Human Immunodeficiency Virus Vaccine?

Today, more people living with HIV than ever before have access to life-saving treatment with HIV medicines (called "antiretroviral therapy" or "ART"), which is good for their health. When people living with HIV achieve and maintain viral suppression by taking medication as prescribed, they can stay healthy for many years and greatly reduce their chances of transmitting HIV to their partners. In addition, others who are at high risk for HIV infection may have access to pre-exposure prophylaxis (PrEP), or ART being used to prevent HIV. Yet, unfortunately, in 2015, 39,513 people were diagnosed with HIV infection in the United States, and more than 2.1 million people became newly infected with HIV worldwide. To control and ultimately end HIV globally, we need a powerful array of HIV-prevention tools that are widely accessible to all who would benefit from them.

Vaccines historically have been the most effective means to prevent and even eradicate infectious diseases. They safely and cost-effectively prevent illness, disability, and death. Like smallpox and polio vaccines, a preventive HIV vaccine could help save millions of lives.

Developing safe, effective, and affordable vaccines that can prevent HIV infection in uninfected people is the NIH's highest HIV-research priority given its game-changing potential for controlling and ultimately ending the HIV/AIDS pandemic.

The long-term goal is to develop a safe and effective vaccine that protects people worldwide from getting infected with HIV. However, even if a vaccine only protects some people who get vaccinated, or even if it provides less than total protection by reducing the risk of infection, it could still have a major impact on the rates of transmission and help control the pandemic, particularly for populations at high risk of HIV infection. A partially effective vaccine could decrease the number of people who get infected with HIV, further reducing the number of people who can pass the virus on to others. By substantially reducing the number of new infections, we can stop the epidemic.

Section 40.5

Human Immunodeficiency Virus Treatment as Prevention

This section includes text excerpted from "HIV Treatment as Prevention," HIV.gov, U.S. Department of Health and Human Services (HHS), January 9, 2019.

Treatment as prevention (TasP) refers to taking human immunodeficiency virus (HIV) medication to prevent the sexual transmission of HIV. It is one of the highly effective options for preventing HIV transmission. People living with HIV who take HIV medication daily as prescribed and get and keep an undetectable viral load have effectively no risk of sexually transmitting HIV to their HIV-negative partners.

TasP works when a person living with HIV takes HIV medication exactly as prescribed and has regular follow-up care, including regular viral load tests to ensure their viral load stays undetectable.

Taking Human Immunodeficiency Virus Medication to Stay Healthy and Prevent Transmission

If you have HIV, it is important to start treatment with HIV medication (called "antiretroviral therapy" or ART) as soon as possible after your diagnosis.

If taken every day, exactly as prescribed, HIV medication can reduce the amount of HIV in your blood (also called the "viral load") to a very low level. This is called "viral suppression." It is called "viral suppression" because HIV medication prevents the virus from growing in your body and keeps the virus very low or "suppressed." Viral suppression helps keep you healthy and prevents illness.

If your viral load is so low that it doesn't show up in a standard lab test, this is called having an "undetectable viral load." People living with HIV can get and keep an undetectable viral load by taking HIV medication every day, exactly as prescribed. Almost everyone who takes HIV medication daily as prescribed can achieve an undetectable viral load, usually within six months after starting treatment.

There are important health benefits to getting the viral load as low as possible. People living with HIV who know their status, take HIV medication daily as prescribed, and get and keep an undetectable viral load can live long, healthy lives.

There is also a major prevention benefit. People living with HIV who take HIV medication daily as prescribed and get and keep an undetectable viral load have effectively no risk of sexually transmitting HIV to their HIV-negative partners

Keep Taking Your Human Immunodeficiency Virus Medication to Stay Undetectable

HIV is still in your body when your viral load is suppressed, even when it is undetectable. So, you need to keep taking your HIV medication daily as prescribed. When your viral load stays undetectable, you have effectively no risk of transmitting HIV to an HIV-negative partner through sex. If you stop taking HIV medication, your viral load will quickly go back up.

If you have stopped taking your HIV medication or are having trouble taking all the doses as prescribed, talk to your healthcare provider as soon as possible. Your provider can help you get back on track and discuss the best strategies to prevent transmitting HIV through sex while you get your viral load undetectable again.

How Do We Know Treatment as Prevention Works?

Large research studies with newer HIV medications have shown that treatment is prevention. These studies monitored thousands of male–female and male–male couples in which one partner has HIV and the other does not over several years. No HIV transmissions were observed when the HIV-positive partner was virally suppressed. This means that if you keep your viral load undetectable, there is effectively no risk of transmitting HIV to someone you have vaginal, anal, or oral sex with.

Talk with Your Human Immunodeficiency Virus Healthcare Provider

Talk with your healthcare provider about the benefits of HIV treatment and which HIV medication is right for you. Discuss how frequently you should get your viral load tested to make sure it remains undetectable.

If your lab results show that the virus is detectable or if you are having trouble taking every dose of your medication, you can still protect your HIV-negative partner by using other methods of preventing sexual transmission of HIV such as condoms, safer sex practices, and/

or pre-exposure prophylaxis (PrEP) for an HIV-negative partner until your viral load is undetectable again.

Taking HIV medicine to maintain an undetectable viral load does not protect you or your partner from getting other sexually transmitted diseases (STDs), so talk to your provider about ways to prevent other STDs.

Talk to Your Partner

TasP can be used alone or in conjunction with other prevention strategies. Talk about your HIV status with your sexual partners and decide together which prevention methods you will use. Some states have laws that require you to tell your sexual partner that you have HIV in certain circumstances.

Other Prevention Benefits of Human Immunodeficiency Virus Treatment

In addition to preventing sexual transmission of HIV there are other benefits of taking HIV medication to achieve and maintain an undetectable viral load:

- **It reduces the risk of mother-to-child transmission from pregnancy, labor, and delivery.** If a woman living with HIV can take HIV medication as prescribed throughout pregnancy, labor, and delivery and if HIV medication is given to her baby for four to six weeks after delivery, the risk of transmission from pregnancy, labor, and delivery can be reduced to one percent or less. Scientists don't know if a woman living with HIV who has her HIV under control can transmit HIV to her baby through breastfeeding. While it isn't known if or how much being undetectable or virally suppressed prevents some ways that HIV is transmitted, it is reasonable to assume that it provides some risk reduction.

- **It may reduce HIV transmission risk for people who inject drugs.** Scientists do not yet know whether having a suppressed or undetectable viral load prevents HIV transmission through sharing needles or other injection drug equipment, but it is reasonable to assume that it provides some risk reduction. Even if you are taking HIV medication and are undetectable, use new equipment each time you inject and do not share needles and syringes with other people.

413

Section 40.6

Effective Sexually Transmitted Disease-Prevention Programs for Youth

This section contains text excerpted from the following sources: Text beginning with the heading "Effective Human Immunodeficiency Virus and Sexually Transmitted Disease Prevention Education Programs" is excerpted from "Effective HIV and STD Prevention Programs for Youth: A Summary of Scientific Evidence," HIV.gov, U.S. Department of Health and Human Services (HHS), October 1, 2010. Reviewed February 2019; Text under the heading "A Healthy Start Is Equal to a Smart Start" is excerpted from "Healthy Relationships, Healthy Life: College Workshops Empower Students to Protect Their Own Sexual Health," Centers for Disease Control and Prevention (CDC), July 23, 2018.

Effective Human Immunodeficiency Virus and Sexually Transmitted Disease-Prevention Education Programs

Research shows that well-designed and well-implemented human immunodeficiency virus (HIV) or sexually transmitted disease (STD)-prevention programs can decrease sexual-risk behaviors among students, including:

- Delaying first sexual intercourse

- Reducing the number of sex partners

- Decreasing the number of times students have unprotected sex

- Increasing condom use

A review of 48 research studies found that about two-thirds of the HIV/STD-prevention programs studied had a significant impact on reducing sexual-risk behaviors, including a delay in first sexual intercourse, a decline in the number of sex partners, and an increase in a condom or contraceptive use. Notably, the HIV-prevention programs were not shown to hasten initiation of sexual intercourse among adolescents, even when those curricula encouraged sexually active young people to use condoms. In addition to determining programs that are most effective in reducing sexual health-risk behaviors among youth, scientists also have identified key common attributes among these programs. Effective HIV/STD-prevention programs tend to be those that

- Are delivered by trained instructors

- Are age-appropriate

- Include components on skill-building, support of healthy behaviors in school environments, and involvement of parents, youth-serving organizations, and health organizations

These common traits should guide curriculum development and integration of program activities for HIV/STD-prevention programs in schools and communities.

Youth Asset-Development Programs

A promising approach to HIV prevention seeks to increase the skills of children and adolescents to avoid health risks, including sexual-risk behaviors. Youth asset-development programs, including those conducted in schools, teach youth how to solve problems, communicate with others, and plan for the future. They also help youth develop positive connections with their parents, schools, and communities.

Youth asset-development programs typically address multiple health-risk behaviors and are commonly provided to children and adolescents over a number of years. Evidence indicates that these programs can be associated with long-term reductions in sexual-risk behaviors.

The CDC's Ongoing Efforts to Identify and Implement Effective Human Immunodeficiency Virus and Sexually Transmitted Disease-Prevention Programs for Youth

The Centers for Disease Control and Prevention's (CDC) Division of Adolescent and School Health (DASH) supports rigorous evaluation research and other projects to identify the types of programs and practices that can reduce sexual-risk behaviors among youth:

- DASH has supported the development and evaluation of

  - All About Youth, a randomized, controlled trial testing two HIV/STD education programs for middle school students: one that emphasizes sexual abstinence until marriage, and one that emphasizes abstinence in conjunction with skill-building activities for a condom and contraceptive use.

- Linking Lives, a program designed to build parents' skills to help them reduce sexual health risks among their middle-school children.

- DASH and the CDC's Division of Reproductive Health (DRH) collaborated with partners to publish a systematic review of the growing body of evidence on positive youth-development approaches for reducing HIV, sexually transmitted infections, and unintended pregnancy.

- DASH scientists

  - Analyze research on program effectiveness.

  - Develop guidelines for best practices in school-based HIV prevention.

  - Create tools to help schools implement the guidelines, such as the Health Education Curriculum Analysis Tool (www.cdc.gov/HECAT), which integrates research findings and national health education standards to help school districts select or develop health-education curricula that are most likely to reduce sexual-risk behaviors among the youth they serve.

A Healthy Start Is Equal to a Smart Start

"The idea is to introduce prevention tips before morbidity hits," said David Johnson, a Public Health Advisor (PHA) in the CDCs STD Program's Office of Health Equity (OHE), describing the purpose of the Healthy Relationships sexual-health workshop and course for incoming freshmen. The CDC is working with a growing number of historically Black colleges and universities (HBCUs) to implement this program. HBCUs can have disproportionate numbers of vulnerable populations, such as young, Black heterosexual women and young, Black gay and bisexual men. "With freshmen, you have the opportunity to lay a healthy foundation for those just coming into their own sexual identity," he said. The CDC's STD Program has expanded Healthy Relationships, a program that grew out of a sexual education workshop for medical students at a few HBCUs, into a comprehensive six- to eight-hour course that is required at most of the colleges that offer it. This program aims to reduce health inequities in STDs among students by engaging the stakeholders of the campus community and ultimately impacting school policy. So far, Healthy Relationships has been rolled out at North Carolina Agricultural and Technical University, Morehouse College, Spelman College, Rust College, and Lane College. The

CDC's STD Program is currently working with partners, such as the Links Inc., to engage other colleges and universities in order to bring Healthy Relationships to their campuses.

So what happens in Healthy Relationships workshops? "Real talk"—sound advice delivered in a relatable tone and format that young adults are receptive to—that includes an open and frank discussion of sexuality as a whole. The workshop covers a broad spectrum of topics that include communication skills, consent, sexual and gender identity, birth control, conflict resolution, and everything in between. "We changed the conversation," said Lydia Poromon, a Policy Analyst in the CDC's STD Program. "We connect with them by using language and scenarios that are culturally relatable. We teach them skills that are transferable and applicable to all relationships. We communicate with them rather than talking to or at them. It's empowerment through education."

Section 40.7

Syringe Services Programs

This section includes text excerpted from "Syringe Services Programs," Centers for Disease Control and Prevention (CDC), December 13, 2018.

People who inject drugs can substantially reduce their risk of getting and transmitting HIV, viral hepatitis and other blood-borne infections by using a sterile needle and syringe for every injection. In many jurisdictions, persons who inject drugs can access sterile needles and syringes through syringe services programs (SSPs) and through pharmacies without a prescription. Though less common, access to sterile needles and syringes may also be possible through a prescription written by a doctor and through other healthcare services.

The SSPs, which have also been referred to as syringe exchange programs (SEPs), needle-exchange programs (NEPs) and needle-syringe programs (NSPs) are community-based programs that provide access to sterile needles and syringes free of cost and facilitate safe disposal of used needles and syringes. As described in the Centers for Disease Control and Prevention (CDC) and U.S. Department of Health and Human Services (HHS) guidance, SSPs are an effective component of a comprehensive, integrated approach to HIV prevention among people with infectious diseases (PWID). These programs have also been associated with reduced risk for infection with hepatitis C virus. Most SSPs offer other prevention materials (e.g., alcohol swabs, vials of sterile water, condoms) and services, such as education on safer injection practices and wound care; overdose prevention; referral to substance-use disorder treatment programs, including medication-assisted treatment; and counseling and testing for HIV and hepatitis C. Many SSPs also provide linkage to critical services and programs, such as HIV care, treatment, pre-exposure prophylaxis (PrEP), and post-exposure prophylaxis (PEP) services; hepatitis C treatment and hepatitis A and B vaccinations; screening for other sexually transmitted diseases and tuberculosis; partner services; prevention of mother-to-child HIV transmission; and other medical, social, and mental-health services.

Federal Funding for Syringe Services Programs

The Consolidated Appropriations Act of 2016 includes language in Division H, Sec. 520 that gives states and local communities, under limited circumstances, the opportunity to use federal funds to support certain components of SSPs.

To support the implementation of this change in the law, HHS has released new guidance for state, local, tribal, and territorial health departments that will allow them to request permission to use federal funds to support SSPs. Federal funds can now be used to support a comprehensive set of services, but they cannot be used to purchase sterile needles or syringes for illegal drug injection.

The guidance states that eligible state, local, tribal, and territorial health departments must consult with the CDC and provide evidence that their jurisdiction is experiencing, or at risk for, significant increases in hepatitis infections or an HIV outbreak due to injection drug use.

After receiving a request for determination of need, the CDC will have 30 business days to notify the requestor whether the evidence is sufficient to demonstrate a need for SSPs. When the CDC finds there is sufficient evidence, state, local, tribal, and territorial health departments and other eligible HHS grant recipients may then apply to their respective federal agencies to direct funds to support approved SSP activities. Each federal agency (e.g., CDC, Health Resources and

Services Administration (HRSA), Substance Abuse and Mental Health Services Administration (SAMHSA)) is currently developing its own guidance for its funding recipients regarding which specific programs may apply and its application process.

The CDC Program Guidance for Implementing Certain Components of Syringe Services Programs, 2016 provides specific procedures for CDC-funded grantees. The CDC guidance details which SSP activities can be supported with CDC funds, which relevant CDC cooperative agreements can be used to support SSPs, and the process by which the CDC-funded programs may request to direct resources to implement new or expand existing SSPs for PWID.

Chapter 41

Post/Pre-Exposure Prophylaxis

What Is Post-Exposure Prophylaxis?

PEP stands for "post-exposure prophylaxis." The word "prophylaxis" means to prevent or protect from an infection or disease. PEP involves taking human immunodeficiency virus (HIV) medicines within 72 hours after a possible exposure to HIV to prevent becoming infected with HIV.

PEP should be used only in emergency situations. It is not meant for regular use by people who may be exposed to HIV frequently. PEP is not intended to replace regular use of other HIV prevention methods, such as consistent use of condoms during sex or pre-exposure prophylaxis (PrEP). PrEP is when people at high risk for HIV take a specific HIV medicine daily to prevent getting HIV.

Who Should Consider Taking Post-Exposure Prophylaxis?

PEP might be prescribed for you if you are HIV negative or don't know your HIV status, and in the last 72 hours you:

This chapter contains text excerpted from the following sources: Text under the heading "What Is Post-Exposure Prophylaxis" is excerpted from "Post-Exposure Prophylaxis (PEP)," AIDS*info*, U.S. Department of Health and Human Services (HHS), November 7, 2018; Text under the heading "What Is Pre-Exposure Prophylaxis" is excerpted from "Pre-Exposure Prophylaxis (PrEP)," AIDS*info*, U.S. Department of Health and Human Services (HHS), November 7, 2018.

- Think you may have been exposed to HIV during sex

- Shared needles or drug preparation equipment ("works")

- Were sexually assaulted

In addition, PEP may be prescribed for a healthcare worker following a possible exposure to HIV at work, for example, from a needlestick injury.

What Should I Do If I Think I Was Recently Exposed to Human Immunodeficiency Virus?

If you think you were recently exposed to HIV, contact your healthcare provider immediately or go to an emergency room right away. Your healthcare provider or emergency room doctor will help to decide whether you should receive PEP.

When Should Post-Exposure Prophylaxis Be Started?

PEP must be started within 72 hours (3 days) after possible exposure to HIV. The sooner you start PEP after a possible HIV exposure, the better. According to research, PEP will most likely not prevent HIV infection if it is started later than 72 hours after a person is exposed to HIV.

How Long Is Post-Exposure Prophylaxis Taken For?

PEP involves taking HIV medicines every day for 28 days. You will need to return to your healthcare provider at certain times while taking PEP and after you finish taking PEP for HIV testing and other tests.

What Human Immunodeficiency Virus Medicines Are Used for Post-Exposure Prophylaxis?

The Centers for Disease Control and Prevention (CDC) provides guidelines on recommended HIV medicines for PEP. The CDC guidelines include recommendations for specific groups of people, including adults and adolescents, children, pregnant women, and people with kidney problems. Your healthcare provider or emergency room doctor will determine which medicines you should take as part of PEP.

How Well Does Post-Exposure Prophylaxis Work?

PEP is effective in preventing HIV infection when it's taken correctly, but it's not 100 percent effective. The sooner you start PEP after a possible HIV exposure, the better. While taking PEP, it's important to keep using other HIV prevention methods, such as using condoms with sex partners and using only new, sterile needles when injecting drugs.

Does Post-Exposure Prophylaxis Cause Side Effects?

The HIV medicines used for PEP may cause side effects. The side effects can be treated and aren't life-threatening. If you are taking PEP, talk to your healthcare provider if you have any side effect that bothers you or that does not go away.

PEP medicines may also interact with other medicines that a person is taking (called a drug interaction). Because of potential drug interactions, it's important to tell your healthcare provider about any other medicines that you take.

What Is Post-Exposure Prophylaxis?

PrEP stands for "pre-exposure prophylaxis." The word "prophylaxis" means to prevent or protect from an infection or disease.

Pre-exposure Prophylaxis (PrEP) can help prevent HIV infection in people who don't have HIV but who are at high risk of becoming infected with HIV. PrEP involves taking an HIV medicine called Truvada every day. Truvada contains two HIV medicines (tenofovir disoproxil fumarate (TDF) and emtricitabine) combined in one pill. If a person is exposed to HIV, having the PrEP medicine in the bloodstream can stop HIV from taking hold and spreading throughout the body.

Who Should Consider Taking Pre-Exposure Prophylaxis?

PrEP is for people who don't have HIV but who are at high risk of becoming infected with HIV through sex or injection drug use.

Specifically, the Centers for Disease Control and Prevention (CDC) recommends that PrEP be considered for people who are HIV negative and in an ongoing sexual relationship with an HIV-positive partner. This recommendation also includes anyone who isn't in a mutually monogamous relationship with a partner who recently tested HIV negative, and:

- Is a gay or bisexual man who has had anal sex without using a condom or been diagnosed with a sexually transmitted disease (STD) in the past six months, or

- Is a heterosexual man or woman who does not regularly use condoms during sex with partners of unknown HIV status who are at substantial risk of HIV infection (for example, people who inject drugs or women who have bisexual male partners).

PrEP is also recommended for people who have injected drugs in the past six months and have shared needles or works or been in a drug treatment program in the past six months.

If you think PrEP may be right for you, talk to your healthcare provider.

How Well Does Pre-Exposure Prophylaxis Work?

PrEP is most effective when taken consistently each day. According to the CDC, by using PrEP every day, you can lower your risk of getting HIV from sex by more than 90 percent and from injection drug use by more than 70 percent. Adding other strategies, such as condom use, along with PrEP can reduce a person's risk even further.

Does Pre-Exposure Prophylaxis Cause Side Effects?

Some people taking PrEP may have side effects, like nausea, but these side effects are usually not serious and go away over time. Talk to your healthcare provider if you have any side effect that bothers you or that does not go away.

What Should I Do If I Think Pre-Exposure Prophylaxis Could Help Me?

If you think you may be at high risk for HIV and that you might benefit from PrEP, talk to your healthcare provider. If you and your healthcare provider agree that PrEP may be a good choice for you, the next step is an HIV test to be sure you don't already have HIV. If you are HIV negative and additional tests show that PrEP is likely safe for you, your healthcare provider can give you a prescription for PrEP.

Many health insurance plans cover the cost of PrEP. A commercial medication assistance program is available for people who may need assistance paying for PrEP.

What Happens Once I Start Pre-Exposure Prophylaxis?

Once you start PrEP, you will need to take PrEP every day. Studies have shown that PrEP is much less effective if it is not taken every day.

You should keep using condoms while taking PrEP. While taking PrEP daily can reduce your risk of HIV infection, the continued use of condoms can help reduce your risk even further. PrEP also does not reduce the risk of getting any other STDs.

You must also take an HIV test every three months while taking PrEP, so you'll have regular follow-up visits with your healthcare provider. If you are having trouble taking PrEP every day or if you want to stop taking PrEP, talk to your healthcare provider.

Part Six

Living with Sexually Transmitted Diseases

Chapter 42

Talking about Your Human Immunodeficiency Virus Status

Section 42.1

Just Diagnosed? What's Next?

This section includes text excerpted from "Living with HIV," HIV.gov, U.S. Department of Health and Human Services (HHS), May 15, 2017.

Nowadays, an estimated 1.1 million people are living with human immunodeficiency virus, (HIV) in the United States. Thanks to better treatments, people with HIV are now living longer—and with a better quality of life (QOL)—than ever before. If you are living with HIV, it's important to make choices that keep you healthy and protect others.

Stay Healthy

You should start medical care and begin HIV treatment as soon as you are diagnosed with HIV. Taking medicine to treat HIV, called antiretroviral therapy (ART) is recommended for all people with HIV. Taking medicine to treat HIV slows the progression of HIV and helps protect your immune system. The medicine can keep you healthy for many years and greatly reduces your chance of transmitting HIV to sex partner(s) if taken the right way, every day.

If you're taking medicine to treat HIV, visit your healthcare provider regularly and always take your medicine as directed to keep your viral load (the amount of HIV in the blood and elsewhere in the body) as low as possible.

Do Tell

It's important to disclose your HIV status to your sex and needle-sharing partner(s) even if you are uncomfortable doing it. Communicating with each other about your HIV status allows you and your partners to take steps to keep both of you healthy.

Also, ask your health department about free partner notification services. Health department staff can help find your sex or needle-sharing partner(s) to let them know they may have been exposed to HIV and provide them with testing, counseling, and referrals for other services. These partner notification services will not reveal your name unless you want to work with them to tell your partners.

Many states have laws that require you to tell your sexual partners if you're HIV-positive before you have sex (anal, vaginal, or oral) or tell your needle-sharing partners before you share drugs or needles to inject drugs. In some states, you can be charged with a crime if you don't tell your partner your HIV status, even if your partner doesn't become infected.

Get Support

Receiving a diagnosis of HIV is a life-changing event. But having HIV is by no means a death sentence. Pay attention to your mental health. People can feel many emotions—sadness, hopelessness, and even anger. Allied healthcare providers and social-service providers, often available at your healthcare provider's office, will have the tools to help you work through the early stages of your diagnosis and begin to manage your HIV.

Reduce the Risk to Others

HIV is spread through certain body fluids from an HIV-infected person: blood, semen, preseminal fluid, rectal fluids, vaginal fluids, and breast milk. In the United States, HIV is most often transmitted by having anal or vaginal sex with someone who is HIV-positive without using a condom or taking medicines to prevent or treat HIV. In addition, a mother can pass HIV to her baby during pregnancy, during labor, through breastfeeding, or by prechewing her baby's food.

The higher your viral load, the more likely you are to transmit HIV to others. When your viral load is very low (called "viral suppression," with fewer than 200 copies per milliliter of blood) or undetectable (about 40 copies per milliliter of blood), your chance of transmitting HIV is greatly reduced. However, this is true only if you can stay virally suppressed. One thing that can increase viral load is not taking HIV medicines the right way, every day.

You can also protect your partners by getting tested and treated for other sexually transmitted diseases (STDs). If you have both HIV and some other STD with sores, such as syphilis, your risk of transmitting HIV can be about three times as high as if you didn't have any STD with sores.

Taking other actions, such as using a condom the right way every time you have sex or having your partner(s) take daily (medicine to prevent HIV (called "pre-exposure prophylaxis" or "PrEP") can lower your chances of transmitting HIV even more.

Section 42.2

Whom to Tell about Your Positive Test Result

This section includes text excerpted from "Talking about Your HIV
Status," HIV.gov, U.S. Department of Health and Human
Services (HHS), May 15, 2017.

It's important to share your status with your sex partner(s) and/or
people with whom you inject drugs. Whether you disclose your status
to others is your decision.

Partners

It's important to disclose your human immunodeficiency virus (HIV)
status to your sex partner(s) and anyone you shared needles with,
even if you are not comfortable doing it. Communicating with each
other about your HIV status means you can take steps to keep both
of you healthy.

If you're nervous about disclosing your test result, or you have been
threatened or injured by a partner, you can ask your doctor or the local
health department to help you tell your partner(s) that they might
have been exposed to HIV. This type of assistance is called "partner
notification" or "partner services." Health departments do not reveal
your name to your partner(s). They will only tell your partner(s) that
they have been exposed to HIV and should get tested.

Many states have laws that require you to tell your sexual partners
if you're HIV-positive before you have sex (anal, vaginal, or oral) or tell
your drug-using partners before you share drugs or needles to inject
drugs. In some states, you can be charged with a crime if you don't tell
your partner your HIV status, even if you used a condom or another
type of protection and the partner does not become infected.

Healthcare Providers

Your healthcare providers (doctors, clinical workers, dentists, etc.)
have to know about your HIV status in order to be able to give you the
best possible care. It's also important that healthcare providers know
your HIV status so that they don't prescribe medication for you that
may be harmful when taken with your HIV medications.

Some states require you to disclose your HIV-positive status before
you receive any healthcare services from a physician or dentist. For
this reason, it's important to discuss the laws in your state about

disclosure in medical settings with the healthcare provider who gave you your HIV test results.

Your HIV test result will become part of your medical records so that your doctor or other healthcare providers can give you the best care possible. All medical information, including HIV test results, falls under strict confidentiality laws such as the Health Insurance Portability and Accountability Act's (HIPAA) Privacy Rule and cannot be released without your permission. There are some limited exceptions to confidentiality. These come into play only when not disclosing the information could result in harm to the other person.

Family and Friends

In most cases, your family and friends will not know your test results or HIV status unless you tell them yourself. While telling your family that you have HIV may seem hard, you should know that disclosure actually has many benefits—studies have shown that people who disclose their HIV status respond better to treatment than those who don't.

If you are under 18, however, some states allow your healthcare provider to tell your parent(s) that you received services for HIV if they think doing so is in your best interest.

Employers

In most cases, your employer will not know your HIV status unless you tell them. But your employer does have a right to ask if you have any health conditions that would affect your ability to do your job that pose a serious risk to others. (An example might be a healthcare professional, such as a surgeon, who does procedures in which there is a risk of blood or other body fluids being exchanged.)

If you have health insurance through your employer, the insurance company cannot legally tell your employer that you have HIV. But it is possible that your employer could find out if the insurance company provides detailed information to your employer about the benefits it pays or the costs of insurance.

All people with HIV are covered under the Americans with Disabilities Act (ADA). This means that your employer cannot discriminate against you because of your HIV status as long as you can do your job.

Section 42.3

Partner Communication and Agreements

his section includes text excerpted from "Monogamy,"
Centers for Disease Control and Prevention (CDC),
December 7, 2015. Reviewed February 2019.

Monogamy

If you and your partner are both HIV-negative, agreeing to be in a monogamous relationship can decrease your chances of getting HIV and other sexually transmitted diseases (STD).

But being in a relationship doesn't automatically protect you from HIV. And monogamy works only if both partners are certain they're HIV-negative and stay monogamous. If you and your partner are both HIV-positive, agreeing to be in a monogamous relationship can decrease your chances of getting other STDs or transmitting HIV to an HIV-negative sexual partner.

If you're in a monogamous relationship with someone who has a different HIV status than you, it's important to know that your overall chance of getting or transmitting HIV increases the more times you have sex with your partner. There are more options nowadays than ever before to keep you and your partner healthy and to reduce your chance of getting or transmitting HIV. The more actions you can take, the safer you can be. Actions include using condoms the right way every time you have sex; the HIV-negative partner talking to their healthcare provider about taking medicine daily (to prevent HIV called "preexposure prophylaxis," or "PrEP"); the HIV-positive partner taking medicine to treat HIV (called "antiretroviral therapy" or "ART") the right way, every day; and choosing lower-risk sexual behaviors. Your risk for getting or transmitting HIV is also affected by whether you or your partner has another STD.

What You Can Do

Being in a monogamous relationship can help reduce your risk of getting HIV if you and your partner are HIV-negative. Talk to your partner about monogamy and what you would do if one of you had sex with another person. Be sure that you and your partner understand any agreements you have about sex and communicate about any changes in your HIV status or sexual activity. And, if you're just beginning a monogamous relationship, it's a good idea for both of you to get tested for HIV before you have sex.

If you're in a monogamous relationship with someone whose HIV status is different from yours, it is important to remember that the overall chance of getting or transmitting HIV increases the more times you have sex. Taking one or more of these actions can decrease your risk of getting or transmitting HIV.

- The most important thing an HIV-positive partner can do is to take medicine to treat HIV the right way every day. ART reduces the amount of virus (viral load) in your partner's blood and body fluids. This means that your partner is less likely to transmit HIV to you.

- Choose less-risky sexual behaviors than anal or vaginal sex, such as oral sex.

- Use condoms the right way every time you have sex.

- The HIV-negative partner should talk to their healthcare provider to see if taking PrEP is right for them.

- The HIV-negative partner can talk to their healthcare provider right away (within three days) about taking medicine (called "postexposure prophylaxis," or "PEP") to prevent getting HIV if you might have been exposed to HIV-for example if the condom breaks during sex.

- Get tested and treated for STDs and encourage your partner to do the same.

Talking openly and frequently with your partner about sex can help you make decisions that may decrease your risk of getting or transmitting HIV.

Choosing Partners with the Same Human Immunodeficiency Virus Status

Serosorting can reduce your HIV risk if you know for sure you don't have HIV and your partner is actually HIV-negative. For serosorting to be effective, though, you need to know your own and your sex partner's HIV status, without any doubt. There is a potential risk in this strategy because your sex partners may not know for sure whether they have HIV if they were not tested recently. Even if they were recently tested, they might be in the window period. Also, sometimes your partners may not tell you they have HIV even if they know they have it. Because of these uncertainties, serosorting is less effective than consistent condom use. And even if your partner is HIV-negative, you can still get or transmit other STDs.

What You Can Do

If both you and your partner are HIV-positive, or both you and your partner are HIV-negative, having sex only with each other will eliminate the risk of transmitting HIV. However, if you do not know your HIV status or your partner's HIV status for sure, serosorting increases the risk of getting HIV when compared to using condoms the right way every time you have sex. This is because some people have not been tested recently, or even if tested may be in the window period, or may not tell you they have HIV even if they know they have it. And you can still get or transmit other sexually transmitted diseases (STD) if you serosort.

For serosorting to be effective, you need to:

• Make absolutely sure that you and your partner are both HIV-positive or both HIV-negative.

• Get tested for HIV and encourage your partner to get tested, too.

• Know when you should get an HIV test. If you or your partner had a potential exposure to HIV since the last test, then you may not really know your HIV status and you and your partner need to get tested again. You should use condoms or other prevention strategies until you can be retested.

Other things you can do to reduce the risk of getting or transmitting HIV include:

• Use condoms the right way every time you have sex.

• If you're HIV-negative, take medicine (PrEP).

• If you're HIV-positive, take medicine (ART).

• Choose sexual activities that are at lower risk for HIV than anal or vaginal sex.

Talking openly and frequently with your partner about sex can help you make decisions that may decrease your risk of getting or transmitting HIV.

Negotiated Safety

Negotiated safety is a type of sex agreement HIV-negative couples can use to help reduce the risk of getting HIV and other STDs if they follow the conditions of the strategy. Negotiated safety requires open communication between partners, careful planning and follow through of a shared agreement, and the use of condoms during sex until the required elements for safety are satisfied.

If partners meet all the conditions of a negotiated-safety agreement, it can help prevent them from getting HIV. If conditions are broken, partners can be placed at high risk. If partners can't follow the sex agreement or other aspects of negotiated safety, other prevention methods should be considered instead.

What You Can Do

If you and your partner agree to and follow the negotiated-safety strategy, including following all required conditions, then your risk of getting HIV can be reduced. This requires open communication between partners, careful planning and follow through of a shared agreement, and the use of condoms during sex until the required elements for safety are satisfied. If you don't think you and your partner can satisfy all of the conditions of negotiated safety, there are other things you can do to reduce the risk of getting HIV including:

- Use condoms the right way every time you have sex.

- Throw out the condom right away.

- Take daily medicine to prevent HIV (PrEP).

- Choose sexual activities that are at lower risk for HIV than anal or vaginal sex.

Section 42.4

Dealing with Stigma and Discrimination Associated with Human Immunodeficiency Virus

This section contains text excerpted from the following sources: Text beginning with the heading "What Is Human Immunodeficiency Virus Stigma?" is excerpted from "HIV Stigma Fact Sheet," Centers for Disease Control and Prevention (CDC), June 20, 2018; Text beginning with the heading "Legal Protections for People Living with HIV and AIDS" is excerpted from "Activities Combating HIV Stigma and Discrimination," U.S. Department of Health and Human Services," (HHS), May 20, 2017.

What Is Human Immunodeficiency Virus Stigma?

Human immunodeficiency virus (HIV) stigma is negative attitudes and beliefs about people with HIV. It is the prejudice that comes with labeling an individual as part of a group that is believed to be socially unacceptable.

Here are a few examples:

1. Believing that only certain groups of people can get HIV

2. Making moral judgments about people who take steps to prevent HIV transmission

3. Feeling that people deserve to get HIV because of their choices

What Is Discrimination?

While stigma refers to an attitude or belief, discrimination is the behavior that results from those attitudes or beliefs. HIV discrimination is the act of treating people with HIV differently than those without HIV.

Here are a few examples:

1. A healthcare professional refusing to provide care or services to a person living with HIV

2. Refusing casual contact with someone living with HIV

3. Socially isolating a member of a community because they are HIV positive

What Are the Effects of Human Immunodeficiency Virus Stigma and Discrimination?

HIV stigma and discrimination affect the emotional well-being and mental health of people with HIV. People with HIV often internalize the stigma they experience and begin to develop a negative self-image. They may fear they will be discriminated against or judged negatively if their HIV status is revealed.

"Internalized stigma" or "self-stigma" happens when a person takes in the negative ideas and stereotypes about people with HIV and starts to apply them to themselves. HIV internalized stigma can lead to feelings of shame, fear of disclosure, isolation, and despair. These feelings can keep people from getting tested and treated for HIV.

What Causes Human Immunodeficiency Virus Stigma?

HIV stigma is rooted in a fear of HIV. Many of our ideas about HIV come from the HIV images that first appeared in the early 1980s. There are still misconceptions about how HIV is transmitted and what it means to live with HIV today. The lack of information and awareness combined with outdated beliefs lead people to fear contracting HIV. Additionally, many people think of HIV as a disease that only certain groups get. This leads to negative value judgments about people who are living with HIV.

Legal Protections for People Living with Human Immunodeficiency Virus and Acquired Immunodeficiency Syndrome

Numerous federal laws protect people living with HIV and acquired immunodeficiency syndrome (AIDS) from discrimination. For example, people living with HIV and acquired immunodeficiency syndrome (AIDS) are protected from discrimination under the Americans with Disabilities Act (ADA), a federal act that guarantees equal opportunities in employment, housing, public accommodations, telecommunications, and transportation, and also applies to all local and state government services. People living with HIV and AIDS are also guaranteed protections from housing discrimination under the federal Fair Housing Act (FHA) and are protected from being excluded from federally funded programs under Section 504 of the Rehabilitation Act of 1973. Further, under the Affordable Care Act, people with pre-existing health conditions, including HIV, can no longer be dropped from, denied, or charged more for healthcare coverage, and under the Health Insurance Portability and Accountability Act of 1996 (HIPAA), the privacy and security of individuals' medical records and other health information maintained by HHS-funded programs and services is protected.

Envisioning a Future Free from Stigma and Discrimination

The National HIV/AIDS Strategy: Updated to 2020 calls for a reduction in stigma and elimination of discrimination associated with HIV status and commits to developing an indicator to measure HIV stigma and track progress toward that target. The Strategy identifies several HIV stigma-reduction steps, including mobilizing communities to reduce HIV-related stigma; strengthening the enforcement of civil rights laws; assisting states in protecting people with HIV from violence, retaliation, and discrimination associated with HIV status; and promoting the public leadership of people living with HIV. These actions will help achieve the Strategy's vision that "The United States will become a place where new HIV infections are rare and when they do occur, every person regardless of age, gender, race/ethnicity, sexual orientation, gender identity or socio-economic circumstance, will have unfettered access to high quality, life-extending care, free from stigma and discrimination."

Across the federal government, multiple agencies play a role in enforcing federal civil rights protections, providing technical assistance for carrying out the mandates of the ADA and other laws, and developing and disseminating information about civil rights and protections. While some departments have the authority to enforce these protections, nearly all have the ability to disseminate relevant information about protecting the rights of persons living with HIV and to take steps to confront and reduce HIV-related stigma.

Chapter 43

Sexually Transmitted Diseases Medicines and Vaccines

Chapter Contents

Section 43.1

What Is an Investigational Drug?

This section includes text excerpted from "HIV Overview—What Is an Investigational HIV Drug?" AIDS*info*, U.S. Department of Health and Human Services (HHS), July 9, 2018.

An investigational human immunodeficiency virus (HIV) drug is a drug that is being tested to treat or prevent HIV infection and is not approved by the U.S. Food and Drug Administration (FDA) for general use or sale in the United States. Medical-research studies—also called "clinical trials"—are done to evaluate the safety and effectiveness of an investigational HIV drug.

What Types of Investigational Human Immunodeficiency Virus Drugs Are Being Studied?

Currently, there are investigational drugs for treating and preventing HIV. There are also investigational drugs for treating HIV-related opportunistic infections (OIs). (Opportunistic infections are infections and infection-related cancers that occur more frequently or are more severe in people with weakened immune systems than in people with healthy immune systems.)

How Are Clinical Trials of Investigational Drugs Conducted?

Clinical trials, which are medical-research studies, are conducted in phases. Each phase has a different purpose and helps researchers answer different questions about the investigational drug.

- Phase 1 trials: Researchers test the investigational drug in a small group of people (20 to 80) for the first time. The purpose is to evaluate its safety and identify side effects.

- Phase 2 trials: The investigational drug is administered to a larger group of people (100 to 300) to determine its effectiveness and to further evaluate its safety.

- Phase 3 trials: The investigational drug is administered to large groups of people (1,000 to 3,000) to confirm its effectiveness, monitor side effects, compare it with standard or equivalent treatments, and collect information that will allow the investigational drug to be used safely.

In most cases, an investigational drug must be proven effective and must show continued safety in a Phase 3 clinical trial to be considered for approval by the FDA for sale in the United States. (Some drugs go through the FDA's accelerated approval process and are approved before a Phase 3 clinical trial is complete.) After a drug is approved by the FDA and made available to the public, researchers track its safety in Phase 4 trials to seek more information about the drug's risks, benefits, and optimal use.

How Can I Get Access to an Investigational Human Immunodeficiency Virus Drug?

One way to get access to an investigational HIV drug is by enrolling in a clinical trial that is studying the drug. Another way is through an expanded-access program (EAP). Expanded access involves using an investigational drug outside of a clinical trial to treat a person who has a serious or immediately life-threatening disease and who has no FDA-approved treatment options. Drug companies must have permission from the FDA to make an investigational drug available for expanded access. Talk to your healthcare provider to see if you may qualify to take part in an expanded access program.

Section 43.2

FDA-Approved Medicines

This section includes text excerpted from "HIV Overview—FDA-Approved HIV Medicines," AIDS*info*, U.S. Department of Health and Human Services (HHS), January 15, 2019.

Treatment with human immunodeficiency virus (HIV) medicines is called "antiretroviral therapy" (ART). ART is recommended for everyone with HIV. People on ART take a combination of HIV medicines (called an "HIV treatment regimen") every day. A person's initial HIV regimen generally includes three HIV medicines from at least two different drug classes.

The FDA-approved medicines for treating HIV are listed below.

Table 43.1. FDA-Approved Human Immunodeficiency Virus Medicines

Drug Class	Generic Name (Other Names and Acronyms)	Brand Name	FDA Approval Date
Nucleoside Reverse Transcriptase Inhibitors (NRTIs)			
Nucleoside reverse transcriptase inhibitors (NRTIs) block reverse transcriptase, an enzyme human immunodeficiency virus (HIV) needs to make copies of itself.	abacavir (abacavir sulfate, ABC)	Ziagen	December 17, 1998
	emtricitabine (FTC)	Emtriva	July 2, 2003
	lamivudine (3TC)	Epivir	November 17, 1995
	tenofovir disoproxil fumarate (tenofovir DF, TDF)	Viread	October 26, 2001
	zidovudine (azidothymidine, AZT, ZDV)	Retrovir	March 19, 1987
Non-Nucleoside Reverse Transcriptase Inhibitors (NNRTIs)			
Nonnucleoside reverse-transcriptase inhibitors (NNRTIs) bind to and later alter reverse transcriptase, an enzyme HIV needs to make copies of itself.	doravirine (DOR)	Pifeltro	August 30, 2018
	efavirenz (EFV)	Sustiva	September 17, 1998
	etravirine (ETR)	Intelence	January 18, 2008
	nevirapine (extended-release nevirapine, NVP)	Viramune	June 21, 1996
		Viramune XR (extended release)	March 25, 2011
	rilpivirine (rilpivirine hydrochloride, RPV)	Edurant	May 20, 2011

Table 43.1. Continued

Drug Class	Generic Name (Other Names and Acronyms)	Brand Name	FDA Approval Date
Protease Inhibitors (PIs)			
PIs block HIV protease, an enzyme HIV needs to make copies of itself.	atazanavir (atazanavir sulfate, ATV)	Reyataz	June 20, 2003
	darunavir (darunavir ethanolate, DRV)	Prezista	June 23, 2006
	fosamprenavir (fosamprenavir calcium, FOS-APV, FPV)	Lexiva	October 20, 2003
	ritonavir (RTV)*Although ritonavir is a PI, it is generally used as a pharmacokinetic enhancer as recommended in the Guidelines for the Use of Antiretroviral Agents in Adults and Adolescents Living with HIV and the Guidelines for the Use of Antiretroviral Agents in Pediatric HIV Infection.	Norvir	March 1, 1996
	saquinavir (saquinavir mesylate, SQV)	Invirase	December 6, 1995
	tipranavir (TPV)	Aptivus	June 22, 2005
Fusion Inhibitors			
Fusion inhibitors block HIV from entering the CD4 cells of the immune system.	enfuvirtide (T-20)	Fuzeon	March 13, 2003

Table 43.1. Continued

Drug Class	Generic Name (Other Names and Acronyms)	Brand Name	FDA Approval Date
CCR5 Antagonists			
CCR5 antagonists block CCR5 coreceptors on the surface of certain immune cells that HIV needs to enter the cells.	maraviroc (MVC)	Selzentry	August 6, 2007
Integrase Inhibitors			
Integrase inhibitors block HIV integrase, an enzyme HIV needs to make copies of itself.	dolutegravir (DTG, dolutegravir sodium)	Tivicay	August 13, 2013
	raltegravir (raltegravir potassium, RAL)	Isentress	October 12, 2007
		Isentress HD	May 26, 2017
Post-Attachment Inhibitors			
Post-attachment inhibitors block CD4 receptors on the surface of certain immune cells that HIV needs to enter the cells.	ibalizumab (Hu5A8, IBA, Ibalizumab-uiyk, TMB-355, TNX-355)	Trogarzo	March 6, 2018
Pharmacokinetic Enhancers			
Pharmacokinetic enhancers are used in HIV treatment to increase the effectiveness of an HIV medicine included in an HIV regimen.	cobicistat (COBI)	Tybost	September 24, 2014

Table 43.1. Continued

Drug Class	Generic Name (Other Names and Acronyms)	Brand Name	FDA Approval Date
Combination HIV Medicines			
Combination HIV medicines contain two or more HIV medicines from one or more drug classes.	abacavir and lamivudine (abacavir sulfate / lamivudine, ABC / 3TC)	Epzicom	August 2, 2004
	abacavir, dolutegravir, and lamivudine (abacavir sulfate / dolutegravir sodium / lamivudine, ABC / DTG / 3TC)	Triumeq	August 22, 2014
	abacavir, lamivudine, and zidovudine (abacavir sulfate / lamivudine / zidovudine, ABC / 3TC / ZDV)	Trizivir	November 14, 2000
	atazanavir and cobicistat (atazanavir sulfate / cobicistat, ATV / COBI)	Evotaz	January 29, 2015
	bictegravir, emtricitabine, and tenofovir alafenamide (bictegravir sodium / emtricitabine / tenofovir alafenamide fumarate, BIC / FTC / TAF)	Biktarvy	February 7, 2018
	darunavir and cobicistat (darunavir ethanolate / cobicistat, DRV / COBI)	Prezcobix	January 29, 2015

Table 43.1. Continued

Drug Class	Generic Name (Other Names and Acronyms)	Brand Name	FDA Approval Date
	darunavir, cobicistat, emtricitabine, and tenofovir alafenamide (darunavir ethanolate / cobicistat / emtricitabine / tenofovir AF, darunavir ethanolate / cobicistat / emtricitabine / tenofovir alafenamide, darunavir / cobicistat / emtricitabine / tenofovir AF, darunavir / cobicistat / emtricitabine / tenofovir alafenamide fumarate, DRV / COBI / FTC / TAF)	Symtuza	July 17, 2018
	dolutegravir and rilpivirine (dolutegravir sodium / rilpivirine hydrochloride, DTG / RPV)	Juluca	November 21, 2017
	doravirine, lamivudine, and tenofovir disoproxil fumarate (doravirine / lamivudine / TDF, doravirine / lamivudine / tenofovir DF, DOR / 3TC / TDF)	Delstrigo	August 30, 2018
	efavirenz, emtricitabine, and tenofovir disoproxil fumarate (efavirenz / emtricitabine / tenofovir DF, EFV / FTC / TDF)	Atripla	July 12, 2006
	efavirenz, lamivudine, and tenofovir disoproxil fumarate (EFV / 3TC / TDF)	Symfi	March 22, 2018

Table 43.1. Continued

Drug Class	Generic Name (Other Names and Acronyms)	Brand Name	FDA Approval Date
	efavirenz, lamivudine, and tenofovir disoproxil fumarate (EFV / 3TC / TDF)	Symfi Lo	February 5, 2018
	elvitegravir, cobicistat, emtricitabine, and tenofovir alafenamide (elvitegravir / cobicistat / emtricitabine / tenofovir alafenamide fumarate, EVG / COBI / FTC / TAF)	Genvoya	November 5, 2015
	elvitegravir, cobicistat, emtricitabine, and tenofovir disoproxil fumarate (QUAD, EVG / COBI / FTC / TDF)	Stribild	August 27, 2012
	emtricitabine, rilpivirine, and tenofovir alafenamide (emtricitabine / rilpivirine / tenofovir AF, emtricitabine / rilpivirine / tenofovir alafenamide fumarate, emtricitabine / rilpivirine hydrochloride / tenofovir AF, emtricitabine / rilpivirine hydrochloride / tenofovir alafenamide, emtricitabine / rilpivirine hydrochloride / tenofovir alafenamide fumarate, FTC / RPV / TAF)	Odefsey	March 1, 2016

Table 43.1. Continued

Drug Class	Generic Name (Other Names and Acronyms)	Brand Name	FDA Approval Date
	emtricitabine, rilpivirine, and tenofovir disoproxil fumarate (emtricitabine / rilpivirine hydrochloride / tenofovir disoproxil fumarate, emtricitabine / rilpivirine / tenofovir, FTC / RPV / TDF)	Complera	August 10, 2011
	emtricitabine and tenofovir alafenamide (emtricitabine / tenofovir AF, emtricitabine / tenofovir alafenamide fumarate, FTC / TAF)	Descovy	April 4, 2016
	emtricitabine and tenofovir disoproxil fumarate (emtricitabine / tenofovir DF, FTC / TDF)	Truvada	August 2, 2004
	lamivudine and tenofovir disoproxil fumarate (Temixys, 3TC / TDF)	Cimduo	February 28, 2018
	lamivudine and zidovudine (3TC / ZDV)	Combivir	September 27, 1997
	lopinavir and ritonavir (ritonavir-boosted lopinavir, LPV/r, LPV / RTV)	Kaletra	September 15, 2000

Section 43.3

What Is a Preventative Human Immunodeficiency Virus Vaccine?

This section includes text excerpted from "HIV Overview—
What Is a Preventive HIV Vaccine?" AIDS*info*, U.S. Department of
Health and Human Services (HHS), August 1, 2018.

A preventive human immunodeficiency virus (HIV) vaccine is given to people who do not have HIV, with the goal of preventing HIV infection in the future. The vaccine would teach the person's immune system to recognize and effectively fight HIV in case the person is ever exposed to HIV.

Are There Any U.S. Food and Drug Administration-Approved Preventive Human Immunodeficiency Virus Vaccines?

Currently, no preventive HIV vaccines have been approved by the U.S. Food and Drug Administration (FDA), but research is underway. You must be enrolled in a clinical trial to receive a preventive HIV vaccine.

How Is a Preventive Human Immunodeficiency Virus Vaccine Different from a Therapeutic Human Immunodeficiency Virus Vaccine?

While a preventive HIV vaccine is given to people who do not have HIV, a therapeutic HIV vaccine is given to people who already have HIV. The goal of a therapeutic HIV vaccine is to strengthen a person's immune response to the HIV that is already in the person's body. Researchers are exploring the use of therapeutic HIV vaccines:

• To slow down the progression of HIV infection

• To eliminate the need for antiretroviral therapy (ART) while still keeping undetectable levels of HIV

• As part of a larger strategy to eliminate all HIV from the body

451

Can I Get Human Immunodeficiency Virus from a Preventive Human Immunodeficiency Virus Vaccine?

No, you cannot get HIV from a preventive HIV vaccine. The preventive HIV vaccines being studied in clinical trials do not contain HIV. Of the approximately 30,000 people who have participated in HIV vaccine studies around the world in the last 25 years, no one has gotten HIV from any of the vaccines tested.

Why Is a Preventive Human Immunodeficiency Virus Vaccine Important?

Treatment options for HIV infection have improved a lot over the last 30 years. But HIV medicines can have side effects, can be expensive, and can be hard to access in some countries. Also, some people may develop drug resistance to certain HIV medicines and then must change medicines.

Current prevention tools for HIV, such as using condoms correctly and pre-exposure prophylaxis (PrEP), work well. But researchers believe a preventive HIV vaccine will be the most effective way to completely end new HIV infections.

Section 43.4

Anti-Human Immunodeficiency Virus Drug Acts to Block Human Papillomavirus

This section includes text excerpted from "NIH Researchers Show How Anti-HIV Drug Acts to Block Herpes Virus," National Institutes of Health (NIH), October 20, 2011. Reviewed February 2019.

National Institutes of Health Researchers Show How an Anti-Human Immunodeficiency Virus Drug Acts to Block the Herpes Virus

Researchers discovered that an anti-human immunodeficiency virus (HIV) drug that stops the spread of the genital herpes virus by disabling a key deoxyribonucleic acid (DNA) enzyme of the herpes virus, according to findings by researchers at the National Institutes of Health (NIH) and other institutions.

The findings explain the results of a clinical trial showing that the anti-HIV drug tenofovir, when formulated as a vaginal gel, could reduce the risk of herpes simplex virus (HSV) infections—as well as HIV infections—in women.

Taken orally, tenofovir had been demonstrated to inhibit reproduction of HIV but had not been known to block the genital herpes virus.

"HIV infection is closely associated with herpes viral infection. When people with genital herpes are exposed to HIV, they are more likely to become infected than are people who do not carry the herpes virus," said Leonid Margolis, Ph.D., head of the Section on Intercellular Interactions (ICI) at *Eunice Kennedy Shriver* National Institute of Child Health and Human Development (NICHD) and one of the authors of the study. "Human tissues convert tenofovir to a form that suppresses HIV. We found that this form of tenofovir also suppresses HSV. This discovery may help to identify drugs to treat the two viruses even more effectively."

Discoveries leading to new uses for previously approved drugs have the potential to save millions of dollars, Dr. Margolis said. New drugs typically undergo years of testing for safety and effectiveness before they are approved for patients. Finding new uses for an approved drug increases the value of the initial investment in testing because most of the testing has previously been completed.

The researchers examined individual cells and groups of cells infected with HSV and found that high concentrations of tenofovir prevent the ability of this virus to reproduce. They also confirmed that tenofovir itself did not damage the cells. These tests included the type of cells that line the vagina, which is a target for infection with HSV and HIV.

Tenofovir is converted by cellular enzymes into another chemical form. The researchers found that this form of tenofovir suppresses not only HIV but HSV as well. Specifically, the researchers showed that this active form of tenofovir can disable an enzyme that the virus needs to reproduce.

The researchers also examined the effects of tenofovir in tissue samples. They injected HSV into tonsil and cervix tissue, and then applied tenofovir. They found that, after 12 days, levels of the virus were only 1 to 13 percent of the viral levels of untreated tissue. Tenofovir also blocked viral reproduction in tissue infected with both HIV and HSV simultaneously.

Using tenofovir to treat lab mice infected with the herpes virus also prevented symptoms of the disease and prolonged the animals' survival, the researchers found.

The vaginal gel showed activity against HSV apparently because of the high concentration of tenofovir that it contains. In contrast, when tenofovir is taken orally, tissue levels do not reach sufficient levels to significantly affect HSV.

"When using the gel, the amount of tenofovir on the affected tissues is about 100 times the amount in the body when taking tenofovir in pill form," said Dr. Margolis. "That explains why its antiherpes activity wasn't noticed before. Thus, under proper conditions, an anti-HIV drug becomes an anti-HSV drug."

In previous research, Dr. Margolis's team showed that an anti-HSV drug, acyclovir, is converted inside the infected cells into an anti-HIV drug. They now believe the next step will be to find the form in which such drugs are most potent against both viruses at the same time.

Chapter 44

Starting Human Immunodeficiency Virus Care

Chapter Contents

Section 44.1

Find a Provider

This section includes text excerpted from "Locate an
HIV Care Provider," HIV.gov, U.S. Department of Health
and Human Services (HHS), May 15, 2017.

Locate a Human Immunodeficiency Virus Care Provider

Once you receive a diagnosis of human immunodeficiency virus
(HIV), the most important next step is to get into medical care. Getting into medical care and staying on treatment will help you manage
your HIV effectively and make decisions that can keep you healthy
for many years.

If you received your diagnosis in a healthcare provider's office or
a nonclinical setting (health fair, community organization, or testing
event), you have probably received a lot of information about HIV, its
treatment, and how to stay healthy. Give yourself time to absorb the
information and get into care and on treatment right away. If you do
not have much information, the website HIV.gov is a good place to
begin to familiarize yourself with HIV.

If you received a diagnosis by taking an HIV test at home, it is
important that you take the next steps to make sure the result is
correct. Both manufacturers provide confidential counseling and will
help you with getting the follow-up test done.

How Do You Find a Human Immunodeficiency Virus-Care Provider?

If you have a primary healthcare provider (someone who manages
your regular medical care and annual tests), that person may have
the medical knowledge to treat your HIV. If not, he or she can refer
you to a healthcare provider who is a specialist in providing HIV care
and treatment.

Here are some other services to help you locate HIV providers and
services near you:

- HIV.gov's HIV Testing Sites and Care Services Locator can
  help you find HIV-related services across the United States,
  including HIV medical care, HIV testing, housing assistance,
  and substance-abuse and mental-health services (from HIV.gov).

- State human immunodeficiency virus (HIV) and acquired immunodeficiency syndrome (AIDS) toll-free hotlines are available to help you connect with agencies that can help determine what services you are eligible for and help you get them (from the U.S. Health Resources and Services Administration (HRSA)).

- The Ryan White HIV/AIDS Medical Care Provider Locator can help you locate HIV/AIDS medical care (from the U.S. Health Resources and Services Administration (HRSA)).

- This directory of credentialed HIV-care specialists and members of the American Academy of HIV Medicine (AAHIVM) can help you access HIV practitioners across the country (from the American Academy of HIV Medicine (AAHIVM)).

It is important that you start medical care and begin HIV treatment as soon as possible after you are diagnosed with HIV. Antiretroviral therapy (ART) is recommended for all people with HIV, regardless of how long they've had the virus or how healthy they are. Starting ART slows the progression of HIV and helps protect your immune system. ART, if taken consistently and correctly, can keep you healthy for many years and greatly reduces your chance of transmitting HIV to others.

Most people living with HIV who do not seek medical care eventually receive an AIDS diagnosis. This happens because, if left untreated, HIV will attack the immune system and allow different types of life-threatening infections and cancers to develop. A cure for HIV does not yet exist, but ART can dramatically prolong the lives of many people living with HIV and lower their chances of infecting others.

Types of Providers

Finding a healthcare team that is knowledgeable about HIV care is an important step in managing your care and treatment. If you are able to choose your provider, you should look for someone who has a great deal of experience treating HIV. This matters because the more HIV experience your provider has, the more familiar she or he will be with the full range of current HIV treatment options, as well as the unique issues that come up in HIV care over time.

The kinds of experts that make up your HIV healthcare team will depend on your healthcare needs and the way that the healthcare system, clinic, or office where you receive care is set up. It should also be based on your preferences and what will work best for you. Don't get hung up on finding the perfect provider the first week after you are diagnosed. The most important thing you can do now for your health is to meet with an HIV provider who can order your first lab tests and start HIV treatment as soon as possible. Don't let the search for the perfect doctor slow you down on this. You can change doctors later if you need to. Your HIV healthcare provider should lead your healthcare team. That person will help you determine which HIV medicines are best for you, prescribe ART, monitor your progress, and partner with you in managing your health. He or she can also help put you in touch with other types of providers who can address your needs. Your primary HIV healthcare provider may be a doctor of medicine (MD) or doctor of osteopathic medicine (DO), nurse practitioner (NP), or a physician assistant (PA). Some women may prefer to see an obstetrics and gynecology (OB-GYN) provider who has expertise in HIV/AIDS. On the whole, the patients of providers with more experience in HIV care tend to do better than those who see a provider who only has limited HIV-care experience.

In addition to your HIV healthcare provider, your healthcare team may include other healthcare providers, allied healthcare professionals, and social-service providers who are experts in taking care of people living with HIV.

The types of professionals who may be involved in your HIV care include:

Healthcare Providers

- **Medical doctors (MD or DO):** Healthcare professionals who are licensed to practice medicine

- **Nurse practitioners (NP):** Registered nurses, with specialized graduate education who can diagnose and treat illnesses independently or as part of a healthcare team

- **Physician assistants (PA):** Healthcare professionals who are trained to examine patients, diagnose injuries and illnesses, and provide treatment to patients under the supervision of physicians and surgeons

Allied Healthcare Professionals

- **Nurses:** Healthcare professionals who provide and coordinate patient care as part of a healthcare team.

- **Mental-health providers:** Professionals, such as a counselor, psychologist, or psychiatrist, who provide mental-healthcare in the form of counseling or other types of therapy

- **Pharmacists:** Healthcare professionals who provide prescription medicines to patients and offer expertise in the safe use of prescriptions. Pharmacists may also provide advice on how to lead a healthy life; conduct health and wellness screenings; provide immunizations; and oversee medicines given to patients.

- **Nutritionists/dietitians:** Experts in food and nutrition who advise people on what to eat in order to lead a healthy lifestyle or achieve a specific health-related goal

- **Dentists:** Healthcare professionals who diagnose and treat problems with a person's teeth, gums, and related parts of the mouth. Dentists also provide advice and instruction on taking care of teeth and gums and on diet choices that affect oral health.

Social Service Providers

- **Social workers:** Professionals who help people solve and cope with problems in their everyday lives

- **Case managers:** Professionals who help people find the support and services they need, develop a services plan, and follow-up to make sure that services are provided

- **Substance-use and substance-abuse specialists:** Counselors who provide advice, treatment, and support to people who have problems with substance use

Patient Navigators

There are a number of different types of navigators who are trained and culturally sensitive workers who provide support and guidance to people by helping them "navigate" through the healthcare system. For example, navigators could be healthcare workers, social workers, those who work for community-based organizations, or peers.

Take Charge of Your Care
How Can You Work Best with Your Healthcare Team

HIV treatment is most successful when you actively take part in your medical care. That means taking your HIV medications every time, at the right time, and in the right way; keeping your medical appointments, and communicating honestly with your healthcare provider. This can be achieved when you:

- Keep all of your medical appointments. There are many tools you can use to help you remember and prepare for your appointments. You can:

  - Use a calendar to mark your appointment days.

  - Set reminders on your phone.

  - Download a free app from the Internet to your computer or smartphone that can help remind you of your medical appointments. Search for "reminder apps" and you will find many choices.

  - Keep your appointment card in a place where you will see it often, such as on a mirror, or on your refrigerator.

- Ask a family member or friend to help you remember your appointment.

- Be prepared for your medical appointments. Before an appointment, write down questions or concerns you want to discuss with your healthcare provider. Be prepared to write down the answers you receive during your visit.

- If you can't keep a scheduled appointment, contact your provider to let them know, and make a new appointment as soon as possible.

- Communicate openly and honestly with your healthcare providers. Your healthcare provider needs to have the most accurate information to manage your care and treatment.

- Keep track of your medical services. You may have multiple healthcare providers working on your healthcare team. Keep records of your lab results, medical visits, appointment dates and times, medicines and medicine schedules, and care and treatment plans.

- Update your contact information. Make sure your healthcare providers have your correct contact information (telephone number, address, and e-mail address) and let them know if any contact information changes.

Section 44.2

What to Expect at Your First Human Immunodeficiency Virus Care Visit

This section includes text excerpted from "What to Expect at Your First HIV Care Visit," HIV.gov, U.S. Department of Health and Human Services (HHS), May 15, 2017.

Living with HIV can be challenging at times. Partnering with your healthcare provider will help you manage your health and HIV care. During your medical appointments, your healthcare provider may:

- Conduct medical exams to see how HIV is affecting your body.

- Ask you questions about your health history.

- Take a blood sample to check your Cluster of Differentiation 4 (CD4) count and viral load.

- Look for other kinds of infections or health problems that may weaken your body, make your HIV infection worse, or prevent your treatment from working as well as possible.

- Give you immunizations, if you need them.

- Discuss, prescribe, and monitor your HIV medicines, including when and how to take them, possible side effects, and continued effectiveness.

- Discuss strategies that will help you follow your HIV-treatment plan and maintain your treatment.

- Help identify additional support you may need, such as finding a social worker, case manager, or patient navigator; finding an HIV support group; finding support services for mental-health or substance-use issues, or finding support services for transportation or housing.

- Ask you about your sex partner(s) and discuss ways to protect them from getting HIV.

- Ask you about your plans, or your partner's plans, for getting pregnant.

Talk regularly with your healthcare provider about how you are feeling and communicate openly and honestly. Tell your healthcare provider about any health problems you are having so that you can get proper treatment. Discuss how often you should expect to attend medical visits. Staying informed about HIV care and treatment advances and partnering with your healthcare provider are important steps in managing your health and HIV care.

What Tests Can Help Monitor Your Human Immunodeficiency Virus Infection?

Your healthcare provider will use blood tests to monitor your HIV infection. The results of these blood tests, which measure the amount of HIV virus and the number of CD4 cells in your blood, will help you and your healthcare provider understand how well your HIV treatment is working to control your HIV infection. These test results will also help your healthcare provider decide whether he or she should make changes to your treatment.

These blood tests include regular CD4 counts and viral-load tests. Read about these tests below.

Cluster of Differentiation 4 Count

CD4 cells, also called "T-cells," play an important role in your body's ability to fight infections. Your CD4 count is the number of CD4 cells you have in your blood. When you are living with HIV, the virus attacks and lowers the number of CD4 cells in your blood. This makes it difficult for your body to fight infections.

Typically, your healthcare provider will check your CD4 count every 3 to 6 months. A normal range for a CD4 cell count is 500 cells to 1,600 cells per cubic millimeter of blood (you may see this written as "cells/mm3"). A low CD4 cell count means you are at higher risk of developing opportunistic infections. These infections take advantage of your body's weakened immune system and can cause life-threatening illnesses. A higher CD4 cell count means that your HIV treatment is working and controlling the virus. As your CD4 count increases, your body is better able to fight infection. If you have a CD4 count of fewer than 200 cells per cubic millimeter of blood, you will be diagnosed as having AIDS.

Viral-Load Test

Your viral load is the amount of HIV in your blood. When your viral load is high, you have more HIV in your body, and your immune system is not fighting HIV as well.

When you take a viral-load test, your healthcare provider looks for the number of HIV virus particles in a milliliter of your blood. These particles are called "copies."

The goal of HIV treatment is to help move your viral load down to undetectable levels. In general, your viral load will be declared "undetectable" if it is under 40 to 75 copies in a sample of your blood. The exact number depends on the lab that analyzes your test.

Your healthcare provider will use a viral-load test to determine your viral load. A viral-load test will:

- Show how well your HIV treatment is controlling the virus, and

- Provide information on your health status.

You should have a viral-load test every three to six months before you start taking a new HIV medicine, and two to eight weeks after starting or changing medicines.

Chapter 45

Taking Care of Yourself

Chapter Contents

Section 45.1

Coping Physically

This section includes text excerpted from "Exercise and Physical Activity," HIV.gov, U.S. Department of Health and Human Services (HHS), January 2, 2019.

Should People Living with Human Immunodeficiency Virus Exercise?

Being human immunodeficiency virus (HIV)-positive is no different from being HIV-negative when it comes to exercise. Regular physical activity and exercise are part of a healthy lifestyle for everyone, including people living with HIV.

What Are the Benefits of Physical Activity?

Physical activity has many important benefits. It can

- Boost your mood
- Sharpen your focus
- Reduce your stress
- Improve your sleep

Physical activity can also help you reduce your risk of developing cardiovascular disease (CVD), high blood pressure (BP), type 2 diabetes, and several types of cancer. These are all health conditions that can affect people living with HIV.

How Much Activity Should You Do?

According to the evidence-based Physical Activity Guidelines (2018), adults need at least 150 to 300 minutes per week of moderate-intensity aerobic activity, such as biking, brisk walking, or fast dancing. Adults also need muscle-strengthening activity, such as lifting weights or doing push-ups, at least two days per week.

If you're living with HIV or have another chronic health condition, talk to your healthcare provider or a physical activity specialist to make sure these guidelines are right for you.

The most important thing is to move more and sit less!

What Types of Activity Are Right for People Living with Human Immunodeficiency Virus?

People living with HIV can do the same types of physical activity and exercise as individuals who do not have HIV.

Physical activity is any body movement that works your muscles and requires more energy than resting. Brisk walking, running, biking, dancing, jumping rope, and swimming are a few examples of physical activity.

Exercise is a type of physical activity that's planned and structured with the goal of improving your health or fitness. Taking an aerobics class and playing on a sports team are examples of exercise. Both are part of living healthy.

Take time to find a fitness routine that you enjoy. You may consider taking part in a group activity that allows you to engage with others. Make it fun, and commit to being physically active regularly.

Section 45.2

Coping Mentally

This section includes text excerpted from "Living with HIV—HIV and Mental Health," AIDS*info*, U.S. Department of Health and Human Services (HHS), January 14, 2019.

What Is Mental Health?

Mental health refers to a person's overall emotional, psychological, and social well-being. Mental health affects how people think, feel, and act. Good mental health helps people make healthy choices, reach personal goals, develop healthy relationships, and cope with stress.

Poor mental health is not the same as mental illness. Mental illnesses include many different conditions—for example, posttraumatic stress disorder (PTSD), bipolar disorder (BD), and schizophrenia. A person can have poor mental health and not have a diagnosed mental illness. Likewise, a person with a mental illness can still enjoy mental well-being.

If you are living with HIV, it's important to take care of both your physical health and your mental health.

Are People with Human Immunodeficiency Virus at Risk for Mental-Health Conditions?

Anyone can have mental-health problems. Mental-health conditions are common in the United States. According to the U.S. Department of Health and Human Services (HHS), in 2014, about one in five American adults experienced a mental-health issue.

However, people with HIV have a higher risk for mental-health conditions than people who do not have HIV. For example, people living with HIV are twice as likely to have depression as people who do not have HIV.

It's important to remember that mental-health conditions are treatable and that people who have mental-health problems can recover.

What Can Cause Mental-Health Problems?

The following factors can increase the risk of mental-health problems:

- Major life changes, such as the death of a loved one or the loss of a job

- Negative life experiences, such as abuse or trauma

- Biological factors that affect genes or brain chemistry

- Family history of mental-health problems

The stress of having a serious medical illness or condition, such as an HIV infection, may also negatively affect a person's mental health. HIV infection and related opportunistic infections can affect the brain and nervous system (NS). This may lead to changes in how a person thinks and behaves. In addition, some medicines used to treat HIV may have side effects that affect a person's mental health.

What Are the Warning Signs of a Mental-Health Problem?

Changes in how a person feels or acts can be a warning sign of a mental-health problem. Potential signs of a mental-health problem include:

- Losing interest in activities that are usually enjoyable
- Experiencing persistent sadness or feeling empty
- Feeling anxious or stressed
- Having suicidal thoughts

If you have any of these signs of a mental-health problem, it's important to get help.

What Should I Do If I Need Help for a Mental-Health Problem?

Talk to your healthcare provider about how you are feeling. Tell them if you are having any problems with drugs or alcohol.

Your healthcare provider will consider whether any of your HIV medicines may be affecting your mental health. They can also help you find a mental-healthcare provider, for example, a psychiatrist or therapist.

Here are additional ways to improve your mental health:

- Join a support group.
- Try meditation, yoga,* or deep breathing to relax.
- Get enough sleep, eat healthy meals, and stay physically active.

Yoga is a mind and body practice with origins in ancient Indian philosophy. The various styles of yoga typically combine physical postures, breathing techniques, and meditation or relaxation.

Part Seven

Additional Help and Information

Chapter 46

Glossary of Terms Related to Sexually Transmitted Diseases

abstinence: Not having sexual intercourse.

acquired immunodeficiency syndrome (AIDS): A disease of the immune system due to infection with HIV (human immunodeficiency virus). HIV destroys the CD4 T lymphocytes (CD4 cells) of the immune system, leaving the body vulnerable to life-threatening infections and cancers. AIDS is the most advanced stage of HIV infection.

adherence: Taking medications exactly as prescribed. Poor adherence to an HIV treatment regimen increases the risk for developing drug-resistant HIV and virologic failure.

antiretroviral therapy (ART): The recommended treatment for HIV infection. ART involves using a combination of three or more antiretroviral (ARV) drugs from at least two different HIV drug classes to prevent HIV from replicating.

bacterial vaginosis (BV): A vaginal infection that develops when there is an increase in harmful bacteria and a decrease in good bacteria in the vagina.

This glossary contains terms excerpted from documents produced by several sources deemed reliable.

biopsy: Removal of tissue, cells, or fluid from the body for examination under a microscope. Biopsies are used to diagnose disease.

cervical cancer: A type of cancer that develops in the cervix. Cervical cancer is almost always caused by the human papillomavirus (HPV), which is spread through sexual contact.

chancroid: A sexually transmitted disease (STD) caused by the bacterium *Haemophilus ducreyi*. Chancroid causes genital ulcers (sores).

chlamydia: A common sexually transmitted disease caused by the bacterium *Chlamydia trachomatis*. Chlamydia often has mild or no symptoms, but if left untreated, it can lead to serious complications, including infertility.

coinfection: When a person has two or more infections at the same time. For example, a person infected with HIV may be coinfected with hepatitis or tuberculosis (TB) or both.

condom: A device used during sexual intercourse to block semen from coming in contact with the inside of the vagina. Condoms are used to reduce the likelihood of pregnancy and to prevent the transmission of sexually transmitted disease, including HIV. The male condom is a thin rubber cover that fits over an erect penis. The female condom is a polyurethane pouch that fits inside the vagina.

dental dam: A thin, rectangular sheet, usually latex rubber, used as a barrier to prevent the transmission of sexually transmitted infections during oral sex.

drug resistance: When a bacteria, virus, or other microorganism mutates (changes form) and becomes insensitive to (resistant to) a drug that was previously effective.

fallopian tubes: Tubes on each side of ovaries to the uterus.

genital warts: A sexually transmitted disease caused by the human papillomavirus (HPV). Genital warts appear as raised pink or flesh-colored bumps on the surface of the vagina, cervix, tip of the penis, or anus.

gonorrhea: A sexually transmitted disease caused by the bacterium *Neisseria gonorrhoeae*. Gonorrhea can also be transmitted from an infected mother to her child during delivery. Gonorrhea often has mild or no symptoms. However, if left untreated, gonorrhea can lead to infertility, spread into the bloodstream, and affect the joints, heart valves, and brain.

hepatitis B virus (HBV) infection: Infection with the HBV. HBV can be transmitted through blood, semen, or other body fluids during sex or injection-drug use. Because HIV and HBV share the same modes of transmission, people infected with HIV are often also coinfected with HBV.

hepatitis C virus (HCV) infection: Infection with the HCV. HCV is usually transmitted through blood and rarely through other body fluids, such as semen. HCV infection progresses more rapidly in people coinfected with HIV than in people infected with HCV alone.

herpes simplex virus 2 (HSV-2) infection: An infection caused by HSV-2 and usually associated with lesions in the genital or anal area. HSV-2 is very contagious and is transmitted by sexual contact with someone who is infected (even if lesions are not visible).

human immunodeficiency virus (HIV): The virus that causes AIDS, which is the most advanced stage of HIV infection. HIV is a retrovirus that occurs as two types HIV-1 and HIV-2. Both types are transmitted through direct contact with HIV-infected body fluids, such as blood, semen, and genital secretions, or from an HIV-infected mother to her child during pregnancy, birth, or breastfeeding (through breast milk).

human papillomavirus (HPV): The virus that causes HPV infection, the most common sexually transmitted infection. There are two groups of HPV types that can cause genital warts and types that can cause cancer. HPV is the most frequent cause of cervical cancer.

injection drug use: A method of illicit drug use. The drugs are injected directly into the body into a vein, into a muscle, or under the skin with a needle and syringe. Blood-borne viruses, including HIV and hepatitis, can be transmitted via shared needles or other drug injection equipment.

molluscum contagiosum: A common, usually mild skin disease caused by the virus molluscum contagiosum and characterized by small white, pink, or flesh-colored bumps with a dimple in the center. Molluscum contagiosum is spread by touching the affected skin of an infected person or by touching a surface with the virus on it. The bumps can easily spread to other parts of the body if someone touches or scratches a bump and then touches another part of the body.

mother-to-child transmission (MTCT): When an HIV-infected mother passes HIV to her infant during pregnancy, labor and delivery, or breastfeeding (through breast milk). Antiretroviral (ARV) drugs are given to HIV-infected women during pregnancy and to their infants after birth to reduce the risk of MTCT of HIV.

opportunistic infection: An infection that occurs more frequently or is more severe in people with weakened immune systems, such as people with HIV or people receiving chemotherapy, than in people with healthy immune systems.

Papanicolaou (Pap) test: A procedure in which cells and secretions are collected from inside and around the cervix for examination under a microscope. Pap test also refers to the laboratory test used to detect any infected, potentially precancerous, or cancerous cells in the cervical cells obtained from a Pap test.

pelvic inflammatory disease (PID): Infection and inflammation of the female upper genital tract, including the uterus and fallopian tubes. Pelvic inflammatory disease is usually due to bacterial infection, including some sexually transmitted diseases, such as chlamydia and gonorrhea. Symptoms, if any, include pain in the lower abdomen, fever, smelly vaginal discharge, irregular bleeding, or pain during intercourse. PID can lead to serious complications, including infertility, ectopic pregnancy (a pregnancy in the fallopian tube or elsewhere outside of the womb), and chronic pelvic pain.

post-exposure prophylaxis (PEP): Short-term treatment started as soon as possible after high-risk exposure to an infectious agent, such as HIV, hepatitis B virus (HBV), or hepatitis C virus (HCV). The purpose of PEP is to reduce the risk of infection. An example of a high-risk exposure is exposure to an infectious agent as the result of unprotected sex.

pubic lice: Also called "crab lice" or "crabs," pubic lice are parasitic insects found primarily in the pubic or genital area of humans.

scabies: An infestation of the skin by the human itch mite (*Sarcoptes scabiei var. hominis*). The microscopic scabies mite burrows into the upper layer of the skin where it lives and lays its eggs. The most common symptoms of scabies are intense itching and a pimple-like skin rash. The scabies mite usually is spread by direct, prolonged, skin-to-skin contact with a person who has scabies.

semen: A thick, whitish fluid that is discharged from the male penis during ejaculation. Semen contains sperms and various secretions. HIV can be transmitted through the semen of a man with HIV.

sexually transmitted disease (STD): An infectious disease that spreads from person to person during sexual contact. Sexually transmitted diseases, such as syphilis, HIV infection, and gonorrhea, are caused by bacteria, parasites, and viruses.

spermicide: A topical preparation or substance used during sexual intercourse to kill sperm. Although spermicides may prevent pregnancy, they do not protect against HIV infection or other sexually transmitted diseases. Irritation of the vagina and rectum that sometimes occurs with use of spermicides may increase the risk of sexual transmission of HIV.

sterility: The inability to get pregnant, or get someone pregnant; often caused by the effects of untreated bacterial infections such as chlamydia or gonorrhea.

syphilis: An infectious disease caused by the bacterium Treponema pallidum, which is typically transmitted through direct contact with a syphilis sore, usually during vaginal or oral sex. Syphilis can also be transmitted from an infected mother to her child during pregnancy. Syphilis sores occur mainly on the genitals, anus, and rectum, but also on the lips and mouth.

transmission: The spread of disease from one person to another.

trichomoniasis: A sexually transmitted disease caused by a parasite.

ulcer: An open lesion on the surface of the skin or a mucosal surface, caused by superficial loss of tissue, usually with inflammation.

vaccination: Giving a vaccine to stimulate a person's immune response. Vaccination can be intended either to prevent a disease (a preventive vaccine) or to treat a disease (a therapeutic vaccine).

vaginal fluid: The natural liquids produced inside a woman's vagina. In an infected person, STDs can be passed when vaginal fluids come in contact with the genital area of a woman's sex partner.

vesicle: A small, fluid-filled bubble, usually superficial, and <0.5cm

virus: A microscopic infectious agent that requires a living host cell in order to replicate. Viruses often cause disease in humans, including measles, mumps, rubella, polio, influenza, and the common cold. HIV is the virus that causes AIDS.

yeast infection: A fungal infection caused by overgrowth of the yeast Candida (usually *Candida albicans*) in moist areas of the body. Candidiasis can affect the mucous membranes of the mouth, vagina, and anus.

Chapter 47

Directory of Organizations That Provide Information about Sexually Transmitted Diseases

Government Agencies That Provide Information about Sexually Transmitted Diseases

Agency for Healthcare Research and Quality (AHRQ)
Office of Communications and Knowledge Transfer (OCKT)
5600 Fishers Ln.
Seventh Fl.
Rockville, MD 20857
Phone: 301-427-1364
Website: www.ahrq.gov

Centers for Disease Control and Prevention (CDC)
1600 Clifton Rd.
Atlanta, GA 30329-4027
Toll-Free: 800-CDC-INFO
(800-232-4636)
Phone: 404-639-3311
Toll-Free TTY: 888-232-6348
Website: www.cdc.gov
E-mail: cdcinfo@cdc.gov

Resources in this chapter were compiled from several sources deemed reliable; all contact information was verified and updated in February 2019.

Federal Trade Commission (FTC)
600 Pennsylvania Ave. N.W.
Washington, DC 20580
Phone: 202-326-2222
Website: www.ftc.gov

Healthfinder.gov
1101 Wootton Pkwy
Rockville, MD 20852
Website: www.healthfinder.gov/
aboutus/contactus.aspx
E-mail: healthfinder@hhs.gov

National Cancer Institute (NCI)
9609 Medical Center Dr.
BG 9609, MSC 9760
Bethesda, MD 20892-9760
Toll-Free: 800-4-CANCER
(800-422-6237)
Phone: 301-435-3848
Website: www.cancer.gov
E-mail: cancergovstaff@mail.nih.
gov

National Center for Complementary and Integrative Health (NCCIH)
9000 Rockville Pike
Bethesda, MD 20892
Toll-Free: 888-644-6226
Toll-Free TTY: 866-464-3615
Website: www.nccih.nih.gov/
tools/contact.htm
E-mail: info@nccih.nih.gov

National Center for Health Statistics (NCHS)
Centers for Disease Control and Prevention (CDC)
3311 Toledo Rd.
Rm. 2217
Hyattsville, MD 20782-2064
Phone: 301-458-4901;
301-458-4001
Website: www.cdc.gov/nchs
E-mail: nhis@cdc.gov

National Institute of Allergy and Infectious Diseases (NIAID)
Office of Communications and Government Relations (OCGR)
5601 Fishers Ln.
MSC 9806
Bethesda, MD 20892-9806
Toll-Free: 866-284-4107
Phone: 301-496-5717
Toll-Free TDD: 800-877-8339
Fax: 301-402-3573
Website: www.niaid.nih.gov/
global/contact-us
E-mail: ocpostoffice@niaid.nih.gov

National Institute of Mental Health (NIMH)
Office of Science Policy, Planning, and Communications (OSPPC)
6001 Executive Blvd.
Rm. 6200, MSC 9663
Bethesda, MD 20892-9663
Toll-Free: 866-615-6464
TTY: 301-443-8431
Toll-Free TTY: 866-415-8051
Fax: 301-443-4279
Website: www.nimh.nih.gov
E-mail: nimhinfo@nih.gov

National Institute of Neurological Disorders and Stroke (NINDS)
NIH Neurological Institute
P.O. Box 5801
Bethesda, MD 20824
Toll-Free: 800-352-9424
Website: www.ninds.nih.gov

National Institute on Aging (NIA)
31 Center Dr., MSC 2292
Bldg. 31, Rm. 5C27
Bethesda, MD 20892
Toll-Free: 800-222-2225
Phone: 301-496-1752
Toll-Free TTY: 800-222-4225
Website: www.nia.nih.gov
E-mail: niaic@nia.nih.gov

National Institutes of Health (NIH)
9000 Rockville Pike
Bethesda, MD 20892
Phone: 301-496-4000
TTY: 301-402-9612
Website: www.nih.gov

National Prevention Information Network (NPIN)
Centers for Disease Control and Prevention (CDC)
Website: www.npin.cdc.gov/
pages/contact-us
E-mail: NPIN-Info@cdc.gov

Office of Minority Health Resource Center (OMHRC)
U.S. Department of Health and Human Services (HHS)
P.O. Box 37337
Washington, DC 20013-7337
Toll-Free: 800-444-6472
TDD: 301-251-1432
Fax: 301-251-2160
Website: www.minorityhealth.
hhs.gov
E-mail: info@minorityhealth.
hhs.gov

Substance Abuse and Mental Health Services Administration (SAMHSA)
5600 Fishers Ln.
Rockville, MD 20857
Toll-Free: 877-SAMHSA-7
(877-726-4727)
Toll-Free TTY: 800-487-4889
Website: www.samhsa.gov/
about-us/contact-us

U.S. Department of Health and Human Services (HHS)
200 Independence Ave. S.W.
Washington, DC 20201
Toll-Free: 877-696-6775
Website: www.hhs.gov

U.S. Food and Drug Administration (FDA)
10903 New Hampshire Ave.
Silver Spring, MD 20993-0002
Toll-Free: 888-INFO-FDA
(888-463-6332)
Website: www.fda.gov

U.S. National Library of Medicine (NLM)
8600 Rockville Pike
Bethesda, MD 20894
Website: www.nlm.nih.gov
E-mail: custserv@nlm.nih.gov

Private Agencies That Provide Information about Sexually Transmitted Diseases

Advocates for Youth
1325 G St. N.W.
Ste. 980
Washington, DC 20005
Phone: 202-419-3420
Fax: 202-419-1448
Website: www.
advocatesforyouth.org

AIDS Healthcare Foundation (AHF)
6255 W. Sunset Blvd.
21st Fl.
Los Angeles, CA 90028
Phone: 323-860-5200
Website: www.aidshealth.org

AIDS.org
Website: www.aids.org

American Cancer Society (ACS)
250 Williams St. N.W.
Atlanta, GA 30303
Toll-Free: 800-ACS-2345
(800-227-2345)
Website: www.cancer.org

American Foundation for AIDS Research (amfAR)
120 Wall St.
13th Fl.
New York, NY 10005-3908
Phone: 212-806-1600
Fax: 212-806-1601
Website: www.amfar.org
E-mail: information@amfar.org

American Medical Association (AMA)
AMA Plaza, 330 N. Wabash Ave.
Ste. 39300
Chicago, IL 60611-5885
Toll-Free: 800-621-8335
Website: www.ama-assn.org

American Sexual Health Association (ASHA)
P.O. Box 13827
Research Triangle Park, NC 27709
Phone: 919-361-8400
Fax: 919-361-8425
Website: www.ashasexualhealth.
org/contact-us/
E-mail: info@ashasexualhealth.
org

American Society for
Colposcopy and Cervical
Pathology (ASCCP)
1530 Tilco Dr.
Ste. C
Frederick, MD 21704
Toll-Free: 800-787-7227
Phone: 301-733-3640
Fax: 240-575-9880
Website: www.asccp.org
E-mail: info@asccp.org

American Society of
Reproductive Medicine
(ASRM)
1209 Montgomery Hwy
Birmingham, AL 35216-2809
Phone: 205-978-5000
Fax: 205-978-5005
Website: www.asrm.org
E-mail: asrm@asrm.org

The Body
Remedy Health Media
461 Fifth Ave.
14th Fl.
New York, NY 10017
Website: www.thebody.com

Cleveland Clinic
9500 Euclid Ave.
Cleveland, OH 44195
Toll-Free: 800-223-CARE
(800-223-2273)
Website: my.clevelandclinic.org

Elizabeth Glaser Pediatric
AIDS Foundation (EGPAF)
1140 Connecticut Ave. N.W.
Ste. 200
Washington, DC 20036
Toll-Free: 888-499-HOPE
(888-499-4673)
Phone: 202-296-9165
Fax: 202-296-9185
Website: www.pedaids.org/
about/contact-us
E-mail: info@pedaids.org

Engender Health
505 Ninth St. N.W.
Ste. 601
Washington, DC 20004
Phone: 202-902-2000
Website: www.engenderhealth.
org
E-mail: info@engenderhealth.org

Foundation for Women's
Cancer (FWC)
230 W. Monroe
Ste. 710
Chicago, IL 60606
Phone: 312-578-1439
Website: www.
foundationforwomenscancer.org
E-mail: FWCinfo@sgo.org

Gay and Lesbian Medical
Association (GLMA)
1133 19th St. N.W.
Ste. 302
Washington, DC 20036
Phone: 202-600-8037
Fax: 202-478-1500
Website: www.glma.org
E-mail: info@glma.org

Gay Men's Health Crisis (GMHC)
307 W. 38th St.
New York, NY 10018-9502
Toll-Free: 800-243-7692
Phone: 212-367-1000
Website: www.gmhc.org

Go Ask Alice!
Website: goaskalice.columbia.edu

Guttmacher Institute
125 Maiden Ln.
Seventh Fl.
New York, NY 10038
Toll-Free: 800-355-0244
Phone: 212-248-1111
Fax: 212-248-1951
Website: www.guttmacher.org

Hepatitis B Foundation
3805 Old Easton Rd.
Doylestown, PA 18902
Phone: 215-489-4900
Fax: 215-489-4920
Website: www.hepb.org
E-mail: info@hepb.org

Hepatitis Foundation International (HFI)
8121 Georgia Ave.
Ste. 350
Silver Spring, MD 20910
Toll-Free: 800-891-0707
Phone: 301-565-9410
Website: www.hepfi.org
E-mail: info@
hepatitisfoundation.org

I Want the Kit (IWTK)
Website: www.iwantthekit.org
E-mail: iwantthekit@jhmi.edu

Immunization Action Coalition (IAC)
2550 University Ave. W.
Ste. 415 N.
Saint Paul, MN 55114
Phone: 651-647-9009
Fax: 651-647-9131
Website: www.immunize.org
E-mail: admin@immunize.org

Kaiser Family Foundation (KFF)
185 Berry St.
Ste. 2000
San Francisco, CA 94107
Phone: 650-854-9400
Fax: 650-854-4800
Website: www.kff.org

National Cervical Cancer Coalition (NCCC)
P.O. Box 13827
Research Triangle Park, NC 27709
Toll-Free: 800-685-5531
Fax: 919-361-8425
Website: www.nccc-online.org
E-mail: nccc@ashasexualhealth.org

National Coalition for LGBT Health
2000 S. St. N.W.
Washington, DC 20009
Phone: 202-232-6749
Fax: 202-232-6750
Website: www.lgbthealth.net
E-mail: info@healthlgbt.org

Planned Parenthood
123 William St.
10th Fl.
New York, NY 10038
Toll-Free: 800-230-PLAN
(800-230-7526)
Website: www.
plannedparenthood.org
E-mail: info@ppnyc.org

Project Inform
25 Taylor St.
San Francisco, CA 94103
Toll-Free: 877-HELP-4-HEP
(877-435-7443)
Phone: 415-558-8669
Fax: 415-558-0684
Website: www.projectinform.org

*Sexuality Information and
Education Council of the
United States (SIECUS)*
1012 14th St. N.W.
Ste. 1108
Washington, DC 20005
Phone: 202-265-2405
Website: www.siecus.org
E-mail: info@siecus.org

Index

Index

HIV testing, *continued*
    preventive services 196
    screening recommendations 308
    statistics 38
"HIV Treatment as Prevention"
    (HHS) 411n
"HIV Vaccines" (HHS) 409n
Home Access HIV-1 Test System,
    overview 331–3
home testing kit, HIV 187
homophobia, HIV 75
"How Do Sexually Transmitted
    Diseases and Sexually Transmitted
    Infections Affect Pregnancy?"
    (NICHD) 291n
"How STDs Impact Women
    Differently from Men" (CDC) 48n
"How the Female Reproductive
    System Works" (OWH) 16n
"How YOU Can Talk. Test. Treat"
    (CDC) 304n
HPV *see also* human papillomavirus
"HPV and Cancer" (NCI) 200n
"HPV Vaccine Information for Young
    Women" (CDC) 211n
human immunodeficiency virus (HIV)
    Affordable Care Act (ACA) 194
    African Americans 74
    alcohol 364
    cervicitis 273
    chancroid 100
    chlamydia 115
    defined 475
    described 57
    global impact 37
    health-fraud scams 347
    immunocompromised persons 256
    investigational drug 442
    life cycle 165
    opportunistic infections 176
    oral sex 357
    post-exposure prophylaxis (PEP) 421
    screening recommendations 308
    statistics 4
    STIs 24
    syphilis 222
    transmission 380
    trichomoniasis 228
    vaccination 451
    vaginitis 299

human papillomavirus (HPV)
    defined 475
    described 66
    genital herpes 138
    genital warts 57
    male circumcision 392
    Pap smear tests 309
    recurrent respiratory papillomatosis
        (RRP) 205
    statistics 34
    STDs 172
    vaccines 409
    women 49
human Papillomavirus (HPV)
    infection
    defined 200
    genital herpes 138
    genital warts 85
    human papillomavirus (HPV)
        vaccine 213
    STDs in women 49
"Human Papillomavirus (HPV)
    Infection" (CDC) 208n
hydrocele, epididymitis 276
hymen, female reproductive
    system 17
hypothalamus, female-sexual
    response 19

I

I Want the Kit (IWTK), website
    address 484
imiquimod, topical therapy 256
immune system
    AIDS 164
    antibodies 184
    chronic hepatitis E 150
    crusted scabies 262
    genital herpes 139
    HIV 57, 83
    molluscum contagiosum 254
    opportunistic infections 176
    vaccine 409
    viral hepatitis 146
    viral load 462
    yeast infections 247
Immunization Action Coalition (IAC),
    contact 484

vaginal itching
   bacterial vaginosis (BV) 65
   douching 371
vaginal odor, douching 371
vaginal opening, depicted 18
vaginal yeast infections
   bacterial vaginosis (BV) 235
   overview 242–7
"Vaginal Yeast Infections"
   (OWH) 242n
"Vaginitis: Condition Information"
   (NICHD) 297n
vasectomy, epididymitis 279
vesicle, defined 477
viral hepatitis
   injection-drug use 376
   overview 146–57
   syringe services programs
      (SSPs) 417
"Viral Hepatitis" (OWH) 146n
viral load
   HIV medications 411
   mother-to-child transmission
      (MTCT) 408
   overview 365–7
"Viral Load" (CDC) 365n
viral strains, viral hepatitis 96
viral suppression
   antiretroviral therapy (ART) 383
   HIV vaccines 409
vomiting
   hepatitis B 68
   neurosyphilis 283
   tabulated *178*
vulva
   human papillomavirus (HPV) 92
   molluscum contagiosum 255
   trichomoniasis 227
   vaginal yeast infection 242
   vaginitis 297

W

warts, symptoms 26
water-soluble lubricant, condom 389
watery skin blisters, genital
   herpes 91

weight loss
   AIDS 164
   HIV 68
   syphilis 223
   tabulated *178*
"What Are Some Types of and
   Treatments for Sexually
   Transmitted Diseases (STDs) or
   Sexually Transmitted Infections
   (STIs)" (NICHD) 89n
"What Are the Best Ways to
   Decrease My Chances of Getting
   or Transmitting HIV?—HIV Risk
   Reduction Tool" (CDC) 380n
"What Is the Link with Infertility?"
   (NICHD) 281n
"What to Expect at Your First HIV
   Care Visit" (HHS) 461n
"What You Need to Know about Sinus
   Disorders" (CDC) 342n
window period, HIV infection 184, 366
womb
   chlamydia 337
   female reproductive system 17
   gonorrhea 90
   pelvic inflammatory disease
      (PID) 85, 285
   vaginitis 297

Y

yeast infection
   bacterial vaginosis (BV) 235
   defined 477
   douching 370
   HIV 68
   vaginitis 298
yellow skin, hepatitis B 68
yellowish-green discharge,
   douching 371
yoga, mental-health problem 469
yogurt, yeast infection 247

Z

zidovudine, tabulated *444*
Zika virus, defined 59

9/19

For Reference

Not to be taken from this room